M. Ponz de Leon   **Colorectal Cancer**

Springer

*Berlin
Heidelberg
New York
Barcelona
Hong Kong
London
Milan
Paris
Tokyo*

Maurizio Ponz de Leon

Colorectal Cancer

With 32 Figures and 17 Tables

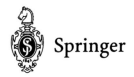 Springer

Dr. Maurizio Ponz de Leon
Department of Internal Medicine,
University of Modena and Reggio Emilia,
Policlinic
Via del Pozzo 71, 41100 Modena, Italy

ISBN 978-3-642-62762-0   ISBN 978-3-642-56008-8 (eBook)
DOI 10.1007/978-3-642-56008-8

Cip Data applied for

Die Deutsche Bibliothek – CIP-Einheitsaufnahme
Ponz de Leon, Maurizio: Colorectal cancer : with 17 tables / Maurizio Ponz de Leon. –
Berlin ; Heidelberg ; New York ; Barcelona ; Hong Kong ; London ; Milan ; Paris ;
Tokyo : Springer, 2002
ISBN 978-3-642-62762-0

This work is subject to copyright. All rights are reserved, whether the whole or part of the material is concerned, specifically the rights of translation, reprinting, reuse of illustrations, recitation, broadcasting, reproduction on microfilm or in any other ways, and storage in data banks. Duplication of this publication or parts thereof is only permitted under the provisions of the German Copyright Law of September 9, 1965, in its current version, and permission for use must always be obtained from Springer-Verlag. Violations are liable for prosecution under the German Copyright Law.

Springer-Verlag Berlin Heidelberg New York
a member of BertelsmannSpringer Science+Business Media GmbH
http://www.springer.de

© Springer-Verlag Berlin Heidelberg 2002

The use of general descriptive names, registered names, trademarks, etc. in this publication does not imply, even in the absence of a specific statement, that such names are exempt from the relevant protective laws and regulations and therefore free for general use.
Product liability: The publishers cannot guarantee the accuracy of any information about the application of operative techniques and medications contained in this book. In every individual case the user must check such information by consulting the relevant literature.

Cover design: Frido Steinen-Broo, Pau, Spain

Printed on acid-free paper   SPIN: 10851885   21/3130/op 5 4 3 2 1 0

Preface

Colorectal cancer continues to be one of the most common human malignancies, afflicting nearly one million individuals in the world every year. The disease can be considered endemic in all Western and industrialized countries, but there are indications that in the near future colorectal neoplasms will become frequent also in populations that at present show a low incidence of the disease.

There is no doubt that tremendous advances have been made in colorectal cancer research, especially in the last 2-3 decades. This applies not only to molecular biology, but also to surgical techniques, anaesthesiology, endoscopic procedures, clinical epidemiology and adjuvant chemotherapy. However, large-scale prevention and the early detection of colorectal malignancies remain difficult tasks, and mass screening can hardly be proposed to the general population. As stressed in other parts of the volume, surgery was the only hope of cure for this disease at the beginning of the twentieth century, and surgery remains at present - in the new millennium - the only option for the majority of affected individuals.

This is not a pessimistic attitude, just an invitation to use common sense and constructive criticism in analysing and interpreting the continuous new advancements of basic and clinical research in colorectal neoplasms.

This critical attitude has been maintained by me throughout the book, an attitude that derives from more than 20 years spent in the study of the main aspects of colorectal tumors, from aetiology to management, from screening and prevention to the new discoveries of molecular biology.

The volume has the limitations but also the advantages of being written by a single author. The main drawback is that presumably some valuable information has not been reported, and some interesting literature has been missed. The main advantages are a uniform style and the attempt to cover the entire topic; of course, the reader will notice some differences from chapter to chapter, and this reflects my personal belief in the clinical and scientific interest of various aspects of the disease.

The book is organized into 14 chapters, which cover the entire field. The first 3 deal with aetiology, pathogenesis and morphology and provide the necessary background for the rest of the volume. Chapters 4 to 9 describe the main clinical features of these neoplasms, including screening, surveillance, chemotherapy, radiotherapy, prevention and prognosis. Then 3 chapters are dedicated to hereditary cancer syndromes (familial adenomatous polyposis, other polyposis of the large bowel and Lynch syndrome), which have been my main scientific interest for many years and represent a remarkable example of how basic research can easily be translated into clinical practice. Chapter 13 deals with carcinoid tumors, while in the last chapter I focus on three main aspects of colorectal cancer research which may assume considerable importance in the new millennium: "The colorectal cancer epidemic", "Gene-environment interaction" and "The care of colorectal cancer patients in the molecular era". My intention is that this volume contains a comprehensive evaluation of the main advances in all these topics.

I hope the volume captures my spirit and the constructive critical attitude; in that way, it may be of help especially to the new generation of investigators who are facing this dreadful disease at the beginning of the new millennium.

Modena, April 2002   Maurizio Ponz de Leon

Acknowledgements

I wish to thank all colleagues and friends who contributed with their criticisms and suggestions to the design and completion of this volume. In particular, thanks are due to the collaborators Prof. Luca Roncucci, Dr.ssa Carmela Di Gregorio, Dr. Piero Benatti, Dr. Antonio Percesepe and Dr. ssa Monica Pedroni, who represent the senior staff of the Colorectal Cancer Study Group of the University of Modena. Dr. Piero Benatti produced most of the figures and graphs appearing in the text, while Dr. ssa Di Gregorio supplied the pathological slides and photographs.

I also wish to thank the junior staff of the Group (Dr. Mirco Menigatti, Dr. ssa Francesca Borghi, Dr. ssa Alessandra Scarselli, Dr. Giovanni Zangardi) for stimulating discussions, and Dorval Ganazzi for informatics support and advice.

The efficient editorial assistance of Dr. J. Heidelmann, Dr. M. Hofman, and Mrs. A. Cerri (Springer Verlag) is gratefully acknowledged.

Finally, I express particular gratitude to Dr. ssa Giuseppina Rossi for the innumerable hours spent in interpreting my handwriting and putting the various chapters into the computer.

Contents

1 The Causes of Colorectal Cancer	1
Introduction	1
Descriptive Epidemiology and Temporal Trends	2
The Environment and Colorectal Cancer	3
Diet and Micronutrients	3
Physical Activity, Obesity and Energy Imbalance	5
Hormonal Factors	6
Smoking and Alcoholic Beverages	6
Inflammatory Bowel Diseases	7
Drugs	7
Colorectal Polyps and the Adenoma-Carcinoma Sequence	8
Familial and Hereditary Factors	10
Familial Colorectal Cancer	10
Hereditary Non-polyposis Colorectal Cancer	11
Familial Adenomatous Polyposis	13
Gene-Environment Interactions	14
Conclusions	14
References	15
2 Pathogenesis of Colorectal Cancer	23
Introduction	23
Main Causes of Colorectal Cancer	24
Pathogenesis of Colorectal Cancer: Different Molecular Pathways for One Disease	25
Sporadic Colorectal Cancer Development (Loss of Heterozygosity Pathway)	26
Tumor Development in FAP and Other Polyposis Syndromes	30
Colorectal Tumorigenesis in HNPCC (Mutator Genes/Microsatellite Instability Pathway)	35
The Mitotic Checkpoint Gene Mutation Pathway	38
Colorectal Cancer Development in Inflammatory Bowel Diseases	38

Tumor Development
Through the I1307 K Mutation of the APC Gene:
Some Clues to Familial Cancer 40
Conclusions 41
References 42

3 Pathology of Colorectal Cancer 49

Introduction 49
The Colorectal Mucosa 50
   Normal Architecture 50
   Cell Proliferation 52
Aberrant Crypts 52
Adenomatous Polyps 54
   Descriptive Epidemiology 54
   Distribution, Size and Multiplicity 55
   Histopathology, Dysplasia
   and "Malignant Polyps" 55
   Adenomas in Familial Adenomatous Polyposis
   and Hereditary Non-polyposis
   Colorectal Cancer 59
   The Adenoma-Carcinoma Sequence 59
   Etiology of Adenomatous Polyps 60
Other Types of Polyps 61
   Hyperplastic, Mixed Polyps
   and Serrated Adenomas 61
   Flat Adenomas 63
   Hamartomatous Polyps 64
   Polyps and Dysplasia
   in Inflammatory Bowel Diseases 65
   Other Benign Tumors 66
Colorectal Carcinoma 66
   Adenoma-Carcinoma Sequence
   Versus "De Novo" Carcinogenesis 66
   Macroscopic Appearance 67
   Histological Features and Grading 67
   Pattern of Metastasis and Staging 69
   Other Tumors of the Large Bowel 70
Conclusions 71
References 72

4 Diagnosis and Clinical Features
of Colorectal Cancer 79

Introduction 79
Clinical Findings: Symptoms and Signs 80

Laboratory Investigations 81
Diagnosis of Colorectal Cancer: Old Methods
and Recent Imaging Techniques 82
    Imaging Studies in Primary Cancer 82
    Imaging Studies in the Diagnosis
    of Recurrent or Metastatic Disease 85
Conclusions 88
References 89

5 Colorectal Cancer Screening and Surveillance ... 95

Introduction 95
Colorectal Cancer Screening
in the General Population 96
    Role of Fecal Occult Blood Testing 97
    Role of Sigmoidoscopy 98
    Role of Colonoscopy and Barium Enema 99
New Screening Procedures
Based on Molecular Analysis 100
Screening in Individuals
with Familial Colorectal Cancer 100
    Understanding the Nature
    of the Familial Risk 101
    Screening Recommendations
    for Individuals with Familial Risk 102
Surveillance After Endoscopic Polypectomy 102
Surveillance After Surgery for Colorectal Cancer .. 103
Surveillance in Patients
with Inflammatory Bowel Disease 104
Surveillance in Hereditary Cancer Syndromes 105
    Familial Adenomatous Polyposis 106
    Hereditary Non-polyposis Colorectal Cancer .. 107
Conclusion: Media, Society
and Colorectal Cancer Screening 108
References 109

6 Prevention and Chemoprevention
of Colorectal Neoplasms 117

Introduction 117
Can We Prevent Colorectal Cancer
with an Appropriate Diet? 118
Can We Prevent Colorectal Cancer
by Modifying Our Lifestyle? 119
Secondary Prevention:
Is the Removal of Adenomas Effective? 120

Colorectal Cancer Prevention
Under Special Conditions 121
Chemoprevention of Colorectal Cancer 123
  General Concepts of Chemoprevention 123
  Main Compounds Used in the Chemoprevention
  of Colorectal Tumors 125
Conclusions 128
References 128

7 Treatment of Colorectal Cancer 135

Introduction 135
Staging Colorectal Neoplasms 136
Treatment of Resectable Colorectal Tumors 137
  Endoscopic Treatment of Malignant Polyps ... 137
  Surgical Treatment of Resectable Tumors
  of the Colon 138
  Surgical Treatment of Resectable Tumors
  of the Rectum 139
  Medical Treatment of Colorectal Tumors 141
  Radiation Treatment of Rectal Cancer 144
  Management of Locally Recurrent Cancer 146
Treatment of Advanced Colorectal Tumors 147
  Surgical Treatment
  of Metastatic Colorectal Cancer 147
  Chemotherapy for Advanced Colorectal Cancer 148
  Toxicity and Cost of Chemotherapy
  in Advanced Colorectal Cancer 151
  Other Treatments
  for Advanced Colorectal Neoplasms 151
Innovative Treatments for Colorectal Cancer 152
Conclusions 154
References 154

8 Survival and Follow-up of Colorectal Cancer 163

Introduction 163
Factors Influencing Colorectal Cancer Survival ... 164
  Gender, Age and Stage at Diagnosis 164
  Morphological and Clinical Indicators 165
  Cell Replication, Nuclear Ploidy
  and Colorectal Cancer Survival 167
  Molecular Markers of Prognosis 168
  Micrometastases and Prognosis 170
Temporal Trends and Ethnic Differences
in Colorectal Cancer Survival 171

Follow-up of Colorectal Cancer Patients 172
  Proposed Surveillance Programs
  After Colorectal Cancer Resection 173
  Controlled Studies Evaluating the Effectiveness
  of Follow-up 174
Conclusions 175
References 175

9 Cancer of the Anal Canal 181

Introduction 181
Epidemiology of Anal Cancer 181
  Descriptive Epidemiology 181
  Risk Factors 182
Clinical Features and Pathology 184
Treatment of Cancer of the Anus 185
  Radiotherapy Alone 185
  Combination Therapy 185
Conclusions 186
References 187

10 Hereditary Non-polyposis Colorectal Cancer
(Lynch Syndrome) 191

Introduction 191
Brief History of HNPCC 191
Epidemiology and Frequency of Lynch Syndrome . . 192
Formal Genetics and the Role of Family History . . 195
Clinical Features of HNPCC 197
  Age at Diagnosis and Preferential Location
  in the Right Colon 198
  Multiple Tumors 199
  Tumor Spectrum 200
Pathology of HNPCC 201
Molecular Biology of HNPCC 202
  DNA Mismatch Repair in Bacteria 203
  Human Mismatch Repair Genes
  in Lynch Syndrome 203
  Microsatellite Instability: the MSI+ Phenotype . . 205
  Microsatellite Instability
  and Cancer Development 206
  Frequency of Mutations in HNPCC Families . . . 207
  New Genes Predisposing to HNPCC 208
Diagnosis of HNPCC 209
  Identification of HNPCC 209
  Suspected HNPCC 210

Genetic Counseling in HNPCC 212
Management and Survival 213
  Treatment and Follow-up 214
  Survival 215
Conclusions 216
References 216

11 Familial Adenomatous Polyposis 225

Introduction 225
Definition and Historical Overview 226
Epidemiology and Formal Genetics 227
Diagnosis, Clinical Features and Morphology 229
  Colorectal Lesions 229
  Extracolonic Manifestations 231
Molecular Biology of FAP 235
  The APC Gene and Its Functions 235
  Genotype-Phenotype Correlations 236
  Methods for Study of the APC Gene 239
Management of Familial Adenomatous Polyposis . . 239
  The Role of Counseling in the Diagnosis
  and Surveillance of Adenomatosis Coli 240
  Surgical Treatment of FAP 241
  Overall Prognosis and Follow-up 243
  Medical Treatment 243
Conclusions 244
References 245

12 Other Polyposis of the Large Bowel 253

Introduction 253
Peutz-Jeghers Syndrome 253
  Clinical Manifestations and Morphology 256
  Molecular Biology of PJS 257
  Management 258
Juvenile Polyposis 259
  Phenotypic Characteristics, Genetics
  and Cancer Risk 259
  Molecular Biology and Genetic Heterogeneity
  of JP 260
  Management of JP 261
Cowden's Disease 261
  Clinical Manifestations and Morphology 261
  Molecular Basis of CD 262
  Management of CD 262
Turcot Syndrome 263

Clinical and Morphologic Aspects of TS 263
Complex Genetic and Molecular Basis of TS ... 263
Management of TS 265
Muir-Torre Syndrome and Other Rare Polyposis .. 265
Clinical and Morphologic Features of MTS ... 265
Molecular Biology of MTS 266
Management of MTS 267
Cronkhite-Canada Syndrome 267
Bannayan-Riley-Ruvalcaba Syndrome 268
Conclusions 268
References 269

13 Carcinoid Tumors of the Large Bowel 275

Introduction 275
Brief History 275
Biology and Pathology of CT 276
Clinical Features of Colorectal CT 277
Diagnosis and Treatment of CT of the Large Bowel 279
Diagnosis of CT 280
Treatment of the Primary Tumor 280
Treatment of Metastatic CT 280
Conclusions 281
References 282

14 Colorectal Cancer at the Beginning of the New Millennium 285

The Colorectal Cancer Epidemic 285
Gene-Environment Interaction 286
Dealing with Colorectal Cancer Patients
in the "Molecular Era" 287
References 288

Subject Index 291

1 The Causes of Colorectal Cancer

Introduction

Colorectal cancer is one of the leading causes of cancer-related morbidity and mortality, responsible for an estimated half a million deaths per year, mostly in Western, well-developed countries [1]. The epidemiology of large-bowel malignancies has generated a lot of interest recently, mainly because the disease provides an excellent model for studying the interactions between specific genes and several environmental factors in its etiology [2].

In contrast to other common malignancies (i.e. pancreas, brain, kidney), the etiology and pathogenesis of which remain virtually unknown, in the last two decades we have gained several new and exciting perspectives on factors predisposing to colorectal cancer. Thus, we now know that a definite fraction – ranging between 1% and 5% of all cases – of colorectal tumors is transmitted from one generation to another in accordance with an autosomal dominant model; this is the case with hereditary non-polyposis colorectal cancer (HNPCC or Lynch syndrome) and of familial adenomatous polyposis (FAP) [3, 4]. Moreover, several environmental factors – including diet, lifestyle, body mass and, perhaps, hormones [5] – are similarly important in the induction and progression of these tumors. In addition, there is compelling evidence that a large fraction of (if not all) colorectal malignancies develops from benign precursor lesions of the large bowel (the adenomatous polyps) and that the systematic removal of polyps may prevent cancer occurrence [6]. Finally, recent developments in molecular biology have greatly increased our understanding of the role of oncogenes, tumor suppressor genes and "mutator" genes in the pathogenesis of colorectal cancer [7, 8].

In the present chapter I propose an updated description of the major factors aetiologically related to colorectal cancer development. One of the main messages is that these tumors cannot be attributed to a single agent (as in the case of smoking and lung cancer), but as a general rule they develop through a close interaction between genetic predisposition (more or less evident) and several environmental factors.

Descriptive Epidemiology and Temporal Trends

According to the World Health Organization [1], approximately 900,000 cases of colorectal malignancies were diagnosed worldwide in 1996, accounting for 8.5% of all new cases of cancer. Crude incidence rates show large variations among countries, ranging from 0.6–5.0 new cases/100,000 per year in several areas in the Third World (such as Senegal, Mexico and India) to 50–70/100,000 in North America, Western Europe, Australia and New Zealand [9]. These differences have usually been attributed to dietary factors, though the possible role of other environmental (or genetic) agents cannot be excluded "a priori". In India, colorectal malignancies occur much more frequently in the wealthy and westernized Parsi population than among Hindus and strictly vegetarian Jains [10]. While rectal cancer appears up to twice as frequently in men as in women, colonic tumors tend to occur with equal frequency in the two sexes. Finally, marked variations in the 5-year survival following the diagnosis of colorectal cancer have been reported; in the USA and in several European countries the 5-year survival is of the order of 50%–55%, as opposed to 30%–35% in many Eastern European countries and, rather curiously, in the UK [11]. The reasons for these differences remain unclear, though, rather intuitively, they should mostly be attributed to different staging at diagnosis.

Migrant studies lend further consistency to the role of environmental factors in the pathogenesis of large-bowel tumors. Thus, changes in incidence and mortality have been reported for migrants from Japan to the USA, or from Eastern Europe to North America [9]. Among immigrants and their descendants, incidence rates tend to approach those of the host country, sometimes within one generation. Moreover, migrants from a higher-risk area – such as Scotland – to an area at relatively lower risk (Australia) show a reduction in risk [12]. The recent and massive immigration from Albania, North Africa and Eastern Europe to the European Community will provide a new opportunity for testing the effect of a different environment on the incidence and mortality associated with colorectal and several other malignancies.

Temporal trends in incidence rates have been more difficult to analyze and interpret. Data from the Connecticut Cancer Registry showed that during the period 1950–1984 colorectal cancer incidence rates tended to increase, at least for men [13]; from the mid-1980s the incidence and mortality rates began to decline, more appreciably for rectal malignancies. The authors suggested that these encouraging figures might reflect improved early detection and removal of precancerous lesions, in particular through an increased use of lower endoscopy and fecal occult blood test. At variance with these results, several European studies showed rising rates of colorectal cancer incidence during the last few decades [5, 14, 15]; similar findings were observed in Japan, where tumors were mostly located in the distal portions of the large bowel. In the specialized Colorectal Cancer Registry of Modena (Italy), incidence rates increased by 12.2% from 1985 to 1997 (Fig. 1.1); according to the authors, improved collection of data, widespread use of colonoscopy (with consequent detection of early and localized tumors before the occurrence of symptoms) and progressive aging of the population might explain the observed findings [16].

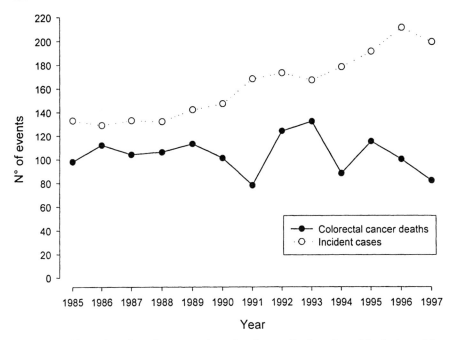

Fig. 1.1. Incidence (number of new cases/years) and mortality (number of deaths/years) for colorectal cancer during the period 1985–1997. Data from the specialized Colorectal Cancer Registry of Modena [16]

Subsite distribution of colorectal malignancies indicated that about 70% of them are localized between the splenic flexure and the lower rectum (distal or left large bowel). Recent studies, however, showed a tendency to a proximal shift of cancer distribution [17, 18]. Although the reasons are unclear, this trend favors the use of colonoscopy (instead of sigmoidoscopy) in the screening and surveillance of high-risk individuals.

The Environment and Colorectal Cancer

The main environmental factors associated with an increased or reduced risk of colorectal malignancies and the main recommendations for primary prevention of these tumors are summarized in Tables 1.1 and 1.2.

Diet and Micronutrients

As with other tumors of the digestive organs, several studies tried to establish a possible link between specific dietary factors and colorectal malignancies. The results of these investigations were frequently discordant, the observed relative

4   The Causes of Colorectal Cancer

Table 1.1. Environmental factors implicated in the etiology of colorectal malignancies

Factors associated with an increased risk	Factors showing a protective role
Diet:	
Meat	Fruit, vegetables
Animal fat	Fiber
Cooking at high temperature	Micronutrients (calcium, folate, antioxidant vitamins)
Lifestyle:	
Low physical activity	High physical activity
Obesity	–
Smoking	–
Alcoholic beverages	–
Diseases:	
Ulcerative colitis	–
Crohn's disease	–
Drugs	
–	Aspirin
–	Sulindac

Table 1.2. Main recommendations for the primary prevention of colorectal malignancies

1. Reduce total fat intake (especially from animal sources) and limit the consumption of meat
2. Include a variety of fresh vegetables, fruit and fiber in the daily diet
3. Avoid sedentary life and perform physical exercise daily
4. Do not smoke and limit consumption of alcoholic beverages
5. Avoid obesity and maintain ideal body weight

risks usually low and of borderline significance, and no strong causative factor could be detected. The effect of individual dietary components is difficult to evaluate, especially in case-control studies, in which individuals are supposed to remember type, frequency and amount of food regularly consumed in previous years; moreover, considering the long biological progression of colorectal neoplasms (from adenomatous polyps to infiltrating carcinoma), the food eaten 20 or 30 years before cancer occurrence could be more important than the diet at the time of diagnosis.

Among individual dietary components, the consumption of red meat and of saturated fat (i.e. from animal sources) seems to be somehow related to an increased risk of colorectal cancer. However, in an analysis of 19 controlled studies [19], J.D. Potter concluded that the data were not entirely convincing, either for saturated/animal fat or for meat/total protein intake. In animal studies, diets containing 40% of the calories as saturated or unsaturated fat are associated with a higher incidence of colorectal tumors than diets with a low fat content [20].

There is a general consensus that diets rich in vegetables and fruit protect against colorectal cancer; this can be due either to their content of fiber or to the presence of various micronutrients [5, 9, 21]. In an analysis of 21 case-control studies, 17 suggested a reduced risk of cancer with a higher consumption of vegetables or fruit [19]. Fiber can protect against colorectal malignancies through various mechanisms including: a decrease in intestinal transit time (which might reduce the contact time of putative carcinogens with mucosal cells); a "bulky" effect with consequent dilution of the luminal content; and the possible interaction with various carcinogens or promoting factors present in the gut lumen. Several micronutrients have been invoked to explain the reduced risk of colorectal neoplasia associated with the consumption of fruit and vegetables, including antioxidant vitamins (A, C and E), flavonoids, protease inhibitors, calcium and folate. Various studies investigated the association between higher intakes of calcium and colorectal cancer development [22–24]; the results, once again, are not consistent, even if most of the evidence suggested some benefit. Calcium supplements might exert a protective effect by reducing the abnormal pattern of cell replication frequently observed in colonic crypts of subjects at increased risk of colorectal cancer [25]. The regular consumption of large doses of antioxidant vitamins (A, C and E) reduced cell replication in the intestinal mucosa [26] and prevented the recurrence of adenomatous polyps [27]; the results, however, were not confirmed by other investigations [29]. Folate intake has also been associated with a reduced risk of both colon and rectal cancer [29]; folate might exert its protective effect by inducing DNA methylation, since DNA hypomethylation seems to be an early step in colorectal tumorigenesis. Further studies, however, did not show any consistent effect of folate (and other micronutrients involved in methyl-group metabolism) on colorectal cancer [30]. Finally, resistant starch might have a protective effect and is at present under investigation in HNPCC family members [19].

Physical Activity, Obesity and Energy Imbalance

Individuals of both sexes in sedentary occupations have an increased risk of colonic tumors, while the risk decreases progressively for jobs requiring a higher level of physical activity; in contrast, no association has been shown between physical activity and cancer of the rectum [31, 32]. The relationship between level of physical activity and risk of colonic neoplasia is fairly consistent and has been reported for occupational activity as well as leisure and total activity [19]: 10 of 11 case-control studies showed an inverse association between physical activity and colon cancer risk. The reasons and the mechanisms whereby physical exercise reduces the susceptibility to large-bowel malignancies remain unclear.

Several clinical investigations suggest that obese individuals are at increased risk of colorectal cancer [33]; however, further studies failed to establish an association between body mass index and risk of colorectal neoplasms [22, 23]. In addition, the increased risk has been found only for the male sex, whereas the available evidence in women is less consistent. It has been suggested [34] that a high physical activity associated with a lean body mass might induce a "metabolic environment" (lower serum insulin, glucose and triacylglycerol levels and, perhaps, lower levels of other hormones and growth factors) which is less suitable for cancer development, especially for tumors of the large bowel and breast. According to this hypothesis, colorectal cancer might be viewed as one more metabolic disorder induced by an energy imbalance [35].

Hormonal Factors

Gastrin stimulates replication of normal colonic epithelial cells [36] and through this mechanism is considered a putative promoter of colorectal tumorigenesis. Several case-control studies failed to establish a consistent association between serum gastrin and colorectal carcinoma [37, 38]; moreover, patients with Zollinger-Ellison syndrome do not seem to be at increased risk for colorectal neoplasms [29]. However, in a recent prospective study [40], serum gastrin above the normal levels was associated with an increased risk for colorectal cancer, with an odds ratio of 3.9; the authors speculated that if this association were causal, then some 8%–9% of all colorectal malignancies might be attributed to high gastrin levels.

Endogenous and exogenous sexual hormones may be elements in the etiology of colorectal tumors. Thus, nuns and nulliparous women seem to be more susceptible to colorectal cancer development, whereas higher parity, early age at first birth and regular use of oral contraceptives might be associated with a reduced risk [41, 42]. However, subsequent investigations failed to reach firm conclusions [23]. Similar inconsistent results were found when investigating the possible association between hormone replacement therapy and colorectal cancer risk [19].

Smoking and Alcoholic Beverages

Colorectal malignancies are usually not included in the long list of tobacco-related neoplasms; however, there are studies indicating a higher risk for colon cancer among cigarette, cigar and pipe smokers [43, 44]. Moreover, Giovannucci and co-workers [45, 46] found in two large cohort studies that for each sex the number of cigarettes smoked during recent years was positively related to the prevalence of adenomatous polyps of the large bowel; the authors concluded that tobacco smoking was related to the risk of colorectal cancer after allowing for an induction period of at least 30–40 years.

Excessive alcohol consumption has been reported to be a risk factor for colorectal neoplasms. Thus, Stocks [47] first reported a slightly elevated risk of colorectal cancer among beer drinkers compared with abstainers. Since then, the association between alcohol consumption and risk of colorectal adenoma or carcinoma has been explored in several cohort and case-control studies, but with controversial results [19]. In 1997, the World Cancer Research Fund concluded that an elevated consumption of alcohol probably increases the risk of colorectal cancer and that this association seems due to total ethanol intake more than to the type of alcoholic beverage [22].

Inflammatory Bowel Diseases

Patients affected by ulcerative colitis are at increased risk for colorectal cancer [48]. Extension of the disease to the various large-bowel segments and duration of active colitis for more than 10 years appear as independent risk factors [49, 50]. The current practice for managing this risk requires lifelong annual colonoscopic surveillance with the collection of several biopsies in order to detect dysplasia or early cancer. It has been suggested that progression towards malignancy in long-lasting ulcerative colitis proceeds in a stepwise fashion of morphological changes, from mild dysplasia to severe dysplasia and eventually cancer [51]. According to this view, several abnormalities – such as aneuploidy, mutations of p53, *ras* and APC genes, as well as chromosomal instability – have been reported in ulcerative colitis [52–54]. It is still unclear whether an appropriate pharmacological treatment (corticosteroids, sulfasalazine, mesalazine) can exert a protective effect.

Whether Crohn's disease represents a risk factor for colorectal cancer is considered less certain. However, various cohort studies reported a significantly increased relative risk of colorectal malignancies among patients affected by Crohn's disease, with risk estimates varying from 4% to 20% according to the age of onset and extent of the disease in the different study populations [55, 56].

Finally, it should be noted that although the risk of cancer in ulcerative colitis or Crohn's disease is of importance for the patient, the burden of colorectal cancer attributable to inflammatory bowel diseases remains negligible. Indeed, data from cancer registries [57] showed that less than 1% of all colorectal malignancies can be related to these diseases.

Drugs

Animal studies showed that aspirin, indomethacin and several other anti-inflammatory compounds (all cyclo-oxygenase 1 or 2 inhibitors) were able to inhibit colorectal tumorigenesis [58, 59]. In humans, most studies focused on aspirin and sulindac. Several case-control and cohort studies suggested that the regular use of aspirin – in moderate doses – is associated with a significantly reduced risk of colorectal adenoma and carcinoma [60, 61]. The daily dose of aspirin effective in lowering the risk of colorectal neoplasia is still uncertain; moreover, before claiming a widespread use of aspirin for colorectal cancer prevention (through specific guidelines or the common mass media), this effect should be balanced against the risk of upper gastrointestinal damage (and bleeding) induced by non-steroidal anti-inflammatory drugs. The administration of standard doses of sulindac to patients with familial adenomatous polyposis induces, in some patients, a dramatic reduction in the number of adenomas of the large bowel [62, 63]. The polyps, however, do not disappear, and in some cases may progress to carcinoma during such therapy [64]; sulindac, therefore, does not seem to be able to change our current practice in the management of adenomatosis coli (i.e. total colectomy with ileorectal anastomosis or restorative proctocolectomy with ileoanal anastomosis), though it might be effective in preventing adenoma recurrence in the remaining rectum after colectomy with ileorectal anastomosis.

Colorectal Polyps and the Adenoma-Carcinoma Sequence

In contrast to neoplasms of many other organs – which develop "de novo" or in the absence of precancerous alterations – there is considerable evidence implicating adenomatous polyps as the precursor lesions of colorectal cancer [2]. Adenomas are well demarcated, circumscribed lumps of epithelial dysplasia and can be classified into three major histological types: tubular, villous and tubulovillous. Colorectal adenomas are rare under the age of 30 years, but their prevalence increases with age, being present in 20%–40% of individuals over the age of 50 years in most Western countries. These lesions can be observed in all segments of the large bowel, but their distribution tends to parallel that of colorectal malignancies, so that about 70% of adenomas are localized in the left colon and rectum [65]. The large majority of adenomatous polyps are less than 1 cm in diameter; larger lesions often show a villous histological pattern and are more frequently associated with malignant changes [66]. Polyps of the large bowel may also be of other types, such as "hamartomatous" (as in juvenile polyposis), "inflammatory" or "hyperplastic"; the biological significance of these lesions remains unclear, and there is no consistent evidence of their evolution towards malignancy [67].

Several lines of evidence suggest that adenomas of the large bowel may become cancerous, and in this respect adenomatous polyps can be viewed as the single most important factor predisposing to colorectal cancer. This does not mean that all polyps undergo malignant changes, neither does it exclude the possibility of "de novo" (i.e. from normal mucosa) colorectal tumorigenesis [68]. The evidence that adenomas may transform into carcinoma can be summarized as follows. First, adenomatous areas are commonly observed in specimens of colorectal carcinoma, and conversely, malignant changes can be seen in approximately 5% of all polyps [69]. Second, in familial adenomatous polyposis – in which the entire large bowel is covered by hundreds of polyps – cancer develops in virtually 100% of untreated patients usually 10–20 years after the appearance of polyps [70]. Third, the National Polyp Study demonstrated that periodic endoscopic surveillance and systematic removal of all polyps of the large bowel reduced the incidence of new colorectal malignancies and lowered the mortality for this type of tumor [71, 72]. Fourth, in a series of 226 subjects in whom colorectal polyps larger than 1 cm could not be excised, a careful follow-up showed the occurrence of 21 invasive carcinomas, with a cumulative risk of cancer at the polyp site after 20 years of 24% [73]. Fifth, the age-specific incidence rate of colorectal adenomas shows a peak of incidence which precedes that of malignant tumors by 5 years [65]; since the malignant transformation of a benign adenoma usually takes years, this pattern of incidence is highly suggestive of a sequence from polyp to cancer. Sixth, several investigations suggested that the risk of colorectal polyps is closely associated with the same environmental factors as those which have been related to the risk of colorectal malignancies, in particular, low physical activity, a high intake of meat (especially red meat) and animal fat, and a low consumption of fruit and vegetables [19, 27]. If adenomatous polyps and cancer share the same aetiological factors, it is likely that they represent two different phases of the same disorder. Finally, recent studies of molecular genetics showed that the same biological alterations – loss of heterozygosity at various chromosomes, mutations of oncogenes and tumor suppressor genes, microsatellite instability – can frequently be detected in either adenomatous polyps or carcinoma of the large bowel [74, 75].

The adenoma-carcinoma sequence provides an excellent model for the study of molecular alterations and the way in which they affect tumor progression [76]. Colorectal tumors progress through a series of recognizable pathological stages. The first of these is probably a hyperproliferative state of colorectal mucosa, with a shift of the replicative zone to the upper portions of the crypts [77, 78]. Clusters of actively replicating cells may undergo clonal expansion and give rise to a small tubular adenoma; this may progress by increasing in size, acquiring cytological atypia, and developing a villous pattern. A further step is the acquisition of malignant behavior, with invasion of the basement membrane and subsequently of the "muscularis mucosae" and muscular wall. Final steps include the infiltration of adjacent tissues and organs and the ability to metastasize to regional lymph nodes and distant organs. This progression, which may require decades for its completion, is accompanied – and probably induced – by several genetic changes, such as (a) hypomethylation of DNA [79], (b) allelic losses at specific chromosomal regions (5q, 17p, 18q) [80], (c) point mutations in the *ras* oncogene [81], (d) reduced expression of the DCC tumor suppressor gene [82], (e) rearrangements in APC and MCC genes [83], and (f) p53 gene mutations [82]. Initially, it was suggested that accumulation rather than the order of molecular alterations was the most important factor in colorectal tumorigenesis [76]. After a careful microallelotyping study of many regions from individual colorectal tumors, Boland et al. [84] proposed that two crucial events could be identified in the progression from normal mucosa to infiltrating colorectal carcinoma. The first is loss of heterozygosity at chromosome 5q and inactivation of the APC gene, which seems to be responsible for the transformation of normal mucosa into small adenoma, thus initiating colorectal tumorigenesis. The second is loss of heterozygosity on 17q, which indicates a key role for the p53 gene in the adenoma to carcinoma transition. Figure 1.2 summarizes the major molecular events implicated in the adenoma-carcinoma sequence.

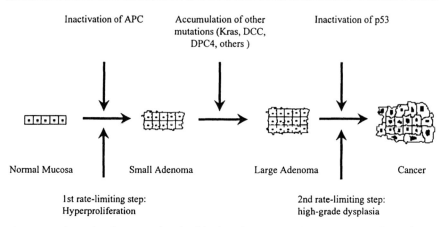

Fig. 1.2. Main molecular events involved in the adenoma-carcinoma sequence [76, 84]

Familial and Hereditary Factors

Our knowledge about hereditary colorectal cancer syndromes has increased remarkably over the past two decades owing to the new opportunities offered by molecular biology and the dedicated efforts of a few pioneers in this exciting field. A detailed analysis of the existing literature on hereditary non-polyposis colorectal cancer (HNPCC or Lynch syndrome) and familial adenomatous polyposis (FAP or adenomatosis coli) is beyond the scope of this chapter; the reader, therefore, is referred to further and more detailed information in the many excellent reviews published in recent years [85–90] and in chapters 10 to 12.

Familial Colorectal Cancer

Some 10%–20% of patients with colorectal cancer have affected first-degree relatives [91, 92], though their family trees do not fulfil the criteria for autosomal monogenic transmission. For these family members, the risk of cancer is about three times higher than that of the general population [93]. The fact that colorectal tumors tend to aggregate in families suggests that even some apparently sporadic forms of cancer may involve a genetic component; however, since no Mendelian pattern of inheritance can be discerned, the most likely type of transmission seems to be multifactorial [94], which implies a close interaction between genes and exogenous factors. As already discussed, several dietary factors together with lifestyle and other conditions are somehow related to colorectal tumors; we might assume that a genetic background (still undefined) determines which individuals in the general population are prone to develop cancer of the large bowel. Subsequently, over the course of many years, exogenous factors may interact with genes in susceptible persons, determining the fraction of them who will become affected. Recently, a specific constitutional mutation of the APC gene (I1307 K, i.e. a transversion of a single base, from thymidine to adenine at codon 1307, which creates a small, hypermutable region of the gene) was identified as a possible cause of familial colorectal cancer in a well-defined ethnic group [95, 96]. This mutation is found in approximately 6% of Ashkenazi Jews, and carriers have an estimated 20% lifetime risk of developing neoplasms of the large bowel. It is unlikely, however, that this mutation contributes to a large fraction of colorectal malignancies in other ethnic groups [97, 98].

Hereditary Non-polyposis Colorectal Cancer

HNPCC, or Lynch syndrome, is an autosomal dominant disease characterized by the early appearance of cancer, usually of the right colon (from caecum to splenic flexure), frequent occurrence of multiple lesions (both synchronous and metachronous), and a striking association with tumors of other organs, in particular the endometrium, urinary tract, ovary, stomach and small bowel [85–90, 99, 100]. In HNPCC, cancers aggregate in each susceptible sibship and are transmitted from one generation to the next ("vertical" transmission) in full accordance with the autosomal monogenic model, usually with high penetrance. Appearance of cancer before the age of 45–50 years is particularly frequent in HNPCC, though this does not exclude the possible occurrence of tumors at an older age. A family tree with all the clinical features of HNPCC is illustrated in Fig. 1.3. Although typical HNPCC families are easily recognizable, in many other

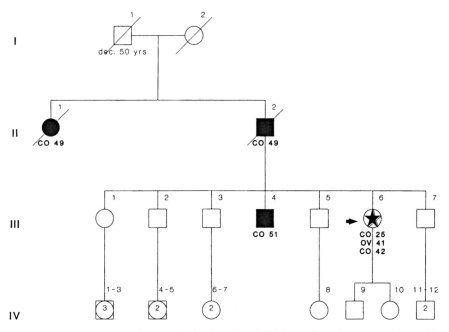

Fig. 1.3. Representative pedigree of a family with a full-blown clinical spectrum of hereditary non-polyposis colorectal cancer

Table 1.3. Revised clinical criteria for the definition of hereditary nonpolyposis colorectal cancer (HNPCC; Amsterdam Criteria II) [102]

1. Presence, in a given family, of at least three relatives with HNPCC-associated malignancy (colorectal cancer, cancer of the endometrium, small bowel, ureter or renal pelvis)
2. One of the affected individuals should be a first-degree relative of the other two
3. At least two successive generations should be affected
4. At least one individual should be diagnosed before the age of 50 years
5. Familial adenomatous polyposis (FAP) should be excluded
6. Tumors should be verified by pathological examination

cases the identification of the disease is much more complex; this is mostly due to the small size of modern families and to the fact that none of the above-mentioned clinical criteria is definitive or discriminatory. According to a panel of experts, the minimum requisites which should be met for a proper definition of HNPCC are the following (Table 1.3): (a) at least three first-degree relatives should have histologically verified cancer in the HNPCC spectrum; (b) adenomatosis coli should be excluded; (c) at least two successive generations should be affected; and (d) in one of the relatives, cancer should be diagnosed before the age of 50 years [101, 102]. Lynch syndrome has been described in many races and populations [103, 104], and its frequency has been estimated to be of the order of 1%–5% of all colorectal malignancies [105–107]. It is likely, however, that many HNPCC families escape clinical diagnosis owing to the poor attention frequently given to the family history of cancer patients; moreover, many kindreds who do not fulfil the standard clinical criteria (Table 1.3) – and who are tentatively labeled as "suspected" HNPCC (or HNPCC-like) – may actually be true HNPCC with incomplete penetrance or variable clinical expressivity [108, 109].

The genetic basis of Lynch syndrome has recently been clarified with the identification of constitutional mutations in a class of genes involved in DNA mismatch repair [110–114]. The function of these genes is to maintain the fidelity of the DNA during cell replication. Malfunctioning (i.e. mutations) of DNA mismatch repair genes renders the genome unstable, and this is particularly evident at "microsatellite loci", short sequences of highly repeating DNA scattered throughout the human genome but usually outside the coding regions [115, 116]. Thus, microsatellite instability is a characteristic feature of genomes that show defects in DNA mismatch repair, as in the case of tumors which develop in Lynch syndrome [117, 118]. The genes that mutate in HNPCC include hMSH2 (from the homologous bacterial gene) on chromosome 2p16; hMLH1 at 3p21; hPMS1 and hPMS2 on chromosomes 2q31 and 7q11, respectively; and hMSH6 at 2p16. A new MED1 gene has recently been identified [119] which might be responsible (when mutated) for Lynch syndrome. The available evidence suggests that hMSH2 and hMLH1 account for most mutations of the mismatch repair genes found to date in HNPCC families [120]. Thus, in a family with a clinical suspicion of Lynch syndrome, this should be confirmed by examining one or more tumors for microsatellite instability, and then by testing the major genes involved in DNA mismatch repair for constitutional mutations. According to most studies, however, mutations of these genes can be found in approximately half of the full-blown HNPCC families and in a lower proportion of suspected HNPCC [121-123]; it is not clear whether this low fraction of positive results should be attributed to mutations which are difficult to detect or to the possible role of other, unknown genes.

Familial Adenomatous Polyposis

FAP (or adenomatosis coli) is a rare autosomal dominant condition caused by mutations in the APC gene [124,125]. The main phenotypic characteristic of FAP is the presence of hundreds or thousands of adenomas in the various tracts of the large bowel; by convention, the clinical diagnosis of FAP can be made when a patient is found to have at least 100 colorectal polyps of various dimensions [126]. Adenomas appear in childhood or early puberty and increase progressively in number and size. When left untreated, one or more of the polyps degenerate into malignancy, usually by the age of 35-45 years, thus some 20 years after the appearance of the polyps. Optimal treatments are total colectomy with ileorectal anastomosis (in this case, polyps tend to recur in the rectal stump, and the patient needs careful endoscopic surveillance) or restorative proctocolectomy with ileoanal anastomosis [127,128]. Patients with FAP may show several extracolonic manifestations including: (a) glandular polyps of the stomach [129], (b) adenomas in the duodenum (especially in the periampullary region, which can evolve into malignancy), jejunum and ileum [130], (c) osteomas of the skull and mandible, (d) congenital hypertrophy of the retinal pigmented epithelium [131, 132], (e) tumors of the soft tissues, such as epidermoid cysts and desmoids [133, 134]. More rarely, FAP patients may develop other cancers, including thyroid tumors, pancreatic cancer or hepatoblastoma [135]. Clinical variants of FAP include Turcot syndrome, in which colorectal polyposis is associated with medulloblastoma and other brain tumors [136, 137], and attenuated familial polyposis, characterized by fewer than 100 synchronous adenomatous polyps in the colorectum [138, 139].

The APC gene has been mapped to chromosome 5q21; the gene encodes a 2843-amino acid protein which plays a role in the cell adhesion process and signal transduction [140-142]. With the most recent techniques [143], germline APC mutations can be detected in up to 70%-90% of FAP patients and families; in most cases, mutations consist of deletions of a few bases leading to stop codons and, thus, to truncated proteins. Genotype-phenotype correlations show that in typical FAP families the majority of these genetic alterations are localized within exon 15 [144], while in attenuated polyposis the mutations are at the 5'-end or at the 3'-end of the gene (exons 1-5) [145]. Moreover, mutations in the central part of the gene (codons 1250-1350) are associated with features of severe polyposis, with the early appearance of polyps and the development of cancer often before the age of 30 years [146, 147]. Some correlations have also been reported between the site of mutations and congenital hypertrophy of the retinal pigmented epithelium [148], multiplicity of extracolonic changes [149] and desmoid tumors [150]. It should be noted that despite these genotype-phenotype correlations, the same mutation can be associated with different clinical features, even within a single family [151]. The most likely explanation for this is the possible existence of modifier genes or environmental factors which can interfere with the APC gene products [152]. In mice, modifiers of the MIN gene (homologous to APC) have recently been identified (MOM1, for modifier of MIN) [153]; whether similar genes (and mechanisms) may explain the phenotypic variability frequently observed in FAP patients and families remains to be elucidated.

Gene-Environment Interactions

The molecular pathway illustrated in Fig. 1.2 was proposed in 1988 [76] and subsequently enriched with new or more detailed information; although we cannot claim that the intimate mechanisms of colorectal tumorigenesis have been completely elucidated, some of the target genes (and proteins) have been identified, and this represents a remarkable advance compared with our knowledge of 15 years ago. Even more important, it is now possible to explore the complex interaction between various environmental factors and the main "protagonists" of colorectal tumor induction and progression.

Thus, for instance, APC gene inactivation seems to play a key role in initiating colorectal tumorigenesis [84]; heterocyclic amines, which are produced by cooking meat at high temperatures, may have a direct effect on APC [154] and have been implicated in the etiology of cancer [155]. Similar mechanisms can reasonably be invoked for the many carcinogens (nitrosamines, polycyclic hydrocarbons, heterocyclic amines) produced during tobacco smoking. The effect of alcohol consumption can be mediated by acetaldehyde, which can form DNA adducts and inhibit DNA repair [19]. Moreover, antioxidant vitamins A, C, E and other bioactive substances (folate, flavonoids) might exert their protective effect by reducing DNA damage [19]. Finally, recent in vitro studies showed that aspirin was able to revert microsatellite instability when added to cultured cells from tumors with marked DNA replication errors [156]. Although these studies are still in their infancy, it is noteworthy that for the first time we are able to establish a hypothetical link between exogenous causes of cancer and the major molecular mechanisms of colorectal tumorigenesis.

Conclusions

There is no doubt that in the last few decades we have learned a lot about the causes and risk factors associated with colorectal neoplasms. Thus, we are now in the position to take preventive measures and to design surveillance programs which might produce a reduction in the incidence and mortality of this common malignancy. The role of family history and of hereditary cancer syndromes became clear, and molecular genetics offers the opportunity to identify individuals and families at high risk for colorectal cancer. However, it should be stressed that molecular screening should be limited to family members of kindreds with a strong clinical suspicion of HNPCC or with clinical features of FAP; there is no evidence that molecular tests can be of any benefit for screening the general population. Case-control and cohort studies showed that a variety of exogenous factors (i.e. meat, animal fat, tobacco smoking, sedentary life) may increase the risk of colorectal cancer, whereas other agents (i.e. physical activity, fruit, vegetables, fiber, micronutrients, non-steroidal anti-inflammatory drugs) may reduce this risk. Many of these factors have also been implicated in the pathogenesis (or the prevention) of other disorders (diabetes mellitus, hypertension, ischaemic heart disease) typical of Western societies and associated with a similar metabolic background. Thus, there is evidence that colorectal cancer can be considered one more metabolic disorder induced by energy imbalance. In other words, colorectal malignancies seem to be one more price that modern society pays for the many advantages (low requirement of physical activity, excess of food and beverages, tobacco smoking) offered by progress and civilization.

References

1. World Health Organization (WHO). The world health report. Geneva (Switzerland): WHO; 1997.
2. Ponz de Leon M. Genetic basis of tumour development. Ital J Gastroenterol 1996; 28: 232–45.
3. Lynch HT, Smyrk T, Lynch J. An update of HNPCC (Lynch syndrome). Cancer Genet Cytogenet 1997; 93:84–99.
4. Lindblom A, Nordenskjöld M. Hereditary cancer. Acta Oncologica 1999; 38:439–47.
5. Wilmink ABM. Overview of the epidemiology of colorectal cancer. Dis Colon Rectum 1997; 40:483–93.
6. Thiis-Evensen E, Hoff GS, Langmark F et al. Population-based surveillance by colonoscopy: effect on the incidence of colorectal cancer. Scand J Gastroenterol 1999; 34:414–20.
7. Lairmore TC, Norton JA. Advances in molecular genetics. Am J Surg 1997; 173: 37–41.
8. Chiang JM, Wu Chou YH et al. K-ras codon 12 mutation determines the polypoid growth of colorectal cancer. Cancer Res 1998; 58:3289–93.
9. Weisburger JH. Causes, relevant mechanisms, and prevention of large bowel cancer. Semin Oncol 1991; 18:316–36.
10. Cancer incidence in the Greater Bombay, by religion and sex, 1973–1978. The Indian Cancer Society, Perel, Bombay, 1985.
11. Sant M, Capocaccia R, Verdecchia A et al. Comparisons of colon-cancer survival among European countries: the Eurocare study. Int J Cancer 1995; 63:43–48.
12. McMichael AJ, McCall MG, Hartshorne JM et al. Patterns of gastrointestinal cancer in European migrants to Australia: the role of dietary change. Int J Cancer 1980; 25:431–7.
13. Chu RC, Tarone RE, Chow WH et al. Temporal patterns in colorectal cancer incidence, survival, and mortality from 1950 through 1990. J Natl Cancer Inst 1994; 86:997–1006.
14. Johansen C, Mellemgaard A, Skow T et al. Colorectal cancer in Denmark 1943–1988. Int J Colorect Dis 1993; 8:42–7.

15. Kemppainen M, Räihä I, Sourander L. A marked increase in the incidence of colorectal cancer over two decades in Southwest Finland. J Clin Epidemiol 1997; 50:147-51.
16. Ponz de Leon M, Benatti P, Percesepe A et al. Epidemiology of cancer of the large bowel - The 12-year experience of a specialized Registry in Northern Italy. Ital J Gastroenterol Hepatol 1999; 31:10-8.
17. Faivre J, Bedenne L, Boutron MC et al. Epidemiological evidence for distinguishing subsites of colorectal cancer. J Epidemiol Community Health 1989; 43:356-61.
18. Beart RW, Melton LJ III, Maruta M et al. Trends in right and left-sided colon cancer. Dis Colon Rectum 1983; 26:393-8.
19. Potter JD. Colorectal cancer: molecules and populations. J Natl Cancer Inst 1999; 91: 91632.
20. Weisburger JH, Wynder EL. Etiology of colorectal cancer with emphasis on mechanisms of action and prevention. In: Devita VT, Hellman S, Rosenberg SA. Important advances in oncology. Lippincott, Philadelphia, 1987; 197-200.
21. Terry P, Giovannucci E, Michaels KB et al. Fruit, vegetables, dietary fiber, and risk of colorectal cancer. J Natl Cancer Inst 2001; 93:525-33.
22. World Cancer Research Fund (WCRF) (Potter JD, Chair). Diet, nutrition and the prevention of cancer: a global perspective. Washington DC: WCRF/American Institute of Cancer Research; 1997.
23. Potter JD, Slattery ML, Bostick RM et al. Colon cancer: a review of the epidemiology. Epidemiol Rev 1993; 15:499-545.
24. Baron JA, Beach M, Mandel JS et al. Calcium supplements for the prevention of colorectal adenomas. Calcium Polyp Prevention Study Group. N Engl J Med 1999; 340: 101-7.
25. Lipkin M, Newmark H. Effect of added calcium on colonic epithelial-cell proliferation in subjects at high risk for familial colonic cancer. N Engl J Med 1985; 313: 1381-4.
26. Paganelli GM, Biasco G, Brandi D et al. Effect of vitamin A, C, and E supplementation on rectal cell proliferation in patients with colorectal adenomas. J Natl Cancer Inst 1992; 84:47-51.
27. Roncucci L, Di Donato P, Carati L et al. Antioxidant vitamins or lactulose for the prevention of the recurrence of colorectal adenomas. Dis Colon Rectum 1993; 36: 227-34.
28. Greenberg ER, Baron JA, Tosteson TD et al. A clinical trial of antioxidant vitamins to prevent colorectal adenoma. N Engl J Med 1994; 331:141-7.
29. Giovannucci E, Rimm EB, Ascherio A et al. Alcohol, low-methionine-low-folate diets and risk of colon cancer in men. J Natl Cancer Inst 1993; 28:276-81.
30. Slattery ML, Schaffer D, Edwards SL et al. Are dietary factors involved in DNA methylation associated with colon cancer? Nutr Cancer 1997; 28:52-62.
31. Thune I, Lund E. Physical activity and risk of colorectal cancer in men and women. Br J Cancer 1996; 73:1134-40.
32. Tavani A, Braga C, La Vecchia C et al. Physical activity and risk of cancers of the colon and rectum: an Italian case-control study. Br J Cancer 1999; 79:1912-6.
33. Singh PN, Fraser GE. Dietary risk factors for colon cancer in a low-risk population. Am J Epidemiol 1998; 148:761-74.
34. McKeown-Eyssen G. Epidemiology of colorectal cancer revisited: serum triglycerides and/or plasma glucose associated with risk? Cancer Epidemiol Biomarkers Prev 1994; 3:687-95.
35. Schoen RE, Tangen CM, Kuller LH et al. Increased blood glucose and insulin, body size, and incident colorectal cancer. J Natl Cancer Inst 1999; 91:1147-54.
36. Sirinek KR, Levine BA, Moyer MP. Pentagastrin stimulates in vitro growth of normal and malignant human colon epithelial cells. Am J Surg 1985; 149:35-9.
37. Seitz JF, Giovannini M, Gouvernet J et al. Elevated serum gastrin levels in patients with colorectal neoplasia. J Clin Gastroenterol 1991; 13:541-5.

38. Kikendall JW, Glass AR, Sobin LH et al. Serum gastrin is not higher in subjects with colonic neoplasia. Am J Gastroenterol 1992; 87:1394–7.
39. Orbuch M, Venzon DJ, Lubenky IA et al. Prolonged hypergastrinemia does not increase the frequency of colonic neoplasia in patients with Zollinger-Ellison syndrome. Dig Dis Sci 1996; 41:604–13.
40. Thorburn CM, Friedman GD, Dickinson CJ et al. Gastrin and colorectal cancer: a prospective study. Gastroenterology 1998; 115:275–80.
41. Fraumeni JF Jr, Lloyd W, Smith EM et al. Cancer mortality among nuns: role of marital status in etiology of neoplastic disease in women. J Natl Cancer Inst 1969; 42: 455–68.
42. McMichael AJ, Potter JD. Reproduction, endogenous and exogenous sex hormones, and colon cancer: a review and hypothesis. J Natl Cancer Inst 1980; 65:1201–7.
43. Giovannucci E. An updated review of the epidemiological evidence that cigarette smoking increases risk of colorectal cancer. Cancer Epidemiol Biomarkers Prev 2001; 10:725–31.
44. Giovannucci E, Colditz GA, Stampfer MJ et al. A prospective study of cigarette smoking and risk of colorectal adenoma and colorectal cancer in U.S. women. J Natl Cancer Inst 1994; 86:192–9.
45. Giovannucci E, Rimm EB, Stampfer MJ et al. A prospective study of cigarette smoking and risk of colorectal adenoma and colorectal cancer in U.S. men. J Natl Cancer Inst 1994; 86:183–91.
46. Slattery ML, Potter JD, Friedman GD et al. Tobacco use and colon cancer. Int J Cancer 1997; 70:259–64.
47. Stocks P. Cancer incidence in North Wales and Liverpool region in relation to habits and environment. Br Emp Cancer Champaign 35th Annual Report 1957; 1:127.
48. Maratka Z, Nedbal J, Kocianova J et al. Incidence of colorectal cancer in proctocolitis: a retrospective study of 959 cases over 40 years. Gut 1985; 26:43–9.
49. Mellemkjaer L, Olsen J, Frisch M et al. Cancer in patients with ulcerative colitis. Int J Cancer 1995; 60:330–3.
50. Ekbom A, Helmick C, Zack M et al. Ulcerative colitis and colorectal cancer: a population-based study. N Engl J Med 1990; 3223:1228–33.
51. Riddell RH, Goldman H, Ransohoff DF et al. Dysplasia in inflammatory bowel disease: standardized classification with provisional clinical applications. Hum Pathol 1983; 11:931–68.
52. Hsieh CJ, Klump B, Holzmann K et al. Hypermethylation of the p16^{INK4a} promoter in colectomy specimens of patients with long-standing and extensive ulcerative colitis. Cancer Res 1998; 58:3942–5.
53. Walsh SV, Loda M, Torres CM et al. p53 and β catenin expression in chronic ulcerative colitis-associated polypoid dysplasia and sporadic adenomas. An immunohistochemical study. Am J Surg Pathol 1999; 23:963–9.
54. Rabinovitch PS, Dziadon S, Brentnall TA et al. Pancolonic chromosomal instability precedes dysplasia and cancer in ulcerative colitis. Cancer Res 1999; 59:5148–53.
55. Glotzer D. The risk of cancer in Crohn's disease. Gastroenterology 1985; 89:438–41.
56. Ekbom A, Helmick C, Zack M et al. Increased risk of large bowel cancer in Crohn's disease with colonic involvement. Lancet 1990; 336:357–9.
57. Ponz de Leon M, Di Gregorio C, Roncucci L et al. Epidemiology of tumours of the colon and rectum: incidence, mortality, survival and familiality in the Health Care District of Modena, 1984–1992. University of Modena, 1995; 1–57.
58. Craven PA, DeRubertis FR. The evolution of cancer of the colon and rectum. Cancer 1992; 36:2251–70.
59. Pollard M, Luckert PH. Indomethacin treatment of rats with dimethylhydrazine-induced intestinal tumors. Cancer Treat Rep 1980; 64:1323–7.
60. Rosenberg L, Louik C, Shapiro S. Nonsteroidal antinflammatory use and reduced risk of large bowel cancer. Cancer 1998; 82:232.

61. Thun MJ, Namboodiri MM, Heath CW Jr. Aspirin use and reduced fatal colon cancer. N Engl J Med 1991; 325:1593-6.
62. Nugent KP, Spigelman AD, Phillips RKS. Tissue prostaglandin levels in familial adenomatous polyposis patients treated with Sulindac. Dis Colon Rectum 1996; 39:659-62.
63. Ladenheim J, Garcia G, Titzer D et al. Effect of Sulindac on sporadic colonic polyps. Gastroenterology 1995; 108:1083-7.
64. Niv Y, Fraser GM. Adenocarcinoma in the rectal segment in familial polyposis coli is not prevented by Sulindac therapy. Gastroenterology 1994; 107:854-7.
65. Ponz de Leon M, Antonioli A, Ascari A et al. Incidence and familial occurrence of colorectal cancer and polyps in a Health-Care district of Northern Italy. Cancer 1987; 62:2848-59.
66. Wilcox GM, Anderson PB, Colacchio TA. Early invasive carcinoma in colonic polyps. Cancer 1986; 57:160-71.
67. Subramony C, Scott-Conner CEH, Skelto D et al. Familial juvenile polyposis. Study of a kindred: evolution of polyps and relationship to gastrointestinal carcinoma. Am J Clin Pathol 1994; 102:91-7.
68. Owen DA. Flat adenoma, flat carcinoma and de novo carcinoma of the colon. Cancer 1996; 77:3-6.
69. Wilcox GM, Beck JR. Early invasive cancer in adenomatous colonic polyps ("Malignant polyps"). Evaluation of the therapeutic options by decision analysis. Gastroenterology 1987; 92:1159-68.
70. Radice P, Cama A, Mariani-Costantini R. Molecular genetics of polyposis and hereditary colorectal cancer. FORUM Trends in experimental and clinical medicine 1996; 6:275-91.
71. O'Brien MJ, Winawer SJ, Zauber AG et al. The National Polyp Study. Patient and polyp characteristics associated with high-grade dysplasia in colorectal adenomas. Gastroenterology 1990; 98:371-9.
72. Bond JH. Interference with the Adenoma-Carcinoma sequence. Eur J Cancer 1995; 31 A:1115-7.
73. Stryker SJ, Wolff BG, Culp CE et al. Natural history of untreated colonic polyps. Gastroenterology 1987; 93:1009-13.
74. Ohnishi T, Tomita N, Monden T et al. A detailed analysis of the role of K-ras gene mutation in the progression of colorectal adenoma. Br J Cancer 1997; 75:341-7.
75. Zauber NP, Sabbath-Solitare M, Marotta SP et al. K-ras mutation and loss of heterozygosity of the adenomatous polyposis coli gene in patients with colorectal adenomas with in situ carcinoma. Cancer 1999; 86:31-6.
76. Vogelstein B, Fearon ER, Hamilton SR et al. Genetic alterations during colorectal-tumor development. N Engl J Med 1988; 319:525-32.
77. Lipkin M, Blattner WE, Fraumeni JF et al. Tritiated thymidine labeling distribution as a marker for hereditary predisposition to colon cancer. Cancer Res 1983; 43:1899-904.
78. Ponz de Leon M, Roncucci L, Di Donato P et al. Pattern of epithelial cell proliferation in colorectal mucosa of normal subjects and of patients with adenomatous polyps or cancer of the large bowel. Cancer Res 1988; 48:4121-6.
79. Goelz S, Vogelstein B, Hamilton S et al. Hypomethylation of DNA from benign and malignant human colon neoplasms. Science 1985; 228:187-90.
80. Vogelstein B, Fearon E, Kern et al. Allelotype of colorectal carcinomas. Science 1989; 244:207-11.
81. Bos J, Fearon ER, Hamilton SR et al. Prevalence of ras gene mutations in human colorectal cancers. Nature 1987; 327:293-7.
82. Cho KR, Vogelstein B. Genetic alterations in the adenoma-carcinoma sequence. Cancer 1992; 70:1727-31.
83. Kinzler K, Nilbert M, Vogelstein B et al. Identification of a gene located at chromosome 5q21 that is mutated in colorectal cancers. Science 1991; 251:1366-70.

84. Boland CR, Sato J, Appelman HD et al. Microallelotyping defines the sequence and tempo of allelic losses at tumour suppressor gene loci during colorectal cancer progression. Nat Med 1995; 1:902-9.
85. Lynch HT, Fusaro RM, Lynch J. Hereditary cancer in adults. Cancer Detection and Prevention 1995; 19:219-33.
86. Lynch HT, Smyrk T. Hereditary Nonpolyposis Colorectal Cancer (Lynch syndrome). Cancer 1996; 78:1149-67.
87. Rodriguez-Bigas MA, Boland CR, Hamilton SR et al. A national Cancer Institute Workshop on Hereditary Nonpolyposis Colorectal Cancer syndrome: meeting highlights and Bethesda guidelines. J Natl Cancer Inst 1997; 89:1758-62.
88. Lynch HT, Watson P, Shaw TG et al. Clinical impact of molecular genetic diagnosis, genetic counseling, and management of hereditary cancer. Part II: hereditary nonpolyposis colorectal carcinoma as a model. Cancer 1999; 86:1637-43.
89. Kinzler KW, Vogelstein B. Lessons from Hereditary Colorectal Cancer. Cell 1996; 87: 159-70.
90. Wallace MH, Phillips KS. Upper gastrointestinal disease in patients with familial adenomatous polyposis. Br J Surg 1998; 85:742-50.
91. Ponz de Leon M, Sassatelli R, Benatti P et al. Identification of Hereditary nonpolyposis colorectal cancer in the general population. The 6-year experience of a population-based registry. Cancer 1993; 71:3493-3501.
92. Carstensen B, Soll-Johanning H, Villadsen E et al. Familial aggregation of colorectal cancer in the general population. Int J Cancer 1996; 68:428-35.
93. Goldgar D, Easton D, Cannon-Albright L et al. Systematic population-based assessment of cancer risk in first-degree relatives of cancer probands. J Natl Cancer Inst 1994; 86:1600-8.
94. Duncan JL, Kyle J. Family incidence of carcinoma of the colon and rectum in North-East Scotland. Gut 1982; 23:169-71.
95. Frayling IM, Beck NE, Ilyas M et al. The APC variants I1307 K and E1317Q are associated with colorectal tumors, but not always with a family history. Proc Natl Acad Sci. 1998; 95:10722-7.
96. Woodage T, King SM, Wacholder S et al. The APC I1307 K allele and cancer risk in a community-based study of Ashkenazi Jews. Nature Genet 1998; 20:62-5.
97. White RL. Excess risk of colon cancer associated with a polymorphism of the APC gene? Cancer Res 1998; 58:4038-9.
98. Stern HS, Viertelhausen S, Hunter AGW et al. APC I1307 K increases risk of transition from polyp to colorectal carcinoma in Ashkenazi Jews. Gastroenterology 2001; 120: 392-400.
99. Fante R, Roncucci L, Di Gregorio C et al. Frequency and clinical features of multiple tumors of the large bowel in general population and in patients with hereditary colorectal carcinoma. Cancer 1996; 77:2013-21.
100. Bellacosa A, Genuardi M, Anti M et al. Hereditary Nonpolyposis Colorectal Cancer: review of clinical, molecular genetics, and counseling aspects. Am J Med Genet 1996; 62:353-64.
101. Vasen HFA, Mecklin JP, Meera Khan P et al. The International Collaborative group on hereditary non-polyposis colorectal cancer (ICG-HNPCC). Dis Colon Rectum 1991; 34:424-5.
102. Vasen HFA, Watson P, Mecklin JP et al and the ICG-HNPCC. New clinical criteria for Hereditary Nonpolyposis Colorectal Cancer (HNPCC, Lynch syndrome) proposed by the International Collaborative Group on HNPCC. Gastroenterology 1999; 116: 1453-6.
103. Lynch HT, Drouhard TJ, Schuelke GS et al. Hereditary nonpolyposis colorectal cancer in a Navajo Indian family. Cancer Genet Cytogenet 1985; 15:209-13.
104. San Jose BA, Navarro NS, Doble F. Hereditary nonpolyposis colorectal cancer: an awareness. JMMS 1989; 25:37-8.

105. Burt RW, Bishop T, Cannon LA et al. Dominant inheritance of adenomatous colonic polyps and colorectal cancer. N Engl J Med 1985; 312:1540-4.
106. Mecklin JP. Frequency of hereditary colorectal carcinoma. Gastroenterology 1987; 93:1021-5.
107. Westlake PJ, Bryant HE, Huchcroft SA et al. Frequency of hereditary nonpolyposis colorectal cancer in Southern Alberta. Dig Dis Sci 1991; 36:1441-7.
108. Benatti P, Sassatelli R, Roncucci L et al. Tumour spectrum in Hereditary non-polyposis colorectal cancer (HNPCC) and in families with "suspected HNPCC". A population-based study in Northern Italy. Int J Cancer 1993; 54:371-7.
109. Wijnen JT, Vasen HFA, Meera Khan P et al. Clinical findings with implications for genetic testing in families with clustering of colorectal cancer. N Engl J Med 1998; 339:511-8.
110. Nicolaides NC, Papadopoulos N, Liu B et al. Mutations of two PMS homologues in hereditary nonpolyposis colon cancer. Nature 1994; 371:75-80.
111. Peltomäki P, Aaltonen LA, Sistonen P et al. Genetic mapping of a locus predisposing to human colorectal cancer. Science 1993; 260:812-2.
112. Liu B, Parsons R, Papadopoulos N et al. Analysis of mismatch repair genes in hereditary non-polyposis colorectal cancer patients. Nat Med 1996; 2:169-74.
113. Papadopoulos N, Nicolaides NC, Wei YF et al Mutation of a *mutL* homolog in hereditary colon cancer. Science 1994; 263:1625-9.
114. Peltomäki P, Vasen HFA, the International Collaborative Group on Hereditary Nonpolyposis Colorectal Cancer. Mutations predisposing to Hereditary Nonpolyposis Colorectal Cancer: database and results of a collaborative study. Gastroenterology 1997; 113:1146-1158.
115. Loeb LA. Microsatellite instability: marker of a mutator phenotype in cancer. Cancer Res 1994; 54:5059-63.
116. Boyer JC, Umar A, Risinger JI et al. Microsatellite instability, mismatch repair deficiency and genetic defects in human cancer cell lines. Cancer Res 1995; 55:6063-70.
117. Aaltonen LA, Peltomaki P, Mecklin JP et al. Replication errors in benign and malignant tumors from Hereditary Nonpolyposis Colorectal Cancer patients. Cancer Res 1994; 54:1645-8.
118. Jass JR, Cottier DS, Jeevaratnam P et al. Diagnostic use of microsatellite instability in hereditary non-polyposis colorectal cancer. Lancet 1995; 346:1200-1.
119. Bellacosa A, Cicchilitti L, Scherpis F et al. MED1, a novel human methyl-CpG-binding endonuclease, interacts with DNA mismatch repair protein MLH1. Proc Natl Acad Sci 1999; 96:3969-74.
120. Viel A, Genuardi M, Capozzi E et al. Characterizaton of MSH2 and MLH1 mutations in italian families with hereditary nonpolyposis colorectal cancer. Genes Chrom Cancer 1997; 18:8-18.
121. Genuardi M, Anti M, Capozzi E et al. MLH1 and MSH2 constitutional mutations in colorectal cancer families not meeting the standard criteria for hereditary nonpolyposis colorectal cancer. Int J Cancer 1998; 75:835-9.
122. Weber TK, Conton W, Petrelli NJ et al. Genomic DNA-based hMSH2 and hMLH1 mutation screening in 32 eastern United States hereditary nonpolyposis colorectal cancer pedigrees. Cancer Res 1997; 57:3798-803.
123. Tannergård P, Lipford J, Kolodner R et al. Mutation screening in the hMLH1 gene in swedish hereditary nonpolyposis colon cancer families. Cancer Res 1995; 55:6092-6.
124. Petersen GM, Boyd PA. Gene tests and counseling for colorectal cancer risk: lessons from familial polyposis. J Natl Cancer Inst 1995; 17:67-71.
125. Groden J, Thliveris A, Samowitz W et al. Identification and characterization of the familial adenomatous polyposis coli gene. Cell 1991; 66:589-600.
126. Haggitt RC, Reid BJ. Hereditary gastrointestinal polyposis syndromes. Am J Surg Pathol 1986; 10:871-87.
127. Nance FC. Management strategies for familial adenomatous polyposis. Ann Surg 1993; 217:99-100.

128. Ziv Y, Church JM, Oakley JR et al. Surgery for the teenager with familial adenomatous polyposis: ileo-rectal anastomosis or restorative proctolectomy? Int J Colorect Dis 1995; 10:6-9.
129. Utsunomiya J, Iwama T. Adenomatosis coli in Japan. In: Winawer S, Schottenfeld D, Sherlock P. Colorectal Cancer: Prevention, Epidemiology and Screening. New York, Raven Press, 1980; 83-95.
130. De Pietri S, Sassatelli R, Roncucci L et al. Clinical and biologic features of adenomatosis coli in Northern Italy. Scand J Gastroenterol 1995; 30:771-9.
131. Berk T, Cohen Z, McLeod RS et al. Congenital hypertrophy of the retinal pigment epithelium as a marker for familial adenomatous polyposis. Dis Colon Rectum 1988; 31:253-7.
132. Lyons LA, Lewis RA, Strong LC et al. A genetic study of Gardner syndrome and congenital hypertrophy of the retinal pigment epithelium. Am J Hum Genet 1988; 42:290-6.
133. Heiskanen I, Järvinen HJ. Occurrence of desmoid tumours in familial adenomatous polyposis and results of treatment. Int J Colorect Dis 1996; 11:157-62.
134. Lewis JJ, Boland PJ, Leung DHY et al. The enigma of desmoid tumors. Ann Surg 1999; 229:866-73.
135. Bülow C, Bülow S and the Leeds Caste Polyposis Group. Is screening for thyroid carcinoma indicated in familial adenomatous polyposis? Int J Colorect Dis 1997; 12: 240-2.
136. Kikuchi T, Rempel SA, Rutz HP et al. Turcot's syndrome of glioma and polyposis occurs in the absence of germ line mutations of exons 5 to 9 of the p53 gene. Cancer Res 1993; 53:957-61.
137. Matsui T, Hayashi N, Yao K et al. A father and son with Turcot's syndrome: evidence for autosomal dominant inheritance. Report of two cases. Dis Colon Rectum 1998; 41:797-801.
138. Dobbie Z, Spycher M, Hürliman R et al. Mutational analysis of the first 14 exons of the adenomatous polyposis coli (APC) gene. Eur J Cancer 1994; 30 A:1709-13.
139. Pedemonte S, Sciallero S, Gismondi V et al. Novel germline APC variants in patients with multiple adenomas. Gene Chrom Cancer 1998; 22:257-67.
140. Bodmer WF, Bailey CJ, Bodmer J et al. Localization of the gene for familial adenomatous polyposis on chromosome 5. Nature 1987; 328:614-9.
141. Kinzler KW, Nilbert MC, Su LK et al. Identification of FAP locus gene from chromosome 5q12. Science 1991; 253:661-5.
142. Moon RT, Miller JR. The APC tumor suppressor protein in development and cancer. Trends Genet 1997; 13:256-8.
143. Laken SJ, Papadopoulos N, Petersen GM et al. Analysis of masked mutations in familial adenomatous polyposis. Proc Natl Acad Sci 1999; 96:2322-6.
144. Joslyn G, Carlson M, Thliveris A et al. Identification of deletion mutations and three new genes at the familial polyposis locus. Cell 1991; 66:601-13.
145. Olschwang S, Laurent-Pulg P, Groden J et al. Germ-line mutations in the first 14 exons of the adenomatous polyposis coli (APC) gene. Am J Hum Genet 1993; 52: 273-9.
146. Leggett BA, Young JP, Biden K et al. Severe upper gastrointestinal polyposis associated with sparse colonic polyposis in a familial adenomatous polyposis family with an APC mutation at codon 1520. Gut 1997; 41:518-21.
147. Ponz de Leon M, Benatti P, Percesepe A et al. Clinical features and genotype-phenotype correlations in 41 italian families with Adenomatosis Coli. Ital J Gastroenterol Hepatol 1999; 31:850-60.
148. Nugent KP, Phillips RKS, Hodgson SV et al. Phenotypic expression in familial adenomatous polyposis: partial prediction by mutation analysis. Gut 1994; 35:1622-3.
149. Giardiello FM, Petersen GM, Piantadosi S et al. APC gene mutations and extraintestinal phenotype of familial adenomatous polyposis. Gut 1997; 40:521-5.

150. Gebert JF, Dupon C, Kadmon M et al. Combined molecular and clinical approaches for the identification of families with familial adenomatous polyposis coli. Ann Surg 1999; 229:350-61.
151. Presciuttini S, Gismondi V, Scarcello E et al. Different expressivity of two adjacent mutations of the APC gene. Tumori 1999; 85:28-31.
152. MacPhee M, Chepenik KP, Liddell RA et al. The secretory phospholipase A2 gene is a candidate for the *Mom1* locus, a major modifier of APC^{Min}-induced intestinal neoplasia. Cell 1995; 81:957-66.
153. Moser AR, Luongo C, Gould KA et al. Apc^{Min}: a mouse model for intestinal and mammary tumorigenesis. Eur J Cancer 1995; 31 A:1061-4.
154. McMichael AJ, Potter JD. Host factors in carcinogenesis: certain bile-acid metabolic profiles that selectively increase the risk of proximal colon cancer. J Natl Cancer Inst. 1985; 75:185-91.
155. Sugimura T, Sato S. Mutagens-carcinogenes in foods. Cancer Res 1983; 43:2415-21.
156. Rüschoff J, Wallinger S, Dietmaier W et al. Aspirin suppresses the mutator phenotype associated with hereditary nonpolyposis colorectal cancer by genetic selection. Proc Natl Acad Sci 1998; 95:11301-6.

2 Pathogenesis of Colorectal Cancer

Introduction

Despite the new technological advancements in early diagnosis and therapeutic strategies, the clinical outcome of patients with colorectal malignancies has changed relatively little over the past 50 years [1, 2]. This concept clearly underlines the need for new therapeutic approaches based on a greater understanding of the molecular basis of these tumors.

During the last 2-3 decades of the past century, several exciting advances have been made regarding factors predisposing to colorectal cancer. For instance, it has been shown that a definite fraction of these tumors is truly hereditary and, thus, transmitted from one generation to the next in accordance with an autosomal dominant model [3, 4]. Similarly, several environmental factors – mostly related to diet and lifestyle – have been identified which seem to play a certain role in colorectal cancer development [5]. Moreover, there is evidence that adenomatous polyps represent the natural precursor of intestinal malignancies, and that their systematic removal may prevent cancer occurrence [6].

Traditionally, colorectal cancer development has been viewed as an ordered process in which three main phases could be discerned: initiation, promotion and progression [7]. The recent explosion of molecular biology provided definite proof that stable alterations in the structure or sequence of DNA (mutations) represent the initiating event in tumorigenesis; these are followed by an uncontrolled expansion of the neoplastic clones which characterizes tumoral growth [8]. Several classes of genes have been identified (oncogenes, tumor suppressor genes, mutator genes) the alterations of which seem to be crucially important both in the initiation and in the promotion/progression of human tumors [9, 10]. Thus, it is now clear that cancer results from a series of genetic alterations leading to the progressive and irreversible loss of normal control of cell growth and differentiation. These concepts apply virtually to all malignancies but are particularly evident in colorectal carcinoma, where the ordered sequence "normal mucosa – small adenoma – large adenoma – cancer" may allow the characterization of genetic changes in each phase of tumor progression [11]. It is therefore possible to explore in great detail the complex interaction between various environmental factors and the molecular events leading to colorectal neoplasia.

In chapter 1 I focused on the main aetiological factors implicated in colorectal cancer development. In this chapter – after a brief introduction on the main causes of intestinal tumors – I aim to analyze the main pathogenetic pathways leading to colorectal neoplasms under different clinical conditions. The main message is that the same apparent phenotypic manifestations (cancer) may result from different molecular alterations and, presumably, from different "environment-gene interactions". These new concepts might be of relevance for the early diagnosis, surveillance and treatment of patients with colorectal cancer.

Main Causes of Colorectal Cancer

Most colorectal malignancies develop from pre-existing adenomas [12]; these are well demarcated lumps of dysplastic epithelium which can be classified into various histological types. The lesions can be found in all segments of the large bowel, and their frequency increases with age [1]. The large majority of adenomatous polyps are less than 1 cm in diameter; larger lesions may show a villous pattern on histology and are more frequently associated with malignant changes. There is clinical, epidemiological and experimental evidence clearly indicating that adenomatous polyps represent the natural precursor of carcinoma; this, however, does not mean that all polyps evolve into cancer and does not rule out the possibility of "de novo" carcinogenesis (i.e. from apparently flat mucosa). Indeed, a recent paper [13] underlines the potential role of flat lesions (which can be overlooked at endoscopy) as a frequent source of malignancy. Moreover, the passage from normal mucosa to adenoma may involve further steps, such as aberrant crypt foci (ACF), which are viewed as possible precursors of adenomatous lesions and cancer. ACF consist of large and thick intestinal crypts with various degrees of nuclear atypia or dysplasia [14]. ACF can easily been observed in methylene blue-stained specimens of colon from animals treated with a carcinogen [15], as well as in the apparently normal mucosa of patients with colorectal cancer [16].

Although the International Classification of Diseases for Oncology distinguishes colonic and rectal neoplasms, a more recent view [17] suggests that we are dealing with three different types of colorectal malignancies: cancer of the right colon, of the left colon and of the rectum. This new classification is mainly based on the following clues: (1) tumors at these three sites tend to occur with specific incidence rates in different areas of the world, thus suggesting the existence of different causative agents; (2) neoplasms of various colorectal subsites show a specific age and sex relationship (for example, tumors of the right colon tend to be more frequent in women, while tumors of the rectum are more frequent in men); (3) temporal trends show a shift of incidence between proximal (increasing) and distal colonic tumors, again suggesting the existence of different aetiological and risk factors.

Among the various environmental factors, several dietary components – such as animal fat, beef meat and alcoholic beverages – low physical activity, overweight and smoking are somehow related to an increased risk of colorectal cancer. In contrast, fruit, vegetables, unabsorbable fiber, antioxidant vitamins

(A, C and E in particular), calcium, folate, physical exercise and anti-inflammatory drugs (especially aspirin and sulindac) seem to show a protective effect [1, 5] and are actually under evaluation for the chemoprevention of these tumors [18]. Patients with ulcerative colitis – especially when long-lasting and involving the entire large bowel – show a markedly increased risk for colorectal malignancies [19].

Finally, familial and hereditary factors are closely related to the risk of large bowel cancer. Among colorectal cancer patients, 10%–20% have affected first-degree relatives, and for these family members the risk of cancer is about three times higher than in the general population [20]. In addition, two major hereditary colorectal cancer syndromes have been described and characterized at the molecular level [21, 22].

Hereditary nonpolyposis colorectal cancer (HNPCC or Lynch syndrome) is an autosomal dominant disease featuring an early occurrence of cancer (usually of the right colon), frequent development of multiple lesions, and a striking association with neoplasms of other organs (especially endometrium, urinary tract, ovary and small bowel). The genetic basis of HNPCC has recently been clarified with the identification of germline mutations in a class of genes involved in DNA mismatch repair [23, 24].

Familial adenomatous polyposis (FAP, or adenomatosis coli) is an autosomal dominant disorder characterized by the presence of hundreds or thousands of polyps of various dimensions distributed along the large bowel and by several other extracolonic manifestations, including adenomas in the stomach and small intestine, desmoid tumors, retinal spots, osteomas, supernumerary teeth and, more rarely, hepatoblastomas and thyroid cancer [25, 26]. The gene responsible for the disease when mutated (called APC, for adenomatous polyposis coli) has recently been mapped (chromosome 5q21) and sequenced [27, 28]; the gene encodes a 2843-amino acid protein which plays a role in the cell adhesion process and signal transduction [29]. Besides FAP, other, rarer forms of hereditary polyposis include Turcot syndrome [30], Peutz-Jeghers disease [31], Cowden disease [32], juvenile polyposis [33], Muir-Torre syndrome [34], Ruvalcaba-Mirhe-Smith disease [35] and Cronkhite-Canada syndrome [36]. For some of these conditions, the genetic basis has recently been characterized, and in some cases this led to the identification of new models of colorectal tumorigenesis (see chapters 11 and 12). Somatic mutations of the *APC* gene are also frequent in sporadic benign and malignant colorectal tumors [27, 33].

Pathogenesis of Colorectal Cancer: Different Molecular Pathways for One Disease

The basic architecture of the large bowel is characterized by glands (crypts) – constituted by columnar and mucinous cells – that are approximately 40–60 cells deep. Under normal conditions, the proliferative zone is confined to the lower portions of the crypts: cells migrate to the upper portions and then are extruded from the mucosal surface; the whole process takes 4–6 days [37]. In the early stages of colorectal tumorigenesis, colonic epithelial cells become unable to repress DNA synthesis during migration from the base to the surface of the crypt and develop an enhanced capacity to proliferate; consequently, the proliferative zone expands, and S-phase cells are distributed throughout the whole length of the gland [38]. Thus, colorectal carcinogenesis begins with a generalized disorder of cell replication and differentiation that antedates, and then accompanies, the development of morphological lesions (aberrant crypt foci, small adenomas, large adenomas and cancer).

Unlike the situation with other common malignancies, colorectal cancer development appears to be an ordered multistep process in which lesions in various stages of progression – from ACF to adenomas of different sizes and, ultimately, to infiltrating carcinoma – can be observed and analyzed. This particular biological behavior provides an excellent system for the study of genetic abnormalities involved in tumor formation. The results of these investigations led to the formulation of a general model for colorectal tumorigenesis, in which the accumulation of genetic changes is responsible for successive waves of clonal expansion that occur during tumor promotion and progression [39] (Fig. 2.1).

Several of these genetic abnormalities have already been identified, while others are under active investigation. The most common include inactivation of tumor suppressor genes, activation of oncogenes (by mutation, overexpression, amplification or other mechanisms), functional or mutational inactivation of a class of genes involved in repairing DNA mismatches (MMR genes) and abnormal DNA methylation. Initially, the accumulation of genetic alterations seemed to be more relevant for tumor formation than their ordered sequence [11]; subsequent studies showed that the occurrence of these lesions may not be casual, and that "rate-limiting" steps could be identified, thus suggesting that a precise ordering of genetic changes can be equally important and, even more relevant, might be different for tumors of different etiology [40].

The available evidence suggests that there are several molecular pathways that can explain the passage from normal mucosa to colorectal carcinoma; this implies the existence of intestinal carcinomas with different biological natures and, possibly, clinical behavior. These new findings confirm the hypothesis of Weisburger and Wynder [17], formulated on the basis of epidemiological observations and before the explosion of molecular biology. Even more important, the existence of different pathways to colorectal carcinoma might allow the development of new approaches targeted to specific molecular steps.

Sporadic Colorectal Cancer Development (Loss of Heterozygosity Pathway)

The large majority of colorectal neoplasms are sporadic tumors. Various cytogenetic observations showed that chromosomes 5q, 17p and 18q were frequently altered in these tumors, in both numerical and structural aspects, while abnormalities of other chromosomes were observed less frequently [41, 42]. These findings are of considerable relevance, since they demonstrate that the simple morphological observation of chromosome structure may provide valu-

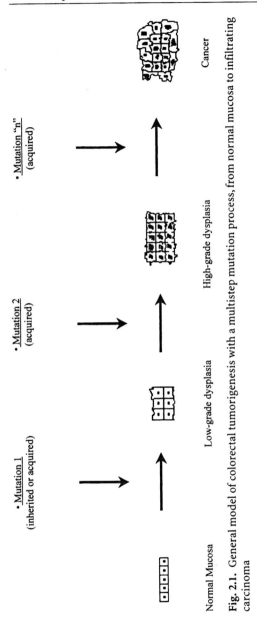

Fig. 2.1. General model of colorectal tumorigenesis with a multistep mutation process, from normal mucosa to infiltrating carcinoma

able information on the presumed localization of genes involved in colorectal tumorigenesis.

Taking advantage of these observations, Vogelstein and collaborators, in a landmark study [11], analyzed *ras* gene mutations and allelic deletions in chromosomes 5, 17 and 18 in 172 colorectal tumors representing various stages of neoplastic development along the adenoma-carcinoma sequence. They showed that the number of genetic changes tended to increase in parallel with the severity of the histological lesions and proposed a model in which accumulated alterations affecting at least the *k-ras* dominant oncogene and several putative tumor suppressor genes (inactivated by allelic loss) could be considered responsible for the progression of colorectal tumors, from normal mucosa to infiltrating carcinoma. Subsequent studies confirmed these preliminary observations and clarified the key role of the APC and MCC genes (both located on chromosome 5q), p53 (chromosome 17p) and DCC genes (chromosome 18q) in colorectal tumorigenesis [43,44], whereas the role of other genetic alterations – such as FHIT gene inactivation [45], SRC gene mutations [49], PPP2R1B gene alterations [50], chromosome 1 deletion [51] and many others – appeared much less clear.

In a detailed microallelotyping study [40], Boland et al. analyzed many regions from individual colorectal neoplasms in order to determine the sequence and timing of the main genetic alterations in colorectal tumor progression. The authors observed loss of heterozygosity (LOH) at chromosome 5q even in small adenomatous polyps and suggested that genetic abnormalities at the APC locus presumably represent the initiating event in the genesis of most sporadic neoplasms. In contrast, LOH at chromosome 17p was usually observed in more advanced lesions – often at the transition from low-grade to high-grade dysplasia – thus suggesting a rate-limiting role for the p53 gene in the evolution from dysplastic adenoma to infiltrating carcinoma.

Our current knowledge about the main molecular events of sporadic colorectal tumorigenesis is illustrated in Fig. 2.2. The most likely initiating event seems to be the somatic inactivation (loss or mutation) of APC, which induces aberrant crypts [52] and polyp formation [40] as a result of the loss of harmony in mucosal cell proliferation, adhesion and migration along the crypt axis. Kinzler and Vogelstein [53] suggested that the APC gene acts as a "gatekeeper" of epithelial cell replication, and that inactivation of this gene is required for net cellular proliferation, since gatekeeper genes are responsible – under normal conditions – for maintaining a constant cell number in renewing cell populations. The APC protein contributes to the regulation of cell-to-cell adhesion through its interaction with β-catenin and E-cadherin, and influences cell migration through its interaction with microtubules [54, 55]; thus, APC-inactivating mutations result in an impairment of the normal adhesion-migration of cells and the transcription of the replicative signal.

The transition from small adenoma to large and dysplastic adenoma involves the accumulation of several genetic changes, many of which remain only partially understood. *K-ras* mutations can be found in 40%–50% of adenomas and carcinomas [56]. DCC gene (for deleted in colorectal carcinoma) losses or mutations are particularly interesting, since DCC encodes a protein with sequence similarities to neural cell adhesion molecules, which indicates a possible role of this gene in regulating cell-environment interactions [57–59]. Deletions of the DPC4 gene are common in colorectal tumors, while missense mutations were found more rarely [46]; the gene has also been implicated in pancreatic carcinogenesis [60]. Finally, changes in the methylation pattern of DNA have frequently been reported in colorectal tumorigenesis [61]; DNA hypermethylation can inhibit the transcrip-

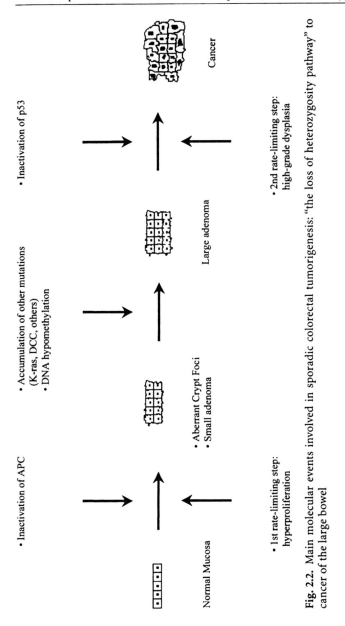

Fig. 2.2. Main molecular events involved in sporadic colorectal tumorigenesis: "the loss of heterozygosity pathway" to cancer of the large bowel

tion of tumor suppressor and of mismatch repair genes, thus providing an alternative explanation for gene inactivation during colonic cancer development [62].

In the final step – from dysplastic adenoma to infiltrating carcinoma – the available evidence indicates a key role for the p53 tumor suppressor gene, which appears to be mutated in the majority of colorectal carcinomas [63, 64]. The p53 gene exhibits several well known as well as hypothetical functions (which are

Table 2.1. The main genes involved in colorectal carcinogenesis (LOH, loss of heterozygosity; PJS, Peutz-Jeghers syndrome; FAP, familial adenomatous polyposis; FJP, familial juvenile polyposis; MSI, microsatellite instability; HNPCC, hereditary nonpolyposis colorectal cancer)

Gene	Chromosomal location	Function	Involved pathway
p53	17p13	Regulation of cell cycle and apoptosis	LOH, PJS, FAP
APC	5q21	"Gatekeeper" of colonic epithelial cell replication	LOH, FAP
K-ras	11p15	Encodes a GTPase-activating protein	LOH, FAP (?)
DCC	18q	Regulation of cell-environment interactions	LOH, FAP (?), PJS (?)
STK11	18q13	Encodes a serine/threonine kinase	PJS
SMAD4	18q21	TGFβ signaling pathway	FJP
PTEN	10q23	Encodes a phosphatase	Cowden syndrome
MSH2	2p16	DNA mismatch repair	HNPCC – MSI
MLH1	3p21	DNA mismatch repair	HNPCC – MSI
PMS1	2q31	DNA mismatch repair	HNPCC – MSI
PMS2	7p22	DNA mismatch repair	HNPCC – MSI
MSH6	2p16	DNA mismatch repair	HNPCC – MSI
BUB1	2q12	Control of mitotic check point	Aneuploid tumors

beyond the scope of this review). It encodes a phosphoprotein which binds to specific DNA sequences and activates several target genes. Among genes with known p53-responsive elements are p51, GADD45 Mdm-2 and many others; moreover, various studies identified several proteins with which p53 may interact in vitro, on account of its unique, highly folded DNA binding configuration [65]. Wild-type p53 regulates various phases of the cell cycle and stimulates the DNA repair system; thus, it is not surprising that inactivation of p53 – through mutations of the gene or binding to specific viral or cellular oncoproteins – is closely associated with human tumorigenesis [66] (Table 2.1).

Tumor Development in FAP and Other Polyposis Syndromes

In contrast to patients with sporadic tumors, individuals affected by familial adenomatous polyposis (FAP) inherit a constitutional mutation in one of the alleles of the APC gene [27, 28]. Polyps and other extracolonic manifestations are not present at birth, but usually develop in the second decade of life through the inactivation of wild-type alleles in the mucosal cells of the intestine; when this occurs, adenomas gradually accumulate in the large bowel, in most cases beginning in the recto-sigmoid region [25, 26]. Mutations located in the central portions of the gene (codons 1200–1350) are usually associated with profuse microadenomatosis, with the colon virtually carpeted by thousands of polyps [67, 68]; mutations located within exons 1–4 or in the most distal portions of the gene (around codon 1600) may induce an attenuated type of FAP in which the number of polyps is usually low (50–100) [69, 70]. Whatever the type of mutation and the number of polyps, the development of malignant lesions requires many years, and in most series the average age at cancer diagnosis is around 35 years. Thus, subjects with germline mutations of the APC gene develop adenomatous polyps only upon complete inactivation of the gene; moreover, they do not necessarily develop cancer, but having hundreds or thousands of adenomatous polyps in their large bowel, the probability that one of these lesions evolves into carcinoma is extremely high. In fact, many of the polyps tend to increase in size and to become dysplastic, especially those located in the most distal portions of the large bowel. The transition from small adenoma to large, dysplastic and then infiltrating lesions requires the accumulation of several other genetic events, which do not seem to be different from those described for sporadic tumors (i.e. mutations of *k-ras* and other oncogenes; inactivation of DCC, p53 and related tumor suppressor genes; possible involvement of modifier genes) [71]. The main molecular and morphological events in FAP tumorigenesis are outlined in Fig. 2.3. Involvement of the APC gene in both FAP and sporadic colorectal carcinoma provides further support for the "two-hit" hypothesis of cancer development proposed by Knudson for childhood neoplasms, such as retinoblastoma and Wilms' tumor [72]. For cancer in adults, however, the situation is more complex, and the two-hit sequence may fully explain polyps but not cancer formation; for this, several other genetic alterations are needed, which usually accumulate over the course of many years.

Among the various less frequent polyposis conditions [30–36], Peutz-Jeghers syndrome [31], juvenile polyposis [33] and Cowden disease [32] have recently been characterized at the molecular level with the identification of the genes responsible for the neoplastic phenotype when mutated. Peutz-Jeghers syndrome (PJS) is a rare autosomal dominant disorder characterized by the early appearance of hamartomatous polyps in the small and large bowel and by mucocutaneous melanin spots, especially in the cheeks and around the lips [73]. Initially considered a fairly benign condition, recent studies have shown that patients with PJS are at increased risk of neoplasms of many organs, including the large and small bowel, pancreas, lung, ovary, breast, thyroid and uterus [74]. The gene responsible for PJS, called STK11, has recently been located at 19p13.3 and encodes a novel serine/threonine kinase, the possible functions of which are under active investigation [75, 76]. The development of a colorectal tumor in PJS, therefore, requires a different initiating event (germline mutations in the STK11 gene) and different intermediate lesions (hamartomatous polyps). Gruber et al. [77] recently studied six PJS families in an attempt to identify the molecular basis of the disease and to characterize the various genetic alterations involved in the development of hamartomas and adenocarcinomas. Inactivating STK11 mutations were detected in hamartomas of all families and appear necessary and sufficient to initiate PJS; thus, the evidence suggests that STK11 is a tumor suppressor gene implicated in the earliest phases of the pathogenesis of

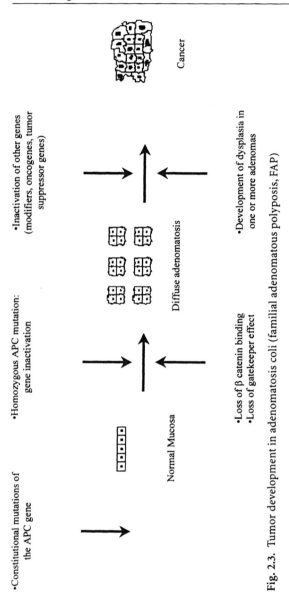

Fig. 2.3. Tumor development in adenomatosis coli (familial adenomatous polyposis, FAP)

hamartomatous polyps and, subsequently, adenocarcinomas. Since no alterations of the APC gene were found, STK11 presumably plays a "gatekeeper" role similar to that of APC in FAP, regulating the development of hamartomas in PJS; moreover, these polyps, previously considered benign, seem to be the precursor lesions of adenocarcinomas. Since none of the 18 tumor samples showed *k-ras* gene mutations, it is likely that alterations of this commonly mutated oncogene are not essential for tumor development in PJS. Loss of heterozygosity on 17p and 18q was detected in adenocarcinomas but not hamartomas; these findings – together with positive immunohistochemical staining for p53 protein – seem to suggest that p53 and presumably other tumor suppressor genes, such as DCC, are involved in a later stage of tumorigenesis in PJS. A tentative pathway to colorectal cancer in PJS is illustrated in Fig. 2.4.

Juvenile polyposis (JP) is a rare disease characterized by the occurrence of multiple juvenile polyps throughout the entire gastrointestinal tract [78]. Almost half of these patients show a strong family history for the trait and features of autosomal dominant transmission (FJP) [79]. Juvenile polyps are considered a subgroup of hamartomas, showing cystically dilated glands, proliferation of stromal elements and an inflammatory infiltrate; since some of these polyps may undergo adenomatous transformation, affected family members show an increased risk for cancer of the gastrointestinal tract [80]. The genetic basis of FJP is at present rather complex and only partially clarified, and available evidence suggests that there is genetic heterogeneity in this syndrome. Constitutional mutation in PTEN, a gene responsible for Cowden disease (see below), has been described in some patients with features of JP [81]; however, it is possible that this represents a phenotypic variant of Cowden disease. More recently, germline mutations in the SMAD4 gene have been found in the majority of patients affected by FJP. The gene is located on chromosome 18q21, appears to be frequently deleted in pancreatic cancer, and encodes a cytoplasmic protein involved in the TGFβ signaling pathway, which mediates growth inhibitory signals from the cell surface to the nucleus [82, 83]. Since not all investigated families and subjects showed germline SMAD4 mutations, it is entirely possible that constitutional mutations in other genes involved in the TGFβ signaling pathway could be present in different families with JP. Despite these preliminary results, the detailed process of cancer development in JP (which also includes pancreatic carcinoma in the disease spectrum) remains to be elucidated.

Cowden syndrome (multiple hamartoma syndrome) is a rare autosomal dominant disease characterized by multiple hamartomas of the skin, oral mucosa, breast, thyroid gland and gastrointestinal tract [84]. The most frequent of these lesions are trichilemmomas of the skin and mucocutaneous papillomatous papules which are present in virtually all patients with Cowden disease (CD). Hamartomatous polyps of the gastrointestinal tract have been reported in 50%–60% of these patients, but their malignant transformation into carcinomas is still questioned. The polyps can be localized anywhere along the gastrointestinal tract and show a wide range of histological features, including typical juvenile polyps, inflammatory polyps, lipomas, ganglioneuromas and lymphoid hyperplasia [85]. Patients with CD are at increased risk for breast and thyroid malignant tumors [86]. The gene responsible for CD when mutated has recently been identified as PTEN/MMAC1 and encodes a dual specificity phosphatase [87]. Germline PTEN mutations have been reported in the large majority of families and patients with CD [88, 89]; moreover, loss of heterozygosity and PTEN deletion were reported in fibroadenomas of the breast, thyroid adenomas and pulmonary hamartomas [89]. From the (limited) evidence available,

34   Pathogenesis of Colorectal Cancer

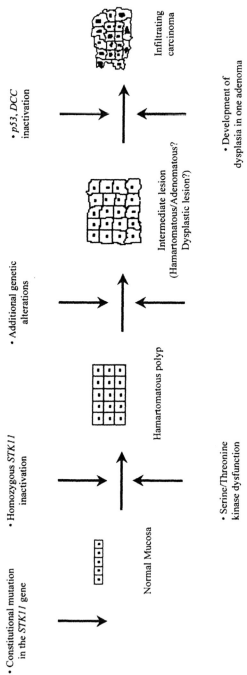

Fig. 2.4. Main genetic alterations involved in Peutz-Jeghers syndrome

it is therefore likely that PTEN behaves as a tumor suppressor gene in CD. Complete inactivation of the gene may lead to hamartomas, other benign tumors and a generalized hyperproliferative status. The development of carcinoma in certain organs (including the colorectum) can be favored by this background, but presumably requires alterations of other genes as well as the interaction with environmental factors.

Colorectal Tumorigenesis in HNPCC
(Mutator Genes/Microsatellite Instability Pathway)

HNPCC (or Lynch syndrome) is an autosomal dominant disorder characterized by the early appearance of malignant tumors predominantly localized in the proximal colon (from caecum to splenic flexure), synchronous and metachronous colorectal neoplasms, and is frequently associated with tumors of other organs [21].

Individuals with Lynch syndrome inherit (or develop) a constitutional mutation in one of the several genes responsible for repairing DNA mismatches. These genes are named hMSH2, hMLH1, hPMS1, hPMS2 and hMSH6/GTBP from the homologous bacterial genes [90-93]. When a somatic mutation inactivates the corresponding wild-type allele, the affected cell - in the colorectal mucosa as well as in the other target organs - tends to accumulate other mutations at a very high rate, and this may enhance the potential for malignant transformation. It should be noted, however, that germline mutations of the DNA mismatch repair genes (called also "mutator genes") can at present be detected in 30%-70% of the investigated families [94-96]. This may reflect an overall low accuracy of the available techniques for detecting mutator gene mutations [97] or to the fact that in some kindreds, chance cancer aggregation may mimic HNPCC, due to the frequency of phenocopies. Alternatively, other unknown genes - either related or unrelated to the DNA mismatch repair - might be responsible for a given fraction of HNPCC.

Inactivation of mutator genes leads to genomic instability, which is particularly evident at microsatellite loci. These are repeated sequences of DNA that are distributed throughout the human genome, most commonly $(A)n/(T)n$ and $(CA)n/(GT)n$. The function of microsatellites is unknown, but they are particularly useful in linkage studies, owing to their high degree of polymorphism [98, 99]. The large majority of tumors from HNPCC patients shows microsatellite instability (MSI) in most of the loci; MSI is also present in 10%-15% of sporadic colorectal malignancies. Thus, mutations in the genes associated with the phenotypic expression of Lynch syndrome are responsible for genomic instability through a generalized defect in the replication/repair processes.

The sequence of events that leads to colorectal cancer development in HNPCC is illustrated in Fig. 2.5. The initial event is a constitutional mutation in one of the several DNA mismatch repair genes; they behave like tumor suppressor genes, so that in the heterozygote state cells have approximately normal DNA repair activity, but loss or mutation of the wild-type allele (i.e. inactivation of the

36 Pathogenesis of Colorectal Cancer

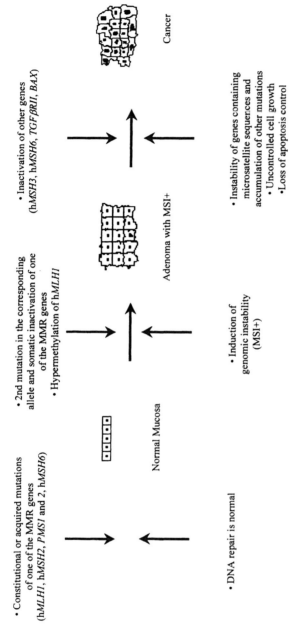

Fig. 2.5. The mismatch repair pathway to colorectal cancer: "the mutator which mutates other mutators"

gene) results in cells with defective repair activity. Such cells develop a "mutator phenotype" [100] and accumulate mutations at a very high rate, with the consequence that polyps occur in the large bowel of these patients. Adenomatous polyps in HNPCC are usually larger than sporadic polyps, show features of aggressive lesions (villous pattern and high-grade dysplasia) more often and tend to appear at an early age [101–103]. Thus, there are reasons to believe that the sequence adenoma-carcinoma is accelerated in HNPCC, and the frequent occurrence of "interval cancers" (i.e. malignant tumors that develop during endoscopic surveillance, in the interval between two successive controls) lends further support to this hypothesis [104, 105].

But how does cancer occur in HNPCC or, in other words, what are the crucial additional mutations which induce the malignant transformation of a large adenoma? Although neoplasms with MSI may accumulate mutations in genes commonly involved in colorectal tumorigenesis (such as *k-ras* or p53), there is evidence indicating a key role of less common mutations. Thus, it has been shown that 90% or more of MSI cancers show alterations of the TGF-βII receptor gene [106]; this gene inhibits the growth of colonic epithelial cells, and thus, when the receptor is inactivated, cell replication is not inhibited, and this may lead to uncontrolled growth and eventually to cancer. The TGF-βII receptor gene contains a short microsatellite of ten consecutive A bases, which are prone to mismatch errors in MSI tumors; for this reason the receptor might be susceptible to mutations in HNPCC tumors. Moreover, other mismatch repair genes – such as MSH3, MSH6 and MLH1 – contain short repeated sequences and are frequently mutated in MSI tumors [107, 108], thus contributing to the malignant transformation in HNPCC. This event led Perucho and collaborators to state that in their model of carcinogenesis "the mutator (the gene with germline mutation) mutates other mutators (the mismatch repair genes mutated at a somatic level due to microsatellite instability)" [109]. Finally, mutations of several other genes – such as BAX, which controls apoptosis – have also been frequently reported in HNPCC [110]. Comparing Fig. 2.2 with Fig. 2.5, it is interesting to note that despite a similar morphologic sequence of events (normal mucosa, adenomas of various size and infiltrating carcinoma), the molecular mechanisms underlying sporadic and hereditary carcinogenesis are somehow different.

A subset of apparently sporadic colorectal neoplasms (10%–15% of the total) show microsatellite instability. These tumors are frequently located in the proximal colon, often exhibit a mucinous histological type, and tend to appear at an advanced age [111]. Pedigree analysis is not consistent with HNPCC but may show some non-specific cancer aggregation. In these cases, mutator genes (especially MSH2 and MLH1) can be somatically inactivated by mutations or other epigenetic mechanisms [112], and various immunohistochemical studies demonstrate loss of expression of DNA mismatch repair genes (mainly MLH1). Recent studies showed that the main cause of mutator gene inactivation in this subset of sporadic tumors is the hypermethylation of MLH1 promoter region [113], which leads to a decreased expression of the gene, both at the RNA and protein levels. Therefore, hypermethylation-associated silencing of MLH1 results in deficiency of DNA mismatch repair gene activity in a relevant number of sporadic colorectal carcinomas and may represent the initiating event of tumorigenesis [114]. The result of this epigenetic event is the development of a mutator phenotype which can be associated with alterations of the same genes implicated in the pathogenesis of colorectal cancer, such as MSH2, MSh6, TGF-βII receptor and BAX (Fig. 2.5). This new pathway to sporadic colorectal cancer shows many similarities to tumor occurrence in Lynch syndrome and represents a model of interaction between epigenetic and truly genetic events in cancer development. Thus, aberrant methylation of MLH1 - and possibly other genes - is likely to be one of the earliest events in tumorigenesis and may represent an important clue in the etiology of cancer of the right colon [115].

The Mitotic Checkpoint Gene Mutation Pathway

As already discussed, most tumors occurring in Lynch syndrome and a definite proportion of sporadic neoplasms show defective DNA repair of mismatched bases; as a consequence of this alteration, these tumors exhibit an increased mutation rate at the nucleotide level and widespread microsatellite instability [98, 99]. However, MSI is not the only kind of genomic instability commonly observed in human tumors, since in approximately 70% of colorectal carcinomas - and in the majority of other cancer types - chromosomal instability (CI) can also be detected, and in this case aneuploidy will be observed, using flow cytometry or other techniques [116].

In a recent investigation [117] Cahill and collaborators attempted to establish the molecular basis of this chromosomal instability: they evaluated the hBUB1 gene, the human homologue of a gene that controls mitotic checkpoint and chromosome segregation in yeast. The results of these studies revealed not only that CI was consistently associated with a loss of function of mitotic checkpoint but, more importantly, that in some cases this mitotic control was lost owing to mutational inactivation of the hBUB1 gene (localized to chromosome 2q12-14 by fluorescence in situ hybridization). Thus, it is likely that in at least a fraction of aneuploid tumors, alterations of the BUB1 gene lead to some derangement of the chromosomal segregation apparatus during mitosis, with consequent deviation from the (normal) diploid status. Aneuploidy, in turn, may increase the loss of other cancer-related genes, thus favoring the gradual transformation of precursor lesions into infiltrating carcinoma. This new model of colorectal carcinogenesis is schematically illustrated in Fig. 2.6; if the working hypothesis is confirmed, then we might consider acquired aneuploidy as a specific driving force in tumor progression, rather than a simple epiphenomenon of neoplastic diseases [118].

Colorectal Cancer Development in Inflammatory Bowel Diseases

Individuals affected by ulcerative or Crohn colitis are at increased risk of colorectal malignancies [119, 120]. The extent of the disease and duration of active colitis lasting more than 10 years appear to be independent risk factors. The

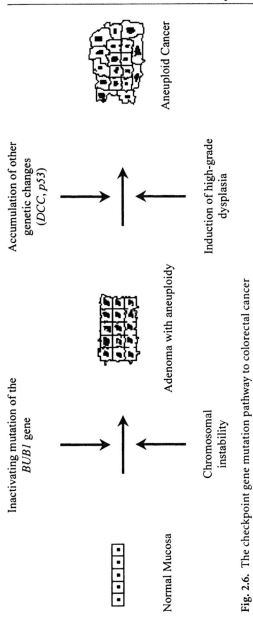

Fig. 2.6. The checkpoint gene mutation pathway to colorectal cancer

current approach for controlling this risk requires lifelong annual colonoscopic surveillance with multiple biopsies, in order to detect severe dysplasia or early carcinoma. In fact, it has been suggested that progression towards malignancy in long-standing colitis proceeds in a stepwise fashion of morphological alterations, from mild dysplasia to severe dysplasia and eventually to infiltrating carcinoma [121].

One of the earliest abnormalities reported in ulcerative colitis is the increased cell turnover rate. Using autoradiography or, more recently, other markers of cell proliferation (such as bromodeoxyuridine, PCNA or Ki67), several studies showed the presence of proliferating cells in the upper third of colonic crypts and along the luminal surface, thus indicating the existence of a failure in the mechanisms repressing DNA synthesis during cell migration from the fundus to the surface [122, 123]. This alteration may represent a physiological reaction to the mucosal inflammatory damage but can also be viewed as the first expression of the proneness of the mucosa towards neoplastic transformation.

Several other abnormalities have been reported in the colorectal mucosa of patients with long-standing ulcerative colitis. These include mutations of oncogenes and tumor suppressor genes (such as p53, K-ras and, less frequently, others) [124, 125], microsatellite and chromosomal instability [126, 127], occasional reduced expression of mutator genes [128] and hypermethylation of the promoter region of genes (such as p16) involved in cell cycle regulation [129]. Ulcerative and Crohn colitis are characterized by repetitive cycles of acute inflammation and mucosal regeneration; as recently suggested by Lyda et al. [130], inflammatory cells may generate free radicals and other metabolites which could induce oxidative DNA damage involving base substitutions, DNA strand breaks, sister chromatid exchanges and mutations of several cancer-related genes. The increased cell replication observed in colorectal mucosa of these patients [122, 123] may further increase the susceptibility of the target cells to various alterations. If the actively replicating cells fail to repair DNA damage, the accumulated mutations would be passed to daughter cells, thus inducing clonal expansion and leading to the development of dysplastic changes and eventually invasive carcinoma. In conclusion, tumor development in inflammatory bowel diseases is presumably related to many of the molecular changes already discussed; with our present knowledge, however, these events cannot be ordered in a well defined pathway.

Tumor Development Through the I1307K Mutation of the APC Gene: Some Clues to Familial Cancer

Table 2.1 summarizes the main genes more closely related to colorectal tumorigenesis. Many of these genes can be mutated in the germline cells and represent – as already discussed and illustrated in Figs. 2.2 to 2.6 – the initiating event of hereditary colorectal cancer syndromes (HNPCC, FAP and related polyposis). However, these account for a small fraction of the colorectal cancer burden, between 1% and 5% of all cases [131], while 10%–20% of patients with tumors of the large bowel have other first-degree relatives affected by cancer (of the colorectum and of other organs) though their family tree does not fulfil the criteria for hereditary cancer syndromes. For these "familial" cases, the risk of cancer is about 3 times that of the general population [132–134], which contrasts with the much higher risk existing in the case of autosomal dominant transmission. Since no Mendelian pattern may explain cancer aggregation in these familial cases, the most likely type of transmission seems to be multifactorial, which implies a close interaction between the genes and environmental factors.

Familial colorectal cancer represents a challenge for at least three reasons: first, in contrast to hereditary tumors, familial cases are extremely more common, and their appropriate control might save thousand of lives, especially in well developed countries; second, the recognition of familial cases can be difficult for many reasons, including the small size of most modern families and the poor attention paid to family history, especially when this is not impressive; third, due to our limited knowledge, there is a relative lack of appropriate guidelines for cancer prevention and surveillance in familial cases.

Recent studies, however, offer some clues towards a better understanding of familial colorectal cancer. Laken et al. [135] reported a constitutional mutation in the APC gene (T to A, at codon 1307) which could be detected in 6% of Ashkenazi Jews and in about 28% of Ashkenazi Jews with colorectal cancer. The mutation (I1307 K) does not alter the function of the encoded protein, but substitutes an AAAAAAAA tract for the AAATAAAA which is normally present at this position; $(A)_8$ is a short microsatellite, and like other microsatellite sequences can be hypermutable, thus causing an increased predisposition to cancer. It is possible that this mutation contributes to a large fraction of colorectal tumors in other ethnic groups [136, 137]. Moreover, these findings might be of relevance as a model for understanding familial cancer; in fact, subtler or unconventional mutations of known genes might be responsible for this increased risk, in this case creating a highly mutable hotspot which is prone to further mutational events, due to the well-known instability of microsatellites.

In a recent editorial, R.L. White [138] underscored the concept of "strongly" and "weakly" predisposing alleles. The former include truncating mutations of APC, which lead to FAP, alterations of mutator genes, that are responsible for Lynch syndrome, or mutations of BRCA1 and 2, associated with hereditary breast cancer [139, 140]. The I1307 K mutation is an example of weakly predisposing alleles, which might be much more common than the strongly predisposing mutations, and can account for a significant fraction of those cancers that are at present attributed to "familial" factors.

Conclusions

There is no doubt that our knowledge of the pathogenesis of colorectal tumors has increased remarkably over the past 2-3 decades. Basil Morson [141] first started the ball rolling by proposing the adenoma-carcinoma sequence and by providing evidence in support of this model. Bert Vogelstein [11] continued the process when he and his co-workers suggested that an accumulation of genetic events was responsible for the passage from small to large adenoma and eventually to carcinoma. The third step was provided by the many investigators who mapped and cloned the genes responsible for FAP and HNPCC when mutated. The available evidence suggests that there are several pathways to colorectal cancer, and it is likely that additional pathways will be discovered in the next few years. Different pathways may mean different tumors, and this reminds me of the hypothesis Weisburger and Wynder presented many years ago [17]. However, tumors with a different biology might also have different and more effective preventive measures, clinical approaches and therapeutic strategies. Thus, our hope for the future is that this enormous body of knowledge accumulated in the last part of the century will be translated into a better control of this common malignancy from the beginning of the new millennium.

References

1. Ponz de Leon M, Roncucci L. The cause of colorectal cancer. Digest Liver Dis 2000; 32:426–39.
2. Chu KC, Tarone KE, Chow WH et al. Temporal patterns in colorectal cancer incidence, survival, and mortality from 1950 through 1990. J Natl Cancer Inst 1994; 86:997–1006.
3. Lynch HT, Smyrk T, Lynch J. An update of HNPCC (Lynch Syndrome). Cancer Genet Cytogenet 1997; 93:84–99.
4. Radice P, Cama A, Mariani-Costantini R. Molecular genetics of polyposis and hereditary colorectal cancer. FORUM Trends in experimental and clinical medicine 1996; 6: 275–91.
5. Potter JD. Colorectal cancer: molecules and populations. J Natl Cancer Inst 1999; 91: 916–32.
6. Newcomb PA, Norfleet RG, Storer BE et al. Screening sigmoidoscopy and colorectal cancer mortality. J Natl Cancer Inst 1992; 84:1572–5.
7. Weinberg RA. Oncogenes, antioncogenes, and the molecular bases of multistep carcinogenesis. Cancer Res 1989; 49:3713–21.
8. Ponz de Leon M. Genetic basis of tumour development. Ital J Gastroenterol 1996; 28: 232–45.
9. Hussain SP, Harris CC. Molecular epidemiology of human cancer: contribution of mutation spectra studies of tumor suppressor genes. Cancer Res 1998;
10. Peltomäki P. Genetic basis of Hereditary Nonpolyposis Colorectal Carcinoma (HNPCC). Ann Med 1994; 26:215–9.
11. Vogelstein B, Fearon ER, Hamilton SR et al. Genetic alterations during colorectal-tumor development. N Engl J Med 1988; 319:525–32.
12. Kalus M. Carcinoma and adenomatous polyps of the colon and rectum in biopsy and organ tissue culture. Cancer 1972; 30:972–82.
13. Rembacken BJ, Fujii T, Cairns A et al. Flat and depressed colonic neoplasms: a prospective study of 1000 colonoscopies in the UK. The Lancet 2000; 355:1211–4.
14. Roncucci L, Stamp D, Medline A et al. Identification and quantification of aberrant crypt foci and microadenomas in the human colon. Hum Pathol 1991; 22:287–94.
15. Di Gregorio C, Losi L, Fante R. Histology of aberrant crypt foci in the human colon. Histopathology 1997; 31:491.
16. Takayama T, Katsuki S, Takahashi Y et al. Aberrant crypt foci of the colon as precursors of adenoma and cancer. N Engl J Med 1998; 339:1277–84.
17. Weisburger JH, Wynder EL. Etiology of colorectal cancer with emphasis on mechanisms of action and prevention. In: Devita VT, Hellman S, Rosenberg SA. Important advances in oncology. Lippincott, Philadelphia, 1987; 197–200.
18. Schatzin A, Kelloff G. Chemo- and dietary prevention of colorectal cancer. Eur J Cancer 1995; 31 A:1198–204.
19. Mařatka Z, Nebdal J, Kociánová J et al. Incidence of colorectal cancer in proctocolitis: a retrospective study of 959 cases over 40 years. Gut 1985; 26:43–9.

References 43

20. Ponz de Leon M, Antonioli A, Ascari A et al. Incidence and familial occurrence of colorectal cancer and polyps in a Health-Care district of Northern Italy. Cancer 1987; 62:2848-59.
21. Lynch HT, Smyrk T. Hereditary Nonpolyposis Colorectal Cancer (Lynch syndrome). Cancer 1996; 78:1149-67.
22. Baba S. Recent advances in molecular genetics of colorectal cancer. World J Surg 1997; 21:678-87.
23. Rhyu MS. Molecular mechanisms underlying Hereditary Nonpolyposis Colorectal Carcinoma. J Natl Cancer Inst 1996; 88:240-51.
24. Bellacosa A, Genuardi M, Anti M et al. Hereditary Nonpolyposis Colorectal Cancer: review of clinical, molecular genetics, and counseling aspects. Am J Med Genet 1996; 62:353-64.
25. Naylor EW, Lebenthal E. Gardner's syndrome. Recent development in research and management. Dig Dis Sci 1980; 25:945-59.
26. Wallace MH, Phillips KS. Upper gastrointestinal disease in patients with familial adenomatous polyposis. Br J Surg 1998; 85:742-50.
27. Moon RT, Miller JR. The APC tumor suppressor protein in development and cancer. Trends Genet 1997; 13:256-8.
28. Heinimann K, Müllhaupt B, Weber W et al. Phenotypic differences in familial adenomatous polyposis based on APC gene mutation status. Gut 1998; 43:675-9.
29. Behrens J, Jerchow BA, Würtelev M et al. Functional interaction of an Axin Homolog Conductin, with β-catenin, APC, and GSK3β. Science 1998; 280:596-9.
30. Hamilton SR, Lui B, Parsons RE et al. The molecular basis of Turcot's syndrome. N Engl J Med 1995; 332:839-47.
31. Spigelman AD, Arese P, Phillips RKS. Polyposis: the Peutz-Jeghers syndrome. Br J Surg 1995; 82:1311-4.
32. Weary PE, Gorlin RJ, Gentry WC et al. Multiple hamartoma syndrome (Cowden's disease). Arch Derm 1972; 106:682-90.
33. Subramony C, Scott-Conner CEH, Skelto D et al. Familial juvenile polyposis. Study of a kindred: evolution of polyps and relationship to gastrointestinal carcinoma. Am J Clin Pathol 1994; 102:91-7.
34. Hall NR, Murday VA, Chapman P et al. Genetic linkage in Muir-Torre syndrome to the same chromosomal region as Cancer Family Syndrome. Eur J Cancer 1994; 30 A:180-2.
35. Haggitt RC, Reid BJ. Hereditary gastrointestinal polyposis syndromes. Am J Surg Pathol 1986; 10:871-87.
36. Hanzawa M, Yoshikawa N, Tezuka T et al. Surgical treatment of Cronkhite-Canada syndrome associated with protein-losing enteropathy. Dis Colon Rectum 1998; 41: 932-4.
37. Lipkin M, Blattner WE, Fraumeni JF et al. Tritiated thymidine labeling distribution as a marker for hereditary predisposition to colon cancer. Cancer Res 1983; 43:1899-904.
38. Deschner EE, Godbold J, Lynch HT. Rectal epithelial cell proliferation in a group in young adults. Cancer 1988; 61:2286-90.
39. Fearon ER, Vogelstein B. A genetic model for colorectal tumorigenesis. Cell 1990; 61: 759-67.
40. Boland CR, Sato J, Appelman HD et al. Microallelotyping defines the sequence and tempo of allelic losses at tumour suppressor gene loci during colorectal cancer progression. Nat Med 1995; 1:902-9.
41. Muleris S, Salmon RJ, Dutrillaux AM et al. Characteristics chromosomal imbalances in 18 near-diploid colorectal tumors. Cancer Genet Cytogenet 1987; 29:289-301.
42. Pathak S, Hopwood LV, Highes JI et al. Identification of colon cancer-predisposed individuals: a cytogenetic analysis. Am J Gastroenterol 1991; 86:679-84.
43. Lairmore TC, Norton JA. Advances in molecular genetics. Am J Surg 1997; 173:37-41.
44. Shibata D, Reale MA, Lavin P et al. The DCC protein and prognosis in colorectal cancer. N Engl J Med 1996; 335:1727-32.

45. Thiagalingam S, Lisitsyn NZ, Hamaguchi M et al. Evaluation of the FHIT gene in colorectal cancers. Cancer Res 1996; 56:2936-9.
46. Takagi Y, Kohmura H, Futamura M et al. Somatic alterations of the DPC4 gene in human colorectal cancers in vivo. Gastroenterology 1996; 111:1369-72.
47. Arber N, Hibshoosh H, Moss SF et al. 1996; Increased expression of cyclin D1 is an early event in multistage colorectal carcinogenesis. Gastroenterology. 1996 Mar; 110(3): 669-74 110:669-74.
48. Zhu Y, Richardson JA, Parada LF et al. Smad3 mutant mice develop metastatic colorectal cancer. Cell 1998; 94:703-14.
49. Irby RB, Mao W, Coppola D et al. Activating SRC mutation in a subset of advanced human colon cancers. Nature Genet 1999; 21:187-90.
50. Wang SS, Esplin ED, Li JL et al. Alterations of the PPP2R1B gene in human lung and colon cancer. Science 1998; 282:284-7.
51. Hanash SM. A role for chromosome 1 in colorectal cancer. Gastroenterology 1996; 111: 250-2.
52. Mahmoud NN, Boolbol SK, Bilinki RT et al. APC gene mutation is associated with a dominant-negative effect upon intestinal cell migration. Cancer Res 1997; 57: 5045-50.
53. Kinzler KW, Vogelstein B. Lessons from Hereditary Colorectal Cancer. Cell 1996; 87: 159-70.
54. Korinek V, Barker N, Morin J et al. Constitutive transcriptional activation by a β-catenin-Tcf complex in APC$^{-/-}$ colon carcinoma. Science 1997; 275:1784-7.
55. Rubinfeld B, Albert I, Porfiri E et al. Loss of β-catenin regulation by the APC tumor suppressor protein correlates with loss of structure due to common somatic mutations of the gene. Cancer Res 1997; 57:4624-30.
56. Jervoise H, Andreyev N, Norman AR et al. Kirsten ras mutations in patients with colorectal cancer: the multicenter "RASCAL" study. J Natl Cancer Inst 1998; 90: 675-84.
57. Jen J, Kim H, Piantadosi S et al. Allelic loss of chromosome 18q and prognosis in colorectal cancer. N Engl J Med 1994; 331:213-21.
58. Reale MA, Hu G, Zafar AI et al. Expression and alternative splicing of the Deleted in Colorectal Cancer (DCC) gene in normal and malignant tissues. Cancer Res 1994; 54:4493-501.
59. Cho KR, Fearon ER. DCC: linking tumour suppressor genes and altered cell surface interactions in cancer? Eur J Cancer 1995; 31 A:1055-60.
60. Lovec H, Sewing A, Lucibello FC et al. Oncogenic activity of cyclin D1 revealed through cooperation with H-ras: link between cell cycle control and malignant transformation. Oncogene 1994; 9:323-6.
61. Schmutte C, Yang AS, Nguyen TT et al. Mechanisms for the involvement of DNA methylation in colon carcinogenesis. Cancer Res 1996; 56:2375-81.
62. Ueki T, Toyota M, Sohn T et al. Hypermethylation of multiple genes in pancreatic adenocarcinoma. Cancer Res 2000; 60:1835-9.
63. Han ES, Moyer MP, Naylor S et al. Mutation in the TP53 gene in colorectal carcinoma detected by polymerase chain reaction. Genes Chrom Cancer 1991; 3:313-7.
64. Kahlenberg MS, Stoler DL, Basik M et al. p53 tumor suppressor gene status and the degree of genomic instability in sporadic colorectal cancers. I Natl Cancer Inst 1996; 88:1665-9.
65. Shimamura A, Fisher DE. p53 in life and death. Clin Cancer Res 1996; 2:435-40.
66. Kaelin WG. The emerging p53 gene family. J Natl Cancer Inst 1999; 91:594-8.
67. Vasen HFA, van der Luijt RB, Slors JFM et al. Molecular genetic tests as a guide to surgical management of familial adenomatous polyposis. Lancet 1996; 348:433-5.
68. Ponz de Leon M, Benatti P, Percesepe A et al. Clinical features and genotype-phenotype correlations in 41 italian families with adenomatosis coli. Ital J Gastroenterol Hepatol 1999; 31:850-60.

69. Samowitz WS, Thliveris A, Spirio LN et al. Alternatively spliced adenomatous polyposis coli (APC) gene transcripts that delete exons mutated in attenuated APC. Cancer Res 1995; 55:3732-4.
70. Spirio LN, Samowitz W, Robertson J et al. Alleles of APC modulate the frequency and classes of mutations that lead to colon polyps. Nature Genet 1998; 20:385-8.
71. Powell SM, Zilz N, Beazer-Barclay Y et al. APC mutations occur early during colorectal tumorigenesis. Nature 1992; 359:235-7.
72. Knudson AG. Hereditary cancer, oncogenes, and antioncogenes. Cancer Res 1985; 45:1437-43.
73. Westerman AM, Entius MM, de Baar E et al. Peutz-Jeghers syndrome: 78-year follow-up of the original family. Lancet 1999; 353:1211-5.
74. Giardiello FM, Welsh SB, Hamilton SR et al. Increased risk of cancer in the Peutz-Jeghers syndrome. N Engl J Med 1987; 316:1511-4.
75. Launonen V, Avizienyte E, Loukola A et al. No evidence of Peutz-Jeghers syndrome gene LKB1 involvement in left-sided colorectal carcinomas. Cancer Res 2000; 60:546-8.
76. Dong SM, Kim KM, Kim SY et al. Frequent somatic mutations in serine/threonine kinase 11/Peutz-Jeghers syndrome gene in left-sided colon cancer. Cancer Res 1998; 58:3787-90.
77. Gruber SB, Entius MM, Petersen GM et al. Pathogenesis of adenocarcinoma in Peutz-Jeghers syndrome. Cancer Res 1998; 58:5267-70.
78. Saul SH, Raffensperger E. Juvenile polyposis: intramucosal signet-cell adenocarcinoma arising in a polyp at a gastrojejunostomy site. Surg Pathol 1988; 1:159-64.
79. Longo WE, Touloukian RJ, West AB et al. Malignant potential of juvenile polyposis coli. Report of a case and review of the literature. Dis Colon Rectum 1990; 33:980-4.
80. Walpole IR, Cullity G. Juvenile polyposis: a case with early presentation and death attributable to adenocarcinoma of the pancreas. Am J Med Genet 1989; 32:1-8.
81. Olschwang S, Serova-Sinilnikova OM, Lenoir G et al. PTEN germ-line mutations in juvenile polyposis coli. Nature Genet 1998; 18:12-4.
82. Howe JR, Roth S, Ringold JC et al. Mutations in the SMAD4/DPC4 gene in juvenile polyposis. Science 1998; 280:1086-8.
83. Howe JR, Ringold JC, Hughes JH et al. Direct genetic testing for Smad4 mutations in patients at risk for juvenile polyposis. Surgery 1999; 126:162-70.
84. Starink TM, van der Veen JPW, Arwert F et al. The Cowden syndrome: a clinical and genetic study in 21 patients. Clin Genet 1986; 29:222-33.
85. Lloyd KM, Dennis M. Cowden's disease: a possible new symptom complex with multiple system involvement. Ann Intern Med 1963; 58:136-42.
86. Gorlin RJ, Cohen MM, Levin LS. Hamartoneoplastic syndromes. In "Syndromes of the Head and Neck", Third Ed. New York: Oxfords University Press, 1990; 336-8, 357-61.
87. Li J, Yen C, Liaw D et al. PTEN, a putative protein tyrosine phosphatase gene mutated in human brain, breast and prostate cancer. Science 1997; 275:1943-7.
88. Tsuchiya KD, Wiesner G, Cassidy SB et al. Deletion 10q23.2-q23.33 in a patient with gastrointestinal juvenile polyposis and other features of a Cowden-like syndrome. Genes Chrom Cancer 1998; 21:113-8.
89. Marsh DJ, Dahia PLM, Coulon V et al. Allelic imbalance, including deletion of PTEN/NMAC1, at the Cowden disease locus on 10q22-23, in hamartomas from patients with Cowden syndrome and germline PTEN mutation. Genes Chrom Cancer 1998; 21:61-9.
90. Liu B, Parsons R, Papadopoulos N et al. Analysis of mismatch repair genes in hereditary non-polyposis colorectal cancer patients. Nat Med 1996; 2:169-74.
91. Kolodner RD, Tytell JD, Schmeits JL et al. Germ-line MSH6 mutations in colorectal cancer families. Cancer Res 1999; 59:5068-74.
92. Miyaki M, Konishi M, Tanaka K et al. Germline mutation of MSH6 as the cause of Hereditary Nonpolyposis Colorectal Cancer. Nature Genet 1997; 17:271-2.

93. Boland CR, Sinicrope FA, Brenner DE et al. Colorectal cancer prevention and treatment. Gestroenterology 2000; 118:115-28.
94. Tannergård P, Lipford JR, Kolodner R et al. Mutation screening in the hMLH1 gene in Swedish hereditary nonpolyposis colon cancer families. Cancer Res 1995; 55: 6092-6.
95. Weber TK, Conlon W, Petrelli NJ et al. Genomic DNA-based hMSH2 and hMLH1 mutation screening in 32 eastern United States Hereditary Nonpolyposis Colorectal Cancer pedigrees. Cancer Res 1997; 57:3798-803.
96. Ponz de Leon M, Pedroni M, Benatti P et al. Hereditary colorectal cancer in the general population: from cancer registration to molecular diagnosis. Gut 1999; 45:32-8.
97. Papadopoulos N, Leach FS, Kinzler KW et al. Monoallelic mutation analysis (MAMA) for identifying germline mutations. Nature Genet 1995; 11:99-102.
98. Loeb LA. Microsatellite instability: marker of a mutator phenotype in cancer. Cancer Res 1994; 54:5059-63.
99. Chung DC, Rustgi AK. DNA mismatch repair and cancer. Gastroenterology 1995; 109: 1685-99.
100. Loeb LA. Mutator phenotype may be required for multistage carcinogenesis. Cancer Res 1991; 51:3075-9.
101. Jass JR. Colorectal adenomas in surgical specimens from subjects with Hereditary Nonpolyposis Colorectal Cancer. Histopathology 1995; 27:263-7.
102. Ahlquist DA. Aggressive polyps in Hereditary Nonpolyposis Colorectal Cancer: targets for screening. Gastroenterology 1995; 108:1590-2.
103. Ponz de Leon M, Della Casa G, Benatti P et al. Frequency and type of colorectal tumors in asymptomatic high-risk individuals in families with Hereditary Nonpolyposis Colorectal Cancer. Cancer Epidemiol Biomarkers Prev 1998; 7:639-41.
104. Lynch HT, Fusaro RM, Lynch J. Hereditary cancer in adults. Cancer Detection and Prevention 1995; 19:219-33.
105. Lynch P. If aggressive surveillance in Hereditary Nonpolyposis Colorectal Cancer is now state of the art, are there any challenges left? Gastroenterology 2000; 118:969-77.
106. Parsons R, Myeroff L, Liu B et al. Microsatellite instability and mutations of the transforming growth factor β type II receptor gene in colorectal cancer. Cancer Res 1995; 55:5548-50.
107. Liu B, Nicolaides NC, Markowitz S et al. Mismatch repair gene defects in sporadic colorectal cancers with microsatellite instability. Nature Genet 1995; 9:48-55.
108. Strand M, Earley MC, Crouse GF et al. Mutations in the MSH3 gene preferentially lead to deletions within tracts of simple repetitive DNA in Saccharomyces cervisiae. Proc Natl Acad Sci 1995; 92:10418-21.
109. Perucho M. Microsatellite instability: the mutator that mutates the other mutator. Nature Med 1996; 2:630-1.
110. Yagi OK, Akiyama Y, Nomizu T et al. Proapoptotic gene BAX is frequently mutated in Hereditary Nonpolyposis Colorectal Cncers but not in adenomas. Gastroenterology 1998; 268-74.
111. Salahshor S, Kressner U, Fischer H et al. Microsatellite instability in sporadic colorectal cancer is not an independent prognostic factor. Br J Cancer 1999; 81:190-3.
112. Cunningham JM, Christensen ER, Tester DJ et al. Hypermethylation of the hMLH1 promoter in colon cancer with microsatellite instability. Cancer Res 1998; 58:3455-60.
113. Deng G, Chen A, Hong J et al. Methylation of CpG in a small region of the hMLH1 promoter invariably correlates with the absence of gene expression. Cancer Res 1999; 59: 2029-33.
114. Herman JG, Umar A, Polyak K et al. Incidence and functional consequences of hMLH1 promoter hypermethylation in colorectal carcinoma. Proc Natl Acad Sci 1998; 95: 6870-5.

References

115. Kuismanen SA, Holmberg MT, Salovaara R et al. Genetic and epigenetic modification of MLH1 accounts for a major share of microsatellite-unstable colorectal cancers. Am J Pathol 2000; 156:1773-9.
116. Williams NN, Daly JM. Flow cytometry and prognostic implications in patients with solid tumors. Surgery Gynecology Obstetrics 1990; 171:257-66.
117. Cahill DP, Lengauer C, Yu J et al. Mutations of mitotic checkpoint genes in human cancers. Nature 1998; 392:300-3.
118. Orr-Weaver TL, Weinberg RA. A checkpoint on the road to cancer. Nature 1998; 392:223-4.
119. Ekbom A, Helmick C, Zack M et al. Ulcerative colitis and colorectal cancer: a population-based study. N Engl J Med 1990; 3223:1228-33.
120. Choi PM, Zelig MP. Similarity of colorectal cancer in Crohn's disease and ulcerative colitis: implications for carcinogenesis and prevention. Gut 1994; 35:950-4.
121. Goldman H. Significance and detection of dysplasia in chronic colitis. Cancer 1996; 78:2261-3.
122. Biasco G, Miglioli M, Minarini A et al. Rectal cell renewal as biological marker of cancer risk in ulcerative colitis. In "Precancerous lesions of the gastrointestinal tract", edited by Sherlock P, Morson BD, Barbara L, Veronesi U, Raven Press, New York, 1983; 261-8.
123. Wright CL, Riddell RH. The pathology and politics of dysplasia in ulcerative colitis. Current Opinion in Gastroenterology 1998; 11:4-10.
124. Walsh SV, Loda M, Torres CM et al. P53 and β catenin expression in chronic ulcerative colitis-associated polyposis dysplasia And sporadic adenomas. An immunohistochemical study. Am J Surg Pathol 1999; 23:963-9.
125. Gibson P, Rosella O, Nov R et al. Colonic epithelium is diffusely abnormal in ulcerative colitis and colorectal cancer. Gut 1995; 36:857-63.
126. Heinen CD, Noffsinger AE, Belli J et al. Regenerative lesions in ulcerative colitis are characterized by microsatellite mutation. Genes Chrom Cancer 1997; 19:170-5.
127. Rabinovitch PS, Dziadon S, Brentnall TA et al. Pancolonic chromosomal instability precedes dysplasia and cancer in ulcerative colitis. Cancer Res 1999; 59:5148-53.
128. Cawkwell L, Sutherland F, Murgatroyd H et al. Defective hMSH2/hMLH1 protein expression is seen infrequently in ulcerative colitis associated colorectal cancers. Gut 2000; 46:367-369.
129. Hsieh CJ, Klump B, Holzmann K et al. Hypermethylation of the $p16^{INK4a}$ promoter in colectomy specimens of patients with long-standing and extensive ulcerative colitis. Cancer Res 1998; 58:3942-5.
130. Lyda MH, Noffsinger A, Belli J et al. Multifocal neoplasia involving the colon and appendix in ulcerative colitis: pathological and molecular features. Gastroenterology 1998; 115:1566-73.
131. Mecklin JP. Frequency of hereditary colorectal carcinoma. Gastroenterology 1987; 93:1021-5.
132. Lovett E. Family studies in cancer of the colon and rectum. Br J Surg 1976; 63:13-8.
133. Woolf CM. A genetic study of carcinoma of the large bowel. Am J Hum Genet 1958; 10:42-7.
134. Ponz de Leon M, Sassatelli R, Sacchetti C et al. Familial aggregation of tumors in the three-year experience of a population-based colorectal cancer registry. Cancer Res 1989; 49:4344-8.
135. Laken SJ, Petersen GM, Gruber SB et al. Familial colorectal cancer in Ashkenazim due to a hypermutable tract in APC. Nature Genet 1997; 17:79-83.
136. Lothe RA, Hektoen M, Johnsen H et al. The APC gene I1307 K variant is rare in Norwegian patients with familial and sporadic colorectal or breast cancer. Cancer Res 1998; 58:2923-4.
137. Prior TW, Chadwick RB, Papp AC et al. The I1307 K polymorphism of the APC gene in colorectal cancer. Gastroenterology 1999; 116:58-63.

138. White RL. Excess risk of colon cancer associated with a polymorphism of the APC gene? Cancer Res 1998; 58:4038-9.
139. Warner E, Foulkes W, Goodwin P et al. Prevalence and penetrance of BRCA1 and BRCA2 gene mutations in unselected Ashkenazi Jewish women with breast cancer. J Natl Cancer Inst 1999; 91:1241-7.
140. Osorio A, Barroso A, Martinez B et al. Molecular analysis of the BRCA1 and BRCA2 genes in 32 breast and/or ovarian cancer Spanish families. Br J Cancer 2000; 82: 1266-70.
141. Morson BC, Bussey HJR, Day DW et al. Adenomas of large bowel. Cancer Surv 1983; 2:451-77.

3 Pathology of Colorectal Cancer

Introduction

Colorectal carcinoma represents one of the leading causes of mortality in all Western countries, and there is evidence indicating a progressive rise of its incidence in countries – such as Japan – in which the disease was relatively uncommon until a few decades ago [1, 2]. Dealing with these tumors requires new and rapidly accumulating knowledge of epidemiology, risk factors, molecular genetics, chemoprevention and novel treatments. In addition, researchers should be aware that colorectal tumors encompass a large variety of precancerous and preneoplastic lesions whose importance, in colorectal tumorigenesis, has been partially clarified very recently [3]. These will be the subject of the present chapter.

It is now a "paradigm" that colorectal malignancies develop from adenomatous polyps, and indeed, a great deal of evidence has accumulated indicating that carcinomas of the large bowel arise – in most, if not all cases – from pre-existing, premalignant lesions, especially when associated with dysplastic changes [4]. This, however, is an oversimplification of the reality, since most polyps do not acquire malignant features during their natural history and may also regress or disappear [5]. In addition, the earliest phases of colorectal tumorigenesis presumably start in normal mucosa, with a disorder of cell replication and renewal [6] and with the appearance of clusters of enlarged crypts [7] showing proliferative, biochemical and biomolecular abnormalities.

The colon is an abdominal organ, covered by the peritoneum except for its most distal part, the rectum; its length is of the order of 100–150 cm. As shown in Fig. 3.1, the anatomic terminology of the various colonic tracts corresponds to their configuration and location. The mesocolon and fascial attachments anchor the colon to the posterior abdominal wall. The colorectal mucosa is covered by two layers of circular and longitudinal smooth muscle cells, which are adjacent to serosa and subserosal tissues; contraction of the external longitudinal muscle layer accounts for the appearance of characteristic haustrations along the colon. Blood supply to the colon is derived from branches of the superior mesenteric artery (from caecum to splenic flexure) and the inferior mesenteric artery (descending colon, sigmoid and rectum). The lower rectum is supplied by the middle and inferior rectal arteries, branches of the internal iliac artery. This particular vascularization lends further support to the suggestion that there are three different types of colorectal malignancies: cancer of the right colon (i.e.

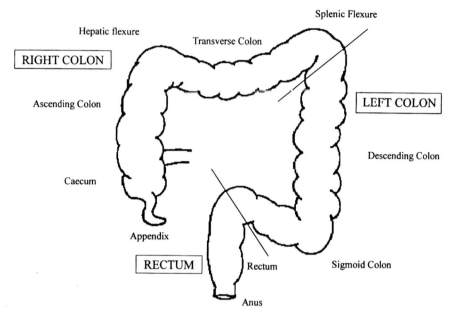

Fig. 3.1. The human large bowel and its subdivision into various segments

neoplasms located from the caecum to the splenic flexure), cancer of the left colon (tumors of the descending, sigmoid and rectosigmoid region) and cancer of the rectum (tumors located within 8 cm from the anal verge) [1, 3]. The large majority of venous blood leaves the colon through the portal system and, thus, reaches the liver – which is the main site of haematogenous metastasis from colorectal cancer; part of the venous blood leaving the rectum reaches the caval system through the haemorrhoidal plexus. Lymphatic flow takes place through channels that parallel the blood vessels and is drained by lymph nodes scattered in the peritoneal folds. The colon is innervated by parasympathetic nerves from mesenteric and pelvic ganglia.

The Colorectal Mucosa

Normal Architecture

The normal colorectal mucosa is constituted by three main elements: epithelium (of the surface and crypts), lamina propria and muscularis mucosae (Fig. 3.2); the last separates the mucosa from the deeper submucosa. The colonic surface epithelium is composed of a single layer of columnar cells which function as a protective barrier between the host and the luminal environment. The two main cellular elements of the epithelium are absorptive cells (responsible for ion and water absorption) and goblet cells (which synthesize, store and secrete mucin); a thin basement membrane (composed of collagen and other proteins) anchors

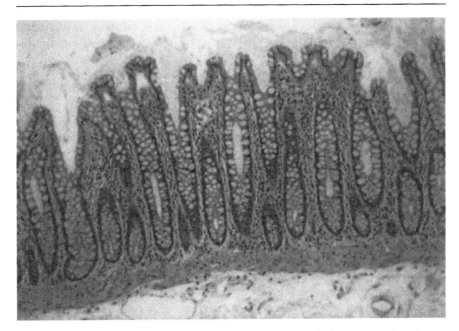

Fig. 3.2. Normal architecture of colorectal mucosa. Epithelial cells, lamina propria and muscularis mucosae are the three fundamental elements (H & E, × 50)

and supports the surface epithelium. A similar single-layer columnar cell epithelium forms the colorectal crypts; in addition to absorptive and goblet cells, crypt epithelium comprises also undifferentiated precursor cells, specialized endocrine cells (containing secretory granules) and rare Paneth cells (pyramid-shaped cells containing eosinophilic secretory granules, whose function remains unclear), especially in the proximal colon.

The lamina propria extends between crypts and reaches the muscularis mucosae; it contains a wide variety of cells – including fibroblasts, lymphocytes, plasma cells, eosinophils, macrophages and mast cells – which are arranged among strands of collagen tissue. Colonic mucosa also contains well-formed gut-associated lymphoid tissue which is responsible for the local defense against harmful agents originating in the gut lumen [8].

The muscularis mucosae is a thin layer of smooth muscle which separates the epithelium and lamina propria from the submucosa. Contraction of the muscularis may alter the shape of the mucosa, thus influencing normal physiological processes (absorption of water and electrolytes, mucin secretion, cell replication).

The submucosa is constituted of the same elements that characterize the lamina propria (such as lymphocytes, that can form lymphatic follicles, fibroblasts, macrophages, mast cells and fibrous tissues). Two neural plexuses are located in the submucosa: one is immediately beneath the muscularis mucosae (Meissner plexus), the second (Auerbach plexus) lies in the deeper part of the submucosa, close to the lamina propria. Vascular elements of the submucosa include arterioles, venules and lymphatic vessels; these submucosal structures may sometimes appear larger or tortuous even in the absence of any colonic abnormality.

Cell Proliferation

The human colonic epithelium is an actively proliferating and self-renewing system; under normal conditions, the replicative zone is confined to the lower 3/4 of the colonic crypts, while it is absent in the upper portions and in the surface epithelium [6]. Thus, cells migrate towards the most superficial regions of the glands and are then extruded from the mucosal surface; the whole process takes 4-6 days [9].

Several lines of evidence suggest that before the appearance of adenomatous polyps other premorphological alterations can be detected in apparently normal mucosa of the colorectal tract; in particular, the process of tumorigenesis may begin with a generalized disorder of cell replication and differentiation which antedates and accompanies the development of morphological lesions. Thus, in the early stages of colorectal carcinogenesis, epithelial cells become unable to repress DNA synthesis during migration from the lower to the upper portions of the crypt and develop an enhanced capacity to proliferate [10]. As a consequence of this, the proliferative zone expands, and S-phase cells can be observed (with the use of H^3-thymidine, bromodeoxyuridine or more recent techniques) throughout the whole length of the gland [11].

An abnormal pattern of cell replication has been detected in several clinical conditions associated with an increased risk for colorectal malignancies; these include familial adenomatous polyposis [12], individuals with adenomatous polyps of the large bowel (especially when large and multiple) [13], patients with long-standing inflammatory bowel diseases [14], normal individuals older that 65 years [15], and patients with previous intestinal resections for colorectal tumors [16].

Aberrant Crypts

Aberrant crypt foci (ACF) are clusters of abnormal colonic crypts that can be identified on the mucosal surface after methylene-blue staining and observation under low magnification (Fig. 3.3) [17]. These lesions can be induced experimentally in the rat colon, and there is now evidence that they may represent one of the earliest steps in the development of colorectal cancer. Two or more weeks after azoxymethane administration, darkly stained, enlarged and slightly elevated crypt foci can be observed over the background of normal colorectal crypts after staining with an appropriate dye [18]. ACF are relatively rare in colorectal mucosa from normal individuals, but their number increases significantly in the flat mucosa of patients with familial adenomatous polyposis or colorectal malignancies [19].

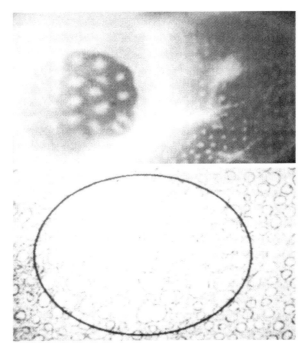

Fig. 3.3. Macroscopic (*upper left*) and microscopic (*lower, in the circle,* × 25) appearance of aberrant crypt foci

The preneoplastic nature of ACF was further supported by the finding of APC gene mutations – one of the earliest events in colorectal tumorigenesis [3] – in minute dysplastic foci of aberrant crypts [20]. A few years later, Losi et al. [21] reported the frequent occurrence of *k-ras* mutations in ACF, and more recently, microsatellite instability could be detected in ACF, over the background of a microsatellite-stable colorectal mucosa [22]. While these molecular alterations favor a possible role of ACF in colorectal cancer development, the mechanisms and the steps through which ACF can progress to macroscopic lesions remain poorly defined [23].

Recently, Di Gregorio and co-workers [24] tried to establish morphological criteria suitable for defining and classifying ACF in histological sections. The authors subdivided ACF into three main groups: group A (approximately 70% of the investigated samples) included ACF whose epithelial cells had regular nuclei, with only mild crowding (but no stratification), no mucin depletion and absence of dysplasia; in group B (20%), ACF showed features of hyperplastic polyps, with enlarged and crowded nuclei, absence of stratification, mucin depletion, presence of no more than 3 mitotic figures, and no dysplasia; in group C (8%–10%), the lesions showed enlarged, crowded and stratified nuclei, with loss of polarity, more than 3 mitoses, mucin depletion and definite evidence of dysplasia. The authors suggested that foci in group A should be considered typical ACF, those of group B are similar to hyperplastic polyps, while group C lesions should include microadenomas. It is rather interesting that this accurate analysis allowed the classification of aberrant crypt foci into groups representing sequential steps in colorectal cancer development.

Adenomatous Polyps

Colorectal adenomatous polyps can be defined as well demarcated, circumscribed lumps of epithelial dysplasia, with uncontrolled crypt cell division. Single transformed cells may generate subclones through new mutations, with the possibility of an enhanced growth rate. Most adenomas remain benign and asymptomatic lesions that can be discovered by chance during lower endoscopy; however, a small fraction of these lesions may evolve into malignancy, and there is evidence indicating that the large majority (if not all) of colorectal carcinomas develop from adenomatous polyps [4].

Descriptive Epidemiology

Although colorectal adenomas have been found in almost all races and populations, a marked geographic variation in the frequency of these lesions has been reported. In general terms, the prevalence and distribution of adenomas tend to parallel those of colorectal carcinoma. Thus, adenomatous polyps are rather infrequent in Africa and in some Asian countries (such as Iran and the Philippines), but extremely common in Western countries [4, 25], where they can be found in 50% or more of individuals over the age of 50 years. As for colorectal carcinoma, migrant studies pointed out a probable role of environmental factors in inducing the appearance of adenomatous lesions; indeed, while these lesions are relatively rare in Nigeria, Uganda and other African populations, they are very common in American blacks, with prevalence rates sometimes higher than in whites [26, 27]. Colorectal adenomas are rare under the age of 30 years, but their prevalence increases with increasing age. Although there is no reason to expect a different frequency of polyps by gender, a certain male prevalence has been reported in some series [28], perhaps due to the reluctance of many women to undergo endoscopic investigations. Adenomatous polyps were undoubtedly detected less frequently 40–50 years ago than at present; it cannot be excluded that changes in diet and lifestyle (hyperalimentation and sedentary lifestyle due to well-being and increased economical resources) might be responsible for this increased prevalence; however, it is more likely – at least in our opinion – that the more common observation of these lesions should mostly be attributed to the widespread use of endoscopic procedures and, in general, to the progressively increasing "medicalization" of Western society [29].

Distribution, Size and Multiplicity

Although adenomatous polyps can be observed in all tracts of the large bowel, their anatomical distribution reflects that of colorectal carcinoma; consequently, about 70% of these lesions are located in the left colon (which is the portion more easily accessible to the endoscopist) [30]. Since colonoscopy is gradually replacing sigmoidoscopy as a screening procedure [31], we can anticipate that a significant number of adenomas will be detected in the proximal colon. In both autopsy and endoscopic series, the large majority (70%-80%) of adenomas are less than 1 cm in diameter [4, 32]; larger lesions more often show a villous histological pattern and evidence of dysplasia or malignancy.

The number of adenomas per patient may vary; in approximately half of the subjects these lesions are single, while in the other half multiple lesions can be observed [4]. Multiplicity of adenomas bears an increased risk of dysplasia and cancer; thus, Muto et al. [33] showed that as the number of adenomas per patient increases, so does the fraction of individuals with invasive carcinoma. In addition, in familial adenomatous polyposis – in which the entire colorectal mucosa is carpeted by hundreds or thousand of adenomas – the risk of developing cancer is virtually 100% [34].

Histopathology, Dysplasia and "Malignant Polyps"

The term "polyp" should not be used by itself for histological diagnosis; polyp, in fact, is a clinical description of any circumscribed mass of cells that projects above the surface of the surrounding normal mucosa. Adenomas are well-demarcated lumps of epithelial dysplasia which can be classified into three major histological types: tubular, villous and tubulovillous (Fig. 3.4). These three types, however, are not clearly distinguishable, being only different manifestations of a spectrum of abnormal tissue architecture [35]. An adenoma is pedunculated when it possesses a long or short stalk; sessile adenomas elevate over the background mucosa without any stalk. Small (< 1 cm) adenomas are also known as "diminutive" [36].

Adenomas usually show different grades of dysplasia and should be classified by taking into account the part with the most advanced grade. The word dysplasia is used to describe structural and cytological alterations in the epithelium that predispose an organ to cancer development. These abnormalities show varying degrees of severity, which can be graded into "mild", "moderate" and "severe" dysplasia [35]. It should be stressed that the terminology used for grading varies not only with the organ or tissue under investigation, but also with the personal preference and attitude of the investigator. Notwithstanding these limitations, severe dysplasia in an adenoma is considered a selective marker for an increased risk of cancer, and this is particularly true for lesions greater than 1.0 cm in diameter and with a marked villous component [4]. The definition of different grades of epithelial dysplasia in adenomas is one of the most convincing pieces of evidence of the "adenoma-carcinoma sequence" [37]. It is likely that

56 Pathology of Colorectal Cancer

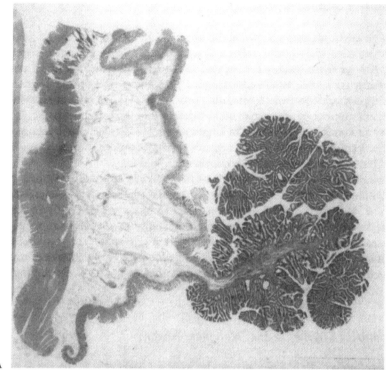

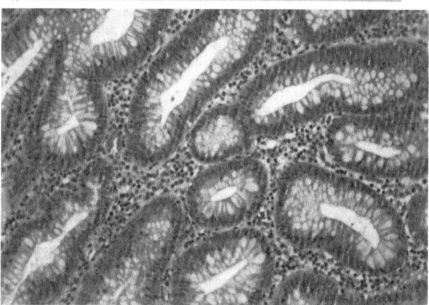

Fig. 3.4 A–C. Microscopic appearance (×5) of a pedunculated tubulovillous adenoma (A). Polystratification of cells and moderate dysplasia are evident (B) (H & E, ×100); villous adenoma (C) (×50). C see p. 57

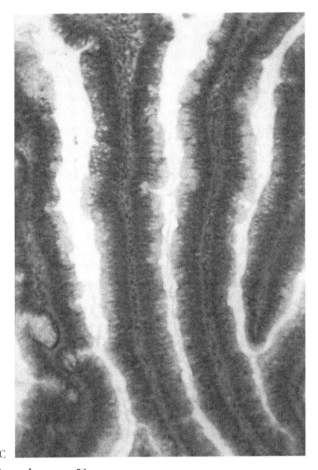

Fig. 3.4 C. Legend see page 56

most (if not all) colorectal carcinomas evolve through stages of increasingly severe epithelial dysplasia before becoming invasive lesions.

An adenoma can be considered "malignant" (Fig. 3.5) when there is evidence that neoplastic cells pass through the muscularis mucosae and infiltrate the submucosa [4]; in this case the definition of "carcinoma developed in adenoma" is appropriate. The literature, however, is rather confusing: definitions such as "carcinoma in situ", "focal carcinoma" or "intramucosal carcinoma" are still common and promote the confusion. For the purposes of cancer registration, these definitions should be avoided and substituted with "severe dysplasia"; in fact, as long as features of malignancy are confined above the muscularis mucosae (i.e. within the mucosa and lamina propria), there is no potential for metastasis, even when tissue and cellular atypia satisfy all the histological criteria for adenocarcinoma. Since there are no lymphatic vessels in the colonic epithelium above the muscularis mucosae, neoplastic cell can metastasize only after crossing

58   Pathology of Colorectal Cancer

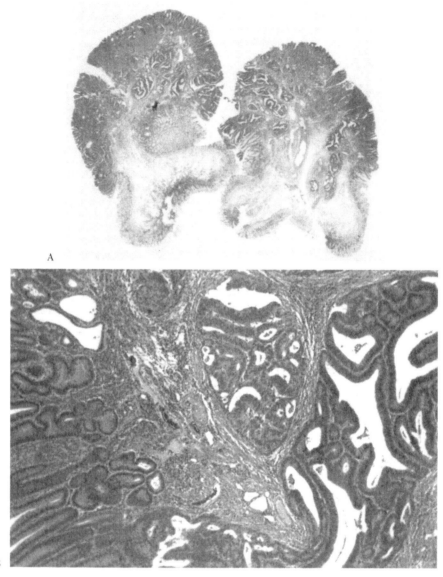

Fig. 3.5 A, B. Microscopic appearance (× 5) of a malignant polyp, with neoplastic cells within the muscularis mucosae and infiltrating the submucosa; residual adenoma on the left (H & E, × 50)

this barrier [37]; therefore, it is more appropriate to restrict the use of the term carcinoma (which implies local invasion and potential for metastasis) to lesions which have invaded the submucosal tissues [38]. However, the terminology is often confusing, and the search for a unifying and clear classification is justified [39].

Adenomas in Familial Adenomatous Polyposis and Hereditary Non-polyposis Colorectal Cancer

Familial adenomatous polyposis (FAP) is an autosomal dominant condition characterized by the presence of at least 100 polyps in the large bowel and by several extracolonic manifestations [40]. Adenomas appear in the second and third decade of life and usually tend to be more numerous in the distal large bowel. In full-blown cases, the entire large bowel is carpeted by thousands of polyps of various dimensions. When the disease is left untreated, cancer develops almost inevitably in the third to fifth decade of life (with a few exceptions). Apart from their number and age of onset, colorectal adenomas in FAP do not show any distinctive aspects or features when compared with the most common sporadic lesions.

Hereditary non-polyposis colorectal cancer (HNPCC or Lynch syndrome) is an inherited condition characterized by early onset colorectal cancer (often before the age of 40 years), preferential location of tumors in the right colon (from the caecum to the splenic flexure), frequency of multiple colorectal malignancies (both synchronous and metachronous) and association with tumors of other organs, especially the endometrium, ovary, stomach and urinary tract [41]. Although the term "non-polyposis" might suggest that adenomas do not occur or are not important in Lynch syndrome, there is evidence that HNPCC patients form adenomas at about the same rate as the general population, that these lesions tend to appear at a younger age, and that adenomas are precursor lesions for malignancy [42]. Moreover, several investigations support the hypothesis that these "hereditary" adenomas might be more "aggressive" than sporadic lesions, in the sense that they are more often large, villous, dysplastic and, consequently, more likely to undergo malignant transformation [43]. The morphological aspect of adenomas in HNPCC does not show any distinctive features; however, adenomatous lesions frequently show microsatellite instability similarly to carcinomas which develop in Lynch syndrome [44, 45]. Whether this molecular finding correlates with the clinical behavior of adenomas in this syndrome remains to be elucidated.

The Adenoma-Carcinoma Sequence

Several lines of evidence indicate that adenomas can develop into carcinomas; this, however, does not imply that all polyps will undergo malignant changes in time, neither does it exclude "de novo" carcinogenesis. Nonetheless, the evidence that adenomas represent the natural precursor of colorectal malignancies is strong and stems from several observations, which can be summarized as follows. First, histological aspects of adenomas are frequently observed in specimens of colorectal carcinoma; in turn, features of malignancy can be seen in approximately 5% of all polyps [46, 47]. Second, in the National Polyp Study, accurate surveillance with systematic removal of all newly detected polyps led to a significant reduction in the expected number of invasive carcinomas [48].

Third, in a series of more than 200 individuals in whom polyps larger than 1 cm could not be removed, clinical follow up showed the development of 21 invasive carcinomas, with a cumulative risk of cancer at the polyp site, after 20 years, of 24% [49]. Fourth, as already discussed, adenomas and malignant tumors tend to have a similar distribution in the various segments of the large bowel, with a maximum frequency in the rectosigmoid region [1, 4, 30]. Fifth, the age-specific incidence rate of colorectal polyps shows an earlier rise than cancer, with a peak of incidence that anticipates that of carcinomas by 5 years [30]; since the malignant transformation of a benign adenoma usually takes years [49], this pattern of incidence speaks in favor of a sequence between adenomatous polyps and cancer. Sixth, both patients with colorectal cancer and individuals with adenomas share a similar increased frequency of site-specific tumors among first-degree relatives [30, 50, 51]. Seventh, recent observations showed that the risk of developing colorectal adenomas is associated with the same environmental factors (diet and lifestyle) which have been related to the risk of colorectal malignancies [52, 53]. Finally, adenomas and carcinomas of the large bowel may show similar molecular alterations, such as activation of oncogenes or inactivation of tumor suppressor genes [3, 54, 55]; this aspect underscores the "evolution" of the concept of the adenoma-carcinoma sequence, from a morphological phenomenon to a complex pathway of biomolecular events presumably induced by (or related to) exogenous and metabolic factors [56].

Etiology of Adenomatous Polyps

Despite numerous studies and many suggestions, the causes of colorectal adenomas remain poorly defined. Two points, however, appear of major importance: first, the causes of these lesions appear to be strictly related to Western society and lifestyle; second, adenomas and carcinomas of the large bowel show basically the same risk profile. Following this line of reasoning, it is not surprising that the development of colorectal adenomas has been directly related to the consumption of meat and animal fat, and to a low level of physical activity; in contrast, vegetables, fruit, fiber and several micronutrients (such as calcium, folate and antioxidant vitamins) seem to have a protective effect [53, 56]. Other factors closely associated with the Western lifestyle – such as smoking and alcohol consumption – have also been implicated in the pathogenesis of colorectal adenomas, but with more conflicting results [50, 57].

Many molecular abnormalities have been reported in colorectal adenomas; these include mutations of oncogenes (such as *k-ras*), inactivation of tumor suppressor genes (such as APC, p53 and DCC) and of mutator genes (those implicated in repairing DNA mismatch, such as MLH1 and MSH2), disturbances of DNA methylation and microsatellite instability. Many of these genetic events may target the transition from normal mucosa to small adenomas, and from these to large adenomas and infiltrating carcinoma. The molecular events implicated in the adenoma-carcinoma sequence have been the subject of various recent reviews to which the reader is referred [3, 56, 58] and are discussed in chapter 2.

Other Types of Polyps

In addition to adenomatous polyps, other types of similar lesions deserve some comments regarding either their frequency (hyperplastic polyps) or their potentially malignant evolution (flat adenomas) or their peculiar histologic features (hamartomas and juvenile polyps).

Hyperplastic, Mixed Polyps and Serrated Adenomas

Hyperplastic polyps are rounded and usually sessile lesions of a few millimeters in diameter showing elongated crypts with a tendency to cystic dilatation (Fig. 3.6). The epithelium consists of a single layer of cells, with no crowding of nuclei or signs of dysplasia [59]. In vitro cell kinetic investigations – together with electron-microscopic studies – suggested that elongation and subsequent infolding of the epithelium should be attributed to an expanded but normally located proliferative zone in the crypt [60]. These lesions are most common in the rectum and sigmoid colon, and become more frequent with increasing age. Macroscopically and at endoscopy they cannot be distinguished from adenomatous polyps.

It is commonly believed that hyperplastic polyps – especially those located in the rectum and sigmoid colon – are absolutely benign lesions which lack any malignant potential. However, there are various reports in the literature in which hyperplastic polyps – especially when distributed in the various tracts of the

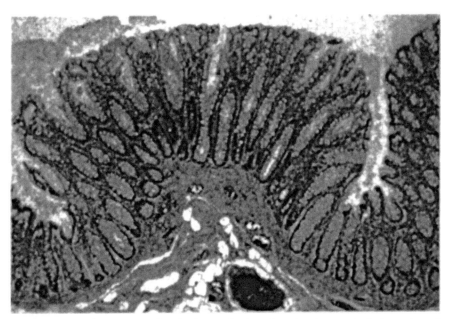

Fig. 3.6. Representative example of a hyperplastic polyp showing marked elongation of crypts (H & E, × 50)

large bowel – can be associated with the development of malignant tumors [6, 62]. As recently suggested by Jass et al. [63], it is likely that in these cases adenomatous changes coexist with hyperplastic features; as an alternative explanation, at least some hyperplastic polyps might carry an intrinsic potential for dysplasia and cancer. Polyps combining features of both hyperplastic and adenomatous lesions are defined as "mixed polyps", and may result from the engulfment of pre-existing hyperplastic polyps by spreading adenoma, stimulation of mucosal hyperplasia at the advancing edge of an adenoma, or the development of an adenoma within a hyperplastic polyp. In these lesions, each component is histologically distinct from the other.

Longacre and Fenoglio-Preiser [64] described the morphologic features of colorectal hyperplastic-adenomatous polyps; these new lesions measured 0.2–7.5 cm and were distributed throughout the colorectum. The general architecture of these polyps was similar to that of hyperplastic polyps, but the cytologic features were different, since surface mitotic activity, nuclear pseudostratification and the nuclear/cytoplasmic ratio were greater than in classic hyperplastic lesions. Moreover, signs of dysplasia were observed in almost 40% of the cases. Since one common feature of these polyps was the presence of a serrated glandular pattern, the authors proposed to call these lesions "serrated adenoma" (Fig. 3.7), in order to stress their neoplastic nature and possible malignant evolution. In line with these observations, recent studies showed various biomolecular alterations in hyperplastic polyps, including *k-ras* and p53 mutations, loss of heterozygosity and microsatellite instability [63, 65, 66].

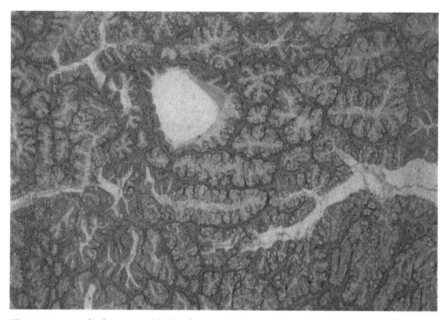

Fig. 3.7. Serrated adenoma, with the characteristic saw-like or dentate aspect of the crypts (H & E, × 50)

In conclusion, hyperplastic polyps should be considered benign lesions with virtually no malignant potential, especially when located in the rectosigmoid region and with a diameter of a few millimeters; however, larger polyps located also in other tracts of the large bowel might retain the capacity to evolve into dysplastic and neoplastic lesions. This might be due to the coexistence of adenomatous changes or to the presence of some intermediate lesion such as serrated adenomas.

Flat Adenomas

Flat adenomas of the large bowel were initially described by Muto and co-workers as slight elevations of the mucosa with a reddish surface which was dome-shaped but rather flat [67, 68]. Histologically, these polyps are tubular, villous or tubulovillous adenomas. Flat adenomas are difficult to detect on routine lower endoscopy, since their shape may change with the degree of air insufflation. Nonetheless, recognition of these lesions is important, since the malignant potential of flat adenomas seems to be considerably higher than that of common sessile or pedunculated polyps of the same size [69], and this provides further biological evidence favoring the adenoma-carcinoma sequence. Studies from Japanese investigators recognized the existence of two main macroscopic variants of flat adenomas, one that is completely flat and the other that shows a central area of depression (depressed adenoma) [70].

Flat adenomas remain a rather controversial topic. In fact, at variance with Japanese colleagues, European and American endoscopists regarded these lesions as rare, and some authors suggested that flat or depressed lesions may only represent an early stage of adenoma formation [71]. Other authors argued that the histologic findings in flat adenomas are not specific and may be mimicked by small adenomas [72]. Rather surprisingly, a recent study showed an elevated frequency (36% of all polyps removed at endoscopy) of flat adenomas in an unselected English population [73]. Most adenomas in this series contained areas of mild or moderate dysplasia, but 31 polyps (10%) were severely dysplastic. The authors emphasized the importance of recognizing flat or depressed lesions in colorectal cancer screening, since most endoscopists usually concentrate on polypoid masses. Thus, it seems that flat adenomas are rather frequent also in Western countries, and that in order to detect them – and for an effective prevention of colorectal cancer – endoscopists should be properly trained.

Along with the existence of sporadic lesions, a "hereditary flat adenoma syndrome" has recently been identified by Lynch and co-workers [74]. The main features of this syndrome include the presence of multiple flat adenomas in the large bowel (usually less than 100), their prevalent distribution in the proximal colon, and the high risk of colorectal cancer, which usually develops after the age of 50 years. The management and surveillance of affected individuals are similar to those recommended to patients with FAP; however, a careful endoscopic follow-up, with removal and histologic examination of all newly developed polyps, may substitute for colectomy in many of these patients [75].

Hamartomatous Polyps

The term "hamartoma" indicates an uncommon polypoid lesion which is observed in two main nosologic entities: Peutz-Jeghers syndrome and juvenile polyposis. The gross appearance of hamartomas does not differ from that of the more common adenomas; they occur in adults as well as in children, are more often pedunculated and located in the rectosigmoid region, vary in size from a few millimeters to several centimeters, and may be single or multiple. Histologically, hamartomas show a complex branching pattern of smooth muscle supporting normal lamina propria and glands; thus, these polyps are basically composed of normal elements indigenous to the site in which they appear, although their general architecture is markedly abnormal. The recognition of misplaced epithelium, presence of multiple normal-appearing cells, lack of nuclear atypia and of lymphatic vessels support the hamartomatous (from the Greek "amartia" = error) origin of these lesions [76].

Peutz-Jeghers syndrome (see chapter 12) is a rare polyposis syndrome characterized by the presence of hamartomatous polyps in the various gastrointestinal tracts (more frequent in the small bowel, followed by the large bowel and stomach), melanin spots on the lips and buccal mucosa, and an autosomal dominant type of genetic transmission [77, 78]. More rarely, hamartomatous lesions can be observed on other mucosal surfaces, such as the respiratory and the urinary tracts [79]. Although hamartomas were usually not included among precancerous lesions, recent studies showed the frequent occurrence of gastrointestinal malignancies in Peutz-Jeghers syndrome; moreover, these patients are prone to the development of tumors of other organs (especially pancreas, breast, lung and ovary) [80, 81]. In line with these observations, various authors documented either the development of adenocarcinoma in hamartomatous polyps [82] or the coexistence of adenomatous and carcinomatous changes in such lesions [83]. Taken together, these findings favor – but not without controversy [81] – the possible existence of a hamartoma-carcinoma – or hamartoma-adenoma-carcinoma-sequence in the large bowel as well as in the stomach and small bowel [84]; it follows that patients with Peutz-Jeghers syndrome should undergo a close follow-up, with the removal of large and/or dysplastic polyps from the accessible sites. Finally, the gene responsible for the disease when mutated has recently been identified and mapped to chromosome 19p [85, 86]. The gene, called LKB1 (or STK11), encodes for a novel serine/threonine kinase whose function is still unknown; inactivating mutations of LKB1 have been detected in most cases of Peutz-Jeghers syndrome, so that the gene should be considered a general cancer-susceptibility gene that predisposes gene carriers to a variety of gastrointestinal and extra-gastrointestinal neoplasms [87].

In juvenile polyposis (chapter 12), hamartomatous lesions may develop in the large bowel (where they are most common), in the stomach and in the small bowel [88]. Histological examination shows dilated and elongated glands with slightly irregular contours and abundant stromal tissue; the glands are lined by normal colonic epithelium, and the stroma is often inflamed and edematous [89]. Mixed polyps can be observed in which hamartomatous and adenomatous areas coexist, and this may explain the frequency of malignant changes reported by some authors [89]. Polyps usually develop during the second and third decade of life, their average diameter is between 1 and 2 cm, and their number varies from 1-2 to 100 or more lesions. Juvenile polyposis may be familial, and in this case an autosomal dominant type of transmission can be recognized [90]. Non-familial cases might be phenocopies or can be due to new mutations in the gene responsible for the disease. Rather interestingly, birth defects (craniomegaly, intellectual handicap, bowel malrotation, cardiac defects and others) are relatively frequent in non-familial polyposis, but rare in familial cases [91]. There are various reports on the occurrence of gastrointestinal malignancies in familial juvenile polyposis. Thus, for instance, in the St. Mark's series, 18 of 87 patients (21%) developed colorectal cancer during the follow-up [89]; it is possible that some hamartomatous lesions naturally evolve into adenoma with various degrees of dysplasia and subsequently undergo malignant transformation. Owing to this risk, colectomy has been advocated as a preventive measure against colorectal neoplasms, especially in patients with numerous polyps [92]; alternatively, close endoscopic surveillance of the large bowel is required. The molecular basis of familial juvenile polyposis has recently been clarified with the identification of the responsible gene - SMAD4 - which appears to be mutated in the majority of these patients [93, 94]. The gene, located at 18q21, encodes a cytoplasmic protein involved in the TGFα signaling pathway.

Polyps and Dysplasia in Inflammatory Bowel Diseases

Patients with ulcerative colitis and Crohn colitis are at increased risk for colorectal malignancies; the risk increases with the duration of the disease and the extent of colorectal involvement [95]. The morphologic basis of tumor occurrence is the development of dysplastic changes in flat mucosa or in polypoid lesions.

In inflammatory bowel disease (IBD), elevated, sessile and reddish nodules - known as pseudopolyps or inflammatory polyps - are often seen in otherwise flat mucosa; these lesions are typically small and multiple and largely composed of granulation tissue, mixed with inflamed and hyperemic mucosa [96]. Dysplasia may grow as a flat lesion or as a dysplasia associated lesion or mass (DALM); DALM has to be distinguished from sporadic adenoma, that is not the consequence of a chronic inflammation but an age-related coincidental finding. The presence of dysplasia in the flat mucosa adjacent to DALM is the criterion for distinguishing DALM from adenoma [96]. The clinical distinction between DALM and sporadic adenoma that may arise in patients with IBD is extremely important. Indeed, the former lesion arises as the result of a chronic inflammatory stimulus in a patient with ulcerative or Crohn colitis, and its presence is an indication for surgery (colectomy); in contrast, the treatment of sporadic adenomas - whether IBD associated or not - remains simple endoscopic polypectomy [97].

Recently, several molecular alterations have been detected in long-standing ulcerative colitis; these include oncogene mutations, inactivations of tumor suppressor genes, loss of heterozygosity, chromosomal and microsatellite instability [98–100]. It is likely that the study of genetic changes will become of use for a further biological characterization of IBD and might represent a useful guide for taking appropriate clinical decisions in the management of these patients.

Other Benign Tumors

Other polyp-like lesions can develop from the proliferative activity of stromal connective, nervous or lymphatic tissue; these include lipomas (which can be recognized by their yellowish color), myomas, fibromas, neurofibromas (type I neurofibromatosis may involve the colon and rectum) and angiomas [101]. The origin of all these lesions is usually submucosal, and their appearance can be similar to that of sessile adenomas, so that for a proper diagnosis, histological examination is required. A possible complication of all these lesions is superficial ulceration, with consequent bleeding. Lymphoid polyps (consisting of lymphatic follicles) can be found in infectious diseases and in inflammatory bowel diseases [102].

Colorectal Carcinoma

Colorectal malignancies continue to be one of the most frequent and life-threatening diseases throughout the world, especially in well-developed and industrialized countries [1]. Their incidence is declining slightly in the USA [103], stable or increasing in most European countries [104], and sharply increasing in Japan and other Eastern countries [105], probably in relation to recent changes in diet and lifestyle. Most of these lesions are adenocarcinomas arising from the columnar surface epithelium; squamous carcinomas can develop from the anal region; melanomas and lymphomas represent rare malignancies of the large bowel, whereas carcinoid tumors (chapter 13) can be found rather frequently, especially in the appendix.

Adenoma-Carcinoma Sequence Versus "De Novo" Carcinogenesis

As already discussed [46–53], most of the available evidence supports the existence of an adenoma-carcinoma sequence whose molecular biology has also been characterized in some detail [54–56]; this, however, does not exclude "a priori" the possibility of de novo colorectal carcinogenesis i.e. the development of cancer from flat mucosa. Some studies tried to address this problem by evaluating the proportion of cancers with adenomatous remnants, which ranged from 0% to 83% [106, 107]. The amplitude of the range reveals the weakness of this approach; in fact, as a carcinoma spreads through the bowel wall, it also expands on the mucosal surface and tends to destroy the previous adenoma. In accordance with this contention, it is not surprising that the proportion of colorectal malignancies with residual adenoma decreases with increasing size of the carcinoma [108]. Two more considerations deserve some comments. First, dysplastic aberrant crypt foci and microadenomas (intramucosal) have been described and previously discussed [17-24]; if carcinoma develops from these minute changes, it may appear as a "de novo" lesion. Second, flat and depressed adenomas do not seem as rare as previously believed [71, 73], and they are difficult to detect during routine endoscopy; it follows that when cancer arises in this particular type of polyp, this may mimic "de novo" tumorigenesis. In conclusion, apparent or real "de novo" carcinogenesis remains a possibility which is supported by a well-grounded biological and morphological basis; this, however, should not discourage endoscopists from removing all colorectal polyps as a screening procedure for the prevention of colorectal carcinoma.

Macroscopic Appearance

Most colorectal malignancies (60%-70%) are located distal to the splenic flexure, particularly in the rectum and sigmoid colon [109]. According to some authors [110, 111], there is a gradual tendency - over the past 20-40 years - towards a more frequent occurrence of these lesions in the proximal colon (from caecum to transverse colon), but it is unclear whether this represents a true biological event or simply the consequence of a wider use of colonoscopy. In hereditary colorectal cancer [40], tumors are preferentially located in the proximal colon.

The gross morphology of colorectal neoplasms includes polyp-like vegetating masses and flat infiltrating lesions, often ulcerated and with slightly raised edges. Vegetating lesions tend to protrude into the lumen and - the symptoms being initially scarce or absent - can reach large dimensions (several centimeters), especially when located in the caecum and ascending colon. Flat lesions form ulcerated plaques which infiltrate the bowel wall and frequently narrow the intestinal lumen, giving symptoms of obstruction. At variance with other tumors, colorectal malignancies may appear spuriously large, also because they can be accompanied by an intense inflammatory reaction [112]. In addition, according to most observations, tumor size was not found to be associated with the clinical outcome or survival [113, 114].

Histological Features and Grading

Most colorectal malignancies (95%) are adenocarcinomas, and in many cases (10%-20%) may show a mucinous component. Mucin can accumulate within tumoral cells or in the glandular lumen (Fig. 3.8). Less frequent histological types include signet-ring cell carcinoma (Fig. 3.9) (about 1%), squamous carcinoma (usually originating from the stratified squamous epithelium of the anal canal), undifferentiated carcinoma and medullary-type adenocarcinoma (solid carcinomas with minimal or no glandular differentiation and slight cellular pleomorphism) [115-117].

68 Pathology of Colorectal Cancer

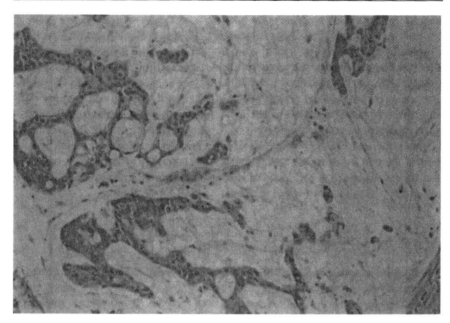

Fig. 3.8. Colorectal carcinoma with a marked accumulation of mucin within tumoral cells and glandular lumen (H & E, × 100)

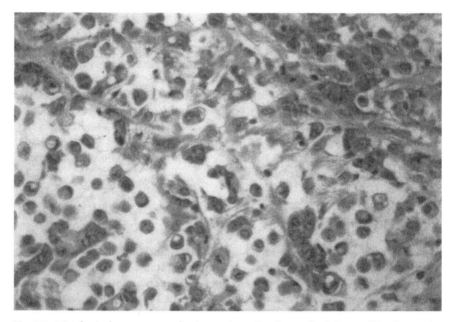

Fig. 3.9. Histological appearance of a signet-ring cell colorectal carcinoma (H & E, × 200)

Colorectal carcinoma can be graded into well differentiated, moderately differentiated and poorly differentiated lesions [115]; in practical terms, this is often an academic exercise with little or no clinical impact. Indeed, there is no consistent evidence that grading may affect survival or serve as a guide in deciding the type of adjuvant chemotherapy or radiotherapy [118, 119]. Other grade-related parameters have been investigated recently; these included nuclear polarity of tumoral cells (discerned versus lost), configuration of tubules (simple versus complex or irregular), pattern of tumor growth (expanding or infiltrating at the tumor edge), lymphocytic infiltration (little to marked), venous and/or lymphatic invasion, and extent of fibrosis (little to extensive) [120, 121]. Some of these parameters - especially venous invasion, pattern of growth and lymphocytic infiltration - have been associated with the clinical outcome in both univariate and multivariate analysis [122, 123]; however, other studies did not confirm these preliminary observations, and the general attitude is to consider all grade-related parameters of little or no help in the management of patients with colorectal cancer [124]. This can be attributed to two main factors: first, grading is essentially a subjective appraisal of a series of histological characteristics and, as such, may show wide interindividual variations. Second, pathological staging at diagnosis in colorectal malignancies is a powerful determinant of the clinical outcome, and a factor which tends to minimize the possible relevance of other prognostic indicators.

Pattern of Metastasis and Staging

In their growth, colorectal malignancies proceed both longitudinally and in depth and tend to infiltrate surrounding organs and tissues. Local extension is particularly evident for tumors of the rectal ampulla, which may infiltrate the bladder, prostate, vagina, uterus, ureters, perineural muscles and pelvic bones. The involvement of the sacral plexus may be particularly painful for the patient [125].

Metastasis to regional lymph nodes can be detected in 30%-50% of the patients at the time of diagnosis. Tumors of the right colon metastasize first to the ileocaecal, right colic and middle colic lymph nodes, and subsequently to the superior mesenteric nodes. Lymph from the left colon is drained from the left colic, sigmoidal and lower mesenteric lymph nodes, where metastasis can develop. Para-aortic lymph nodes can also be a site of metastasis from colorectal malignancies. Rectal tumors tend to metastasize to the superior haemorrhoidal, hypogastric and superficial iliac lymph nodes, whereas the involvement of inguinal lymph nodes can occur only in advanced stages of the disease [126].

The liver is the main site of haematogenous metastasis, which can be detected in 10%-30% of the patients at diagnosis [127]. After the liver, malignant cells can reach and colonize the lung and, more rarely, brain and bone marrow. Recent immunohistochemical and biomolecular studies revealed the presence of cancer cells (single or cluster) in the bone marrow in a relevant proportion (approximately 30%) of patients with advanced colorectal malignancies [128, 129]; similar observations were previously reported for breast cancer [130]. The biological and clinical significance of these findings remain unclear, and follow-up studies are required to make clear whether micrometastases can affect the management and clinical outcome.

Almost 70 years after its original description, Dukes' staging is still commonly used to assess the prognosis and, to some degree, determine the treatment of patients with colorectal cancer [131]. Although this classification was originally limited to three classes (A, B and C), a Dukes' D class was subsequently added to indicate the presence of distant (mostly haematogenous) metastases. In 1986, Hutter and Sobin [132] proposed a "Universal Staging System for Cancer of the Colon and Rectum" and demonstrated that the TNM system could easily be adapted in order to correspond to the Dukes' staging into four main categories. This staging system follows simple physiopathological considerations and partially eliminates ambiguities and confusion consequent to the numerous revisions of the Dukes' procedure [133, 134]. Thus, stage I (Dukes A) tumors invade the submucosa (T1) or the muscular wall (T2), but do not extend beyond this. Stage II (Dukes B) lesions invade through the muscularis propria into the subserosa and pericolic tissues (T3), or infiltrate the visceral peritoneum invading other organs (T4). In stage III tumors there is a metastatic involvement of lymph nodes (N1, 1-3 nodes; N2, more than 3 nodes). Finally, stage IV (Dukes' D) lesions metastasize to the liver, lung or other organs; metastases to the peritoneum and ovary – after perforation of the tumor into the peritoneal cavity – are included in this class.

Other Tumors of the Large Bowel

Carcinoid tumors can be detected throughout the whole gastrointestinal tract, though some 50% of them are commonly found in the appendix [135]. These tumors develop mostly in young adults and are more often entirely asymptomatic; in many cases they represent an occasional finding during examination of the appendix for acute appendicitis. Macroscopically, these tumors appear as small nodules (usually less than 1.5 cm in diameter), yellow-brownish, located between the mucosa and submucosa. At histology, the lesion consists of masses of rounded cells, with a uniform nucleus and acidophilic cytoplasm, separated by an abundant vascular stroma (Fig. 3.10) [136]. In the later phases of its growth, the neoplasm may infiltrate the muscularis propria and the pericolic tissues. Histochemical studies reveal the presence of typical argyrophilic granules in the cytoplasm of tumoral cells.

Apart from carcinoids, other types of neuroendocrine carcinomas can occasionally be detected in the large bowel [137]. The diagnosis of these tumors requires immunohistochemical studies with monoclonal antibodies directed to neuron-specific enolase, human chromogranin A, serotonin, or vasoactive intestinal peptide [138]. With the use of these techniques, many of the cases initially considered as poorly differentiated carcinomas could be reclassified as neuroendocrine tumors [137]. The importance of recognizing neuroendocrine

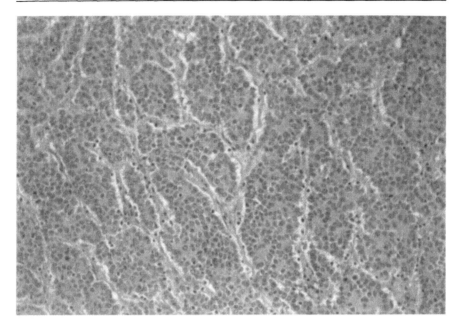

Fig. 3.10. Carcinoid tumor of the appendix (H & E, × 100). Masses of round cells with uniform nucleus and no tendency to glandular formation can be observed

differentiation within a colorectal cancer is that the medical treatment may be different and may include cytotoxic compounds which are usually not employed for adenocarcinomas [139]. In addition, in contrast to carcinoids, neuroendocrine tumors tend to have a poor clinical outcome: in one large series, metastases to lymph nodes or distant sites were present in about 80% of the patients, and the overall 5-year survival was as low as 6% [137].

Non-Hodgkin lymphomas may affect the large bowel, though they are more frequent in the stomach and especially in the small bowel, owing to the abundance of lymphatic tissue [140, 141]. The macroscopic appearance may be that of a mass protruding into the lumen or, less frequently, of a large annular plaque of the intestinal wall. These lesions are softer than common adenocarcinomas, grayish and often ulcerated.

Conclusions

What can be learned from the morphological basis of colorectal tumors? What is the main message? In our opinion, no other malignancy shows such an abundance of preneoplastic and precancerous lesions; in addition, these lesions can be reached and removed quite easily. The situation is far different from that of most malignant tumors affecting humans which usually appear as cancer and not as premalignancies. Thus, at least in theory, colorectal neoplasms might be prevented by interfering with the process of tumorigenesis that begins with an uncontrolled growth in the epithelium, continues with the formation of polyps of various dimensions and eventually, after many years, evolves into malignancy. But even in this phase there is time for intervention, since we know that localized tumors are curable with surgery in the large majority of cases. If many patients still die of colorectal cancer, this is due to a lack of relevant symptoms and to the reluctance of many individuals to undergo appropriate screening. If we can manage to alert the population to the importance of polyps and their removal, colorectal cancer might be prevented and, perhaps, defeated.

References

1. Weisburger JH, Wynder EL. Etiology of colorectal cancer with emphasis on mechanisms of action and prevention. In "Important Advances in Oncology". Edited by Devita VT, Hellman S, Rosenberg SA. Philadelphia: Lippincott, 1987; 197–200.
2. Levi F, Lucchini F, La Vecchia C. Worldwide patterns of cancer mortality, 1985–89. Eur J Cancer Prev 1994; 3:109–43.
3. Ponz de Leon M, Percesepe A. Pathogenesis of colorectal cancer. Dig Liv Dis 2000; 32: 807–21.
4. Morson BC, Bussey HJR, Day DW. Adenomas of large bowel. Cancer Surveys 1983; 3:451–477.
5. Waddell WR, Miesfeld RL. Adenomatous polyposis coli, protein kinases, protein tyrosine phosphatase: the effect of Sulindac. J Surg Oncol 1995; 58:252–6.
6. Lipkin M. Phase 1 and phase 2 proliferative lesions of colonic epithelial cells in diseases leading to colonic cancer. Cancer 1974; 34:878–8.
7. Siu IM, Robinson DR, Schwartz S et al. The identification of monoclonality Cancer Res 1999; 59:63–66.
8. Elson CO, Kagnoff MF, Fiocchi C et al. Intestinal immunity and inflammation: recent progress. Gastroenterology 1986; 91:746–68.
9. Lipkin M, Bell B, Sherlock P. Cell proliferation kinetics in the gastrointestinal tract of man. I. Cell renewal in colon and rectum. J Clin Invest 1963; 42:767–76.
10. Lipkin M, Winawer SJ, Sherlock P. Early identification of individuals at increased risk for cancer of the large intestine. Part II: development of risk factor profile. Clin Bullet 1981; 11:66–74.
11. Deschner EE. Cell proliferation as a biological marker in human colorectal neoplasia. In Colorectal Cancer: prevention, epidemiology and screening. Edited by Winawer S, Schottenfeld D, Sherlock P. New York: Raven Press, 1980; 133–42.
12. Deschner EE, Lipkin M. Proliferative pattern in colonic mucosa in familial polyposis. Cancer 1975; 35:413–8.
13. Ponz de Leon M, Roncucci L, Di Donato P et al. Pattern of epithelial cell proliferation in colorectal mucosa of normal subjects and of patients with adenomatous polyps or cancer of the large bowel. Cancer Res 1988; 48:4121–6.
14. Deschner EE, Winawer SJ, Katz S et al. Proliferative defects in ulcerative colitis patients. Cancer Invest 1983; 1:41–7.
15. Roncucci L, Ponz de Leon M, Scalmati A et al. The influence of age on colonic epithelial cell proliferation. Cancer 1988; 62:2373–7.
16. Scalmati A, Roncucci L, Ghedini G et al. Epithelial cell kinetics in the remaining colorectal mucosa after surgery for cancer of the large bowel. Cancer Res 1990; 50:7937–41.
17. Roncucci L, Medline A, Bruce RW. Classification of aberrant crypt foci and microadenomas in human colon. Cancer Epidemiol Biomarkers Prev 1991; 1:57–60.
18. Bird RP, McLellan EA, Bruce WR. Aberrant crypts, putative precancerous lesions, in the study of the role of diet in the aetiology of colon cancer. Cancer Surv 1989; 8:189–200.

19. Roncucci L, Stamp D, Medline A et al. Identification and quantification of aberrant crypt foci and microadenomas in the human colon. Hum Pathol 1991; 22:287-94.
20. Jen J, Powell SM, Papadopoulos N et al. Molecular determinants of dysplasia in colorectal lesions. Cancer Res 1994; 54:5523-6.
21. Losi L, Roncucci L, Di Gregorio C et al. K-ras and p53 mutations in human colorectal aberrant crypt foci. J Pathol 1996; 178:748-55.
22. Heinen CD, Shivapurkar N, Tang Z et al. Microsatellite instability in aberrant crypt foci from human colons. Cancer Res 1996; 56:5339-41.
23. Shpitz B, Hay K, Medline A et al. Natural history of aberrant crypt foci. A surgical approach. Dis Colon Rectum 1996; 39:763-7.
24. Di Gregorio C, Losi L, Fante R et al. Histology of aberrant crypt foci in the human colon. Histopathol 1997; 30:328-34.
25. Cajucom CC, Barrios GG, Cruz L et al. Prevalence of colorectal polyps in Filipinos. An autopsy study. Dis Colon Rectum 1992; 35:676-80.
26. Williams AO, Chung EB, Agbatra A et al. Intestinal polyps in American negros and Nigerian Africans. Br J Cancer 1975; 31:485-91.
27. Correa P, Strong JP, Reif A et al. The epidemiology of colorectal polyps. Prevalence in New Orleans and international comparison. Cancer 1977; 39:2258-64.
28. Cannon-Albright LA, Bishop DT, Samowitz W et al. Colonic polyps in an unselected population: prevalence, characteristics and associations. Am J Gastroenterol 1994; 89:827-31.
29. Ponz de Leon M, Benatti P, Percesepe A et al. Epidemiology of cancer of the large bowel – The 12-year experience of a specialized Registry in Northern Italy. Ital J Gastroenterol Hepatol 1999; 31:10-8.
30. Ponz de Leon M, Antonioli A, Ascari A et al. Incidence and familial occurrence of colorectal cancer and polyps in a health-care district of Northern Italy. Cancer 1987; 60:2848-59.
31. Imperiale TF, Wagner DR, Lin CY et al. Risk of advanced proximal neoplasms in asymptomatic adults according to the distal colorectal findings. N Engl J Med 2000; 343: 169-74.
32. Anwar S, White J, Hall C et al. Sporadic colorectal polyps: management options and guidelines. Scand J Gastroenterol 1999; 34:4-11.
33. Muto T, Bussey HJRB, Morson BC. The evolution of cancer of the colon and rectum. Cancer 1975; 36:2251-70.
34. Ponz de Leon M, Sassatelli R, Zanghieri G et al. Hereditary adenomatosis of the colon and rectum: clinical features of eight families from Northern Italy. Am J Gastroenterol 1989; 84:906-16.
35. Morson BC, Dowson IM. Gastrointestinal pathology, 2nd ed. Blackwell Scientific, Oxford, 1979.
36. Weston AP, Campbell DR. Diminutive colonic polyps: histopathology. Spatial distribution, concomitant significant lesions, and treatment complications. Am J Gastroenterol 1995; 90:24-8.
37. Fenoglio GM, Lane N. The anatomical precursor of colorectal carcinoma. Cancer 1974; 34:819-23.
38. Decosse JJ. Malignant colorectal polyp. Gut 1984; 25:433-6.
39. Schlemper RJ, Riddell RH, Kato Y et al. The Vienna classification of gastrointestinal epithelial neoplasia. Gut 2000; 47:251-5.
40. Naylor EW, Lebenthal E. Gardner's syndrome; recent development in research and management. Dig Dis Sci 1980; 25:945-59.
41. Lynch HT, Smyrk T. Hereditary nonpolyposis colorectal cancer (Lynch syndrome). An updated review. Cancer 1996; 78:1149-67.
42. Jass JR. Colorectal adenomas in surgical specimens from subjects with hereditary nonpolyposis colorectal cancer. Histopathol 1995; 27:263-7.

43. Ponz de Leon M, Della Casa G, Benatti P et al. Frequency and type of colorectal tumors in asymptomatic high-risk individuals in families with hereditary nonpolyposis colorectal cancer. Cancer Epidemiol Biomarkers Prev 1998; 7:639-41.
44. Peltomaki P. Microsatellite instability as an indicator of hereditary susceptibility to colon cancer. Gastroenterology 1995; 109:2031-3.
45. Iimo H, Jass JR, Simms LA et al. DNA microsatellite instability in hyperplastic polyps, serrated adenomas, and mixed polyps: a mild mutator pathway for colorectal cancer? J Clin Pathol 1999; 52:5-9.
46. Kyzer S, Begin LR, Gordon PH et al. The care of patients with colorectal polyps that contain invasive adenocarcinoma. Endoscopic polypectomy or colectomy? Cancer 1992; 70(8):2044-50.
47. Pollard CW, Nivatvongs S, Rojanasakul A et al. The fate of patients following polypectomy alone for polyps containing invasive carcinoma. Dis Colon Rectum 1992; 35:933-7.
48. Winawer SJ, Zauber AG, O'Brien MJ et al. Randomized comparison of surveillance intervals after colonoscopic removal of newly diagnosed adenomatous polyps. N Engl J Med 1993; 328:901-6.
49. Stryker SJ, Wolff BG, Culp CE et al. Natural history of untreated colonic polyps. Gastroenterology 1987; 93:1009-13
50. Ponz de Leon M, Sassatelli R, Sacchetti C et al. Familial aggregation of tumors in the three-year experience of a population-based colorectal cancer Registry. Cancer Res 1989; 49:4344-8.
51. Ahsan H, Neugut AI, Garbowski GC et al. Family history of colorectal adenomatous polyps and increased risk for colorectal cancer. Ann Inter Med 1998; 128:900-5.
52. Benito E, Obrador A, Stiggelbout A et al. A population-based case-control study of colorectal cancer in Majorca. I. Dietary factors. Int J Cancer 1990; 45:69-76.
53. Kampman E, Giovannucci E, van't Veer P et al. Calcium, vitamin D, dairy foods, and the occurrence of colorectal adenomas among men and women in two prospective studies. Am J Epidemiol 1994; 139:16-29.
54. Vogelstein B, Fearon ER, Hamilton SR et al. Genetic alterations during colorectal-tumor development. N Engl J Med 1988; 319:525-32.
55. Boland CR, Sato J, Appelman HD et al. Microallelotyping defines the sequence and tempo of allelic losses at tumour suppressor gene loci during colorectal cancer progression. Nature Med 1995; 1:902-9.
56. Potter JD. Colorectal cancer: molecules and populations. J Natl Cancer Inst 1999; 91:916-32.
57. Ponz de Leon M, Roncucci L. The cause of colorectal cancer. Digest Liver Dis 2000; 32:426-39.
58. Lairmore TC, Norton JA. Advances in molecular genetics. Am J Surg 1997; 173:37-41.
59. Rex DK, Smith JJ, Ulbright TM et al. Distal colonic hyperplastic polyps do not predict proximal adenomas in asymptomatic average-risk subjects. Gastroenterology 1992; 102:317-9.
60. Hayashi T, Yatani R, Apostol J et al. Pathogenesis of hyperplastic polyps of the colon: a hypothesis based on ultrastructure and in vitro cell kinetics. Gastroenterology 1974; 66:347-56.
61. Bengoechea O, Martinez-Penuela JM, Larrinaga B et al. Hyperplastic polyposis of the colorectum and adenocarcinoma in a 24 year old man. Am J Surg Pathol 1987; 11:323-7.
62. Heng Teoh H, Delahunt B, Isbister WH. Dysplastic and malignant areas in hyperplastic polyps of the large intestine. Pathol 1989; 21:138-42.
63. Jass JR, Ruskiewicz A, Painter D et al. Neoplastic progression occurs through mutator pathways in hyperplastic polyposis of the colorectum. Gut 2000; 47:43-9.
64. Longacre TA, Fenoglio-Preiser CM. Mixed hyperplastic adenomatous polyps/serrated adenomas. Am J Surg Pathol 1990; 14:524-37.

References

65. Otori K, Oda Y, Sugiyama K et al. High frequency of K-ras mutations in human colorectal hyperplastic polyps. Gut 1997; 40:660-3.
66. Lothe RA, Anderson SN, Hofstad B et al. Deletion of lp loci and microsatellite instability in colorectal polyps. Genes Chromosomes Cancer 1995; 14:182-8.
67. Muto T, Kamiya J, Sawada T et al. Morphogenesis of human colonic cancer. Dis Colon Rectum 1983; 26:257-62.
68. Muto T, Kamiya J, Sawada T et al. Small flat adenoma of the large bowel with special reference to its clinicopathologic features. Dis Colon Rectum 1985; 28:847-51.
69. Adachi M, Muto T, Okinaga K et al. Clinicopathologic features of the flat adenoma. Dis Colon Rectum 1991; 34:981-6.
70. Yao T, Tada S, Tsuneyoshi M. Colorectal counterpart of gastric depressed adenoma. A comparison with flat and polypoid adenomas with special reference to the development of pericryptal fibroblasts. Am J Surg Pathol 1994; 18:559-68.
71. Lanspa SJ, Rouse J, Smyrk T et al. Epidemiological characteristics of the flat adenoma of Muto. A prospective study. Dis Colon Rectum 1992; 35:543-46.
72. Samowitz WS, Burt RL. The nonspecificity of histological findings reported for flat adenomas. Hum Pathol 1995; 26:571-3.
73. Rembacken BJ, Fujii T, Cairns A et al. Flat and depressed colonic neoplasms: a prospective study of 1000 colonoscopies in the UK. Lancet 2000; 355:1211-4.
74. Lynch HT, Smyrk T, Lanspa SJ et al. Flat adenomas in a colon cancer-prone kindred. J Natl Cancer Inst 1988; 80:278-82.
75. Lynch HT, Smyrk TC, Watson P et al. Hereditary flat adenoma syndrome: a variant of familial adenomatous polyposis? Dis Colon Rectum 1992; 35:411-21.
76. Giardiello FM, Offerhaus JGA. Phenotype and cancer risk of various polyposis syndromes. Eur J Cancer 1995; 31 A:1085-7.
77. Burdick D, Prior JT, Scanlon GT. Peutz-Jeghers syndrome: a clinicopathological study of a large family with a ten-year follow-up. Cancer 1963; 16:854-67.
78. Foley TR, McGarrity JT, Abt AB. Peutz-Jeghers syndrome: a clinico-pathologic survey of the "Harrisburg family" with a 49-year follow-up. Gastroenterology 1988; 95:1535-40.
79. Sommerhaug RG, Mason T. Peutz-Jeghers syndrome and ureteral polyposis. JAMA 1970; 211:120-2.
80. Giardiello F, Welsh SB, Hamilton SR et al. Increased risk of cancer in the Peutz-Jeghers syndrome. N Engl J Med 1987; 316:1511-4.
81. McGarrity TJ, Kulin HE, Zaino RJ. Peutz-Jeghers syndrome. Am J Gastroenterol 2000; 95:596-604.
82. Miller LJ, Bartholomew LG, Dozois RR et al. Adenocarcinoma of the rectum arising in a hamartomatous polyp in a patient with Peutz-Jeghers syndrome. Dig Dis Sci 1983; 28:1047-51.
83. Perzin KH, Bridge MF. Adenomatous and carcinomatous changes in hamartomatous polyps of the small intestine (Peutz-Jeghers syndrome). Report of a case and review of the literature. Cancer 1982; 49:971-83.
84. Flageole H, Raptis S, Trudel JL et al. Progression toward malignancy of hamartomas in a patient with Peutz-Jeghers syndrome: case report and literature review. Can J Surg 1994; 37:231-6.
85. Hemminki A, Tomlinson I, Markie D et al. Localization of a susceptibility locus for Peutz-Jeghers syndrome to 19p using comparative genomic hybridization and targeted linkage analysis. Nat Genet 1997; 15:87-90.
86. Amos CI, Bali D, Thiel TJ et al. Fine mapping of a genetic locus for Peutz-Jeghers syndrome on chromosome 19p. Cancer Res 1997; 57:3653-6.
87. Jenne DE, Reimann H, Nezu J et al. Peutz-Jeghers syndrome is caused by mutations in a novel serine threonine kinase. Nat Genet 1998; 18:38-43.
88. Woodford-Richens K, Bevan S, Churchman M et al. Analysis of genetic and phenotipic heterogeneity in juvenile polyposis. Gut 2000; 46:656-60.

89. Jass JR, Williams CB, Bussey HJR. Juvenile polyposis – a precancerous condition. Histopathol 1988; 13:619–30.
90. Bussey HJR, Veale AMO, Morson BC. Genetics of gastrointestinal polyposis. Gastroenterology 1978; 74:896–7.
91. Haggitt RC, Reid BJ. Hereditary gastrointestinal polyposis syndromes. Am J Surg Pathol 1986; 10:871–87.
92. Jarvinen H, Franssila KO. Familial juvenile polyposis coli: Increased risk of colorectal cancer. Gut 1984; 25:792–800.
93. Friedl W, Kruse R, Uhlhaas S et al. Frequent 4-bp deletion in exon 9 of the SMAD4/MADH4 gene in familial juvenile polyposis patients. Gene Chromosomes Cancer 1999; 25:403–6.
94. Roth S, Sistonen P, Salovaara R et al. SMAD4 genes in juvenile polyposis. Genes Chromosomes Cancer 1999; 26:54–61.
95. Eaden JA, Abrams KR, Mayberry JF. The risk of colorectal cancer in ulcerative colitis: a meta-analysis. Gut 2001; 48:526–35.
96. Melville DM, Jass JR, Morson BC et al. Observer study of the grading of dysplasia in ulcerative colitis: comparison with clinical outcome. Hum Pathol 1989; 20:1008–14.
97. Skelton AA, Lehman RE, Schrock TR et al. Retrospective review of colorectal cancer in ulcerative colitis at a tertiary center. Arch Surg 1996; 131:806–11.
98. Suzuki H, Harpaz N, Tarmin L et al. Microsatellite instability in ulcerative colitis-associated colorectal dysplasia and cancers. Cancer Res 1994; 54:4841–4.
99. Walsh SV, Loda M, Torres CM et al. p53 and â catenin expression in chronic ulcerative colitis-associated polypoid dysplasia and sporadic adenomas. An immunohistochemical study. Am J Surg Pathol 1999; 23:963–9.
100. Wright CL, Riddell RH. The pathology and politics of dysplasia in ulcerative colitis. Current Opinion Gastroenterol 1998; 14:11–4.
101. Morson BC. Precancerous lesions of the colon and rectum. Classification and controversial issues. JAMA 1962; 179:104–9.
102. Louw JH. Polypoid lesions of the large bowel in children with particular reference to benign lymphoid polyposis. Pediatric Surg 1968; 3:195–209.
103. Troisi RJ, Freedman AN, Devesa SS. Incidence of colorectal carcinoma in the U.S. An update of trends by gender, race, age, subsite, and stage, 1975–1994. Cancer 1999; 85:1670–6.
104. Coleman MP, Demaret E. Cancer registration in the European community. Int J Cancer 1988; 42:339–45.
105. Tamura K, Ishiguro S, Munakata A et al. Annual changes in colorectal carcinoma incidence in Japan. Analysis of survey data on incidence in Aomori Prefecture. Cancer 1996; 78:1187–94.
106. Spratt JS, Ackerman LV, Moyer CA. Relationship of polyps of the colon to colonic cancer. Ann Surg 1958; 148:682–98.
107. Helwig EB. Adenomas and the pathogenesis of cancer of the colon and rectum. Dis Colon Rectum 1959; 2:5–17.
108. Bedenne L, Faivre J, Boutron MC et al. Adenoma-Carcinoma sequence or "de novo" carcinogenesis? A study of adenomatous remnants in a population-based series of large bowel cancers. Cancer 1992; 69:883–8.
109. Ponz de Leon M, Antonioli A, Ascari A et al. Incidence and familial occurrence of colorectal cancer and polyps in a health-care district of Northern Italy. Cancer 1988; 62:2858–59.
110. Nazarian HK, Giuliano AE, Hiatt JR. Colorectal carcinoma: analysis of management in two medical eras. J Surg Oncol 1993; 52:46–9.
111. Sariego J, Byrd ME, Kerstein M et al. Changing patterns in colorectal carcinoma: a 25-year experience. Am Surg 1992; 58:686–91.
112. Talbot IC. Pathology and natural history. In: "Recent results in Cancer Research." Springer-Verlag: Berlin – Heidelberg 1982; 83:59–66.

113. Griffin MR, Bergstrahl EJ, Coffey RJ et al. Predictors of survival after curative resection of carcinoma of the colon and rectum. Cancer 1987; 60:2318-24.
114. Ponz de Leon M, Sant M, Micheli A et al. Clinical and pathologic prognostic indicators in colorectal cancer. A population-based study. Cancer 1992; 69:626-35.
115. Bosman FT. Prognostic value of pathological characteristics of colorectal cancer. Eur J Cancer 1995; 31:1216-1221.
116. Lanza G, Gafà R, Matteuzzi M et al. Medullary-type poorly differentiated adenocarcinoma of the large bowel: a distinct clinicopathologic entity characterized by microsatellite instability and improved survival. J Clin Oncol 1999; 17:2429-38.
117. Sasaki O, Atkin WS, Jass JR. Mucinous carcinoma of the rectum. Histopathol 1987; 11:259-72.
118. Hermanek P, Guggenmoos-Holzmann I, Gall FP. Prognostic factors in rectal carcinoma. A contribution to the further development of tumor classification. Dis Colon Rectum 1989; 32:593-9.
119. Newland RC, Dent OF, Chapuis PH et al. Survival after curative resection of lymph node negative colorectal carcinoma. A prospective study of 910 patients. Cancer 1995; 76:564-71.
120. Jass JR. Lymphocitic infiltration and survival in rectal cancer. J Clin Pathol 1986; 39:585-9.
121. Jass JR, Love SB, Northover JMA. A new prognostic classification of rectal cancer. Lancet 1987; 1303-6.
122. Deans GT, Heatley M, Patterson CC et al. Colorectal carcinoma: importance of clinical and pathological factors in survival. Ann R Coll Surg Engl 1994; 76:59-64.
123. Bokey EL, Chapuis PH, Dent OF et al. Factors affecting survival after excision of the rectum for cancer. Dis Colon Rectum 1997; 40:3-10.
124. Bozzetti F, Mariani L, Miceli R et al. Cancer of the low and middle rectum: local and distant recurrences, and survival in 350 radically resected patients. J Surg Oncol 1996; 62:207-13.
125. Willett CG, Badizadegan K, Ancukiewicz M et al. Prognostic factors in stage T3N0 rectal cancer. Do all patients require postoperative pelvic irradiation and chemotherapy? Dis Colon Rectum 1999; 42:167-73.
126. Sanchez-Cespedes M, Esteller M, Hibi K et al. Molecular detection of neoplastic cells in lymph nodes of metastatic colorectal cancer patients predicts recurrence. Clin Cancer Res 1999; 5:2450-4.
127. Gatta G, Capocaccia R, Sant M et al. Understanding variations in survival for colorectal cancer in Europe: a EUROCARE high resolution study. Gut 2000; 47:533-8.
128. Kanthan R., Loewy J., Kanthan S.C. Skeletal metastases in colorectal carcinomas. A Saskatchewan profile. Dis Colon Rectum 1999; 42:21592-7.
129. Ghossein RA, Bhattacharya S, Rosai J. Molecular detection of micrometastases and circulating tumor cells in solid tumors. Clin Cancer Res 1999; 5:1950-60.
130. Braun S, Pantel K, Müller P et al. Cytokeratin-positive cells in the bone marrow and survival of patients with stage I, II, or III breast cancer. N Engl J Med 2000; 242:525-33.
131. Dukes CE. The classification of cancer of the rectum. J Pathol Bacteriol 1932; 35:323-32.
132. Hutter RVP, Sobin LH. A universal staging system for cancer of the colon and rectum. Let there be light. Arch Pathol Lab Med 1986; 110:367-8.
133. Thebo JS, Senagore AJ, Reinhold DS et al. Molecular staging of colorectal cancer. Dis Colon Rectum 2000; 43:155-62.
134. Chapuis PH, Dixon MF, Fielding LP et al. Staging of colorectal cancer. Int J Colorect Dis 1987; 2:123-38.
135. Spread C, Berkel H, Jewell L et al. Colon carcinoid tumors. A population-based study. Dis Colon Rectum 1994; 37:482-91.
136. Caplin ME, Buscombe JR, Hilson AJ et al. Carcinoid tumour. Lancet 1998; 352:799-805.

137. Saclarides TJ, Szeluga D, Staren ED. Neuroendocrine cancers of the colon and rectum. Results of a ten-year experience. Dis Colon Rectum 1994; 37:635–42.
138. De Bruïne AP, Wiggers T, Beek C et al. Endocrine cells in colorectal adenocarcinomas: incidence, hormone profile and prognostic relevance. Int J Cancer 1993; 54:765–71.
139. Staren ED, Gould VE, Warren WH et al. Neuroendocrine carcinomas of the colon and rectum: a clinicopathologic evaluation. Surg 1988; 104:1080–9.
140. Gray GM, Rosenberg SA, Cooper AD et al. Lymphomas involving the gastrointestinal tract. Gastroenterology 1982; 82:143–52.
141. Fan CW, Changchien CR, Wang JY et al. Primary colorectal lymphoma. Dis Colon Rectum 2000; 43:1277–82.

4 Diagnosis and Clinical Features of Colorectal Cancer

Introduction

Overall 5-year survival and prognosis of colorectal malignancies showed only a slight improvement (10%–20%) over the past 40–50 years [1, 2]. This contrasts with the enormous advances in our knowledge of the pathogenesis of the disease [3, 4], with the existence of new combined adjuvant treatments [5, 6], with the refinement of surgical techniques [7, 8], and with the evidence of lower endoscopy as an effective screening procedure [9, 10].

One of the reasons for the modest increase in survival can be related to the frequent lack of specific symptoms, with a consequent difficulty of early diagnosis of non-invasive neoplasia. The relationship between type of symptoms, their duration and the prognosis of colorectal malignancies has been evaluated in various investigations [11–14]. Although, rather intuitively, early diagnosis should lead to a better control of the disease, the results of these studies indicate that survival seems to be influenced more by the biological behavior of the cancer than by the length of the symptomatic disease. If the early diagnosis of symptomatic subjects results in an insignificant improvement in prognosis, then the detection of tumors in the presymptomatic stage – which at least in part corresponds to premalignancy or locally invasive disease – might offer a better prospect of cure for these patients.

Tremendous advances have recently been achieved in the diagnosis of colorectal tumors, and consequently, a broad range of techniques are available for patients and clinicians. Although one often feels that new technological advances exceed our understanding of how to use them properly, selected approaches are becoming accepted tools in our diagnostic procedures. With a cautiously optimistic attitude, we might foresee that in the near future a major objective should become possible: early diagnosis with accurate preoperative staging, obtained with the least invasive technique.

The purpose of this chapter is twofold: first, to review our current knowledge of the main clinical and laboratory findings of colorectal malignancies, with all their limitations; second, to discuss and analyze the relative contribution of old, relatively new and recent techniques to diagnosing these neoplasms.

Clinical Findings: Symptoms and Signs

At present, some 10%–15% of all patients with colorectal cancer are still hospitalized as an emergency, owing to acute symptoms such as (a) abdominal distension due to colonic obstruction (usually after many days of obstinate constipation), (b) severe abdominal pain due to generalized or localized peritonitis, when the tumor perforates and the intestinal content reaches the peritoneum, (c) massive bleeding from the rectum, owing to ulceration or necrosis of the tumoral mass. These individuals are treated immediately, often with an emergency laparotomy, which provides the correct diagnosis of cancer at surgery, and before any diagnostic procedure.

Another subgroup of individuals with colorectal malignancies are admitted to hospital (or referred to physicians) because of nonspecific symptoms, such as iron-deficiency anemia, anorexia, weight loss and extreme fatigue; in many of these patients, subsequent investigations may disclose metastatic disease in the liver, lung or other organs.

Most of patients with colorectal cancer present with vague abdominal symptoms, such as diffuse or localized abdominal pain, obstinate constipation, episodes of diarrhea, changes in bowel habits, tenesmus or chronic rectal bleeding (especially for distal lesions). Since irritable bowel syndrome, hemorrhoids and constipation are extremely frequent in the Western population [15], it may be difficult – on the basis of clinical presentation – to sort out whether the symptoms reflect an exacerbation of these chronic conditions or may conceal a neoplasm of the large bowel. As a simple rule, all patients with anorectal discomfort or abdominal symptoms lasting more than a few weeks should undergo digital examination of the anorectal region and flexible sigmoidoscopy. However, if we consider that some 30%–40% of colorectal lesions are localized proximally to the splenic flexure, a more appropriate approach should also include colonoscopy [16].

Finally, symptoms may be completely absent, and in a sizeable fraction of patients the tumor represents an occasional finding during abdominal surgery or endoscopic investigations.

In 1977, Irvin and Greaney examined the relationship between the duration of symptoms and the long-term prognosis of colorectal carcinoma [17]; the study included 355 patients undergoing surgical resection of the large bowel during the period 1966 to 1970. These were subdivided into four groups in relation to the symptomatic clinical history (from less than 5 months to more than 12 months). The 5-year survival was of the order of 20%–30% in all four groups; similarly, Dukes' staging at operation was completely unrelated to the interval between onset of symptoms and clinical diagnosis of cancer. The authors concluded that the duration of symptoms had little bearing on the staging and survival of patients with colorectal cancer, and that intuitively only the presymptomatic detection of tumors might improve clinical prognosis.

Similar conclusions were reached by Ponz de Leon et al. in 1988 [14]. In this study, 406 consecutive patients with colorectal neoplasms were evaluated, and the diagnosis was arbitrarily considered "early" when the length of symptomatic disease was less than 2 months and "late" when more than 60 days were required to reach the diagnosis of cancer. Dukes' staging showed that either localized or invasive neoplasms were equally distributed between patients with an early or late diagnosis. Similar findings were also reported by Holliday and Hardcastle in a series of 116 patients with colorectal malignancies [18]. At variance with the above-mentioned studies, Robinson et al. [19] suggested that patients with a delayed diagnosis tended to have more advanced disease, though this was statistically significant only for rectal tumors.

In conclusion, although clinical symptoms cannot be ignored and should alert physicians to a prompt intervention, they are usually of little help for an early diagnosis of colorectal neoplasms. The main reason for this is the common occurrence of bowel disturbances in the general population; consequently, many individuals underestimate that symptoms such as abdominal discomfort, pain or rectal bleeding might also be due to the presence of cancer in the large bowel [20]. The ideal approach is to screen asymptomatic individuals with lower endoscopy in the attempt to remove all premalignant (adenomatous polyps) lesions. The results of the National Polyp Study [21, 22] clearly indicate that such a strategy might lead to a significant reduction of morbidity and mortality for colorectal cancer.

Laboratory Investigations

There are no specific laboratory tests that can indicate or suggest the presence of colorectal malignancies. As a consequence of long-standing rectal bleeding, anemia and low serum iron may occur; these findings are rather nonspecific, though it is good clinical practice – in their presence – to take into consideration the possible existence of an asymptomatic tumoral lesion of the digestive organs [23]. Impairment of liver function tests occurs only in the case of metastatic disease (in the liver) and are of little help for the clinician.

The search for occult blood in the stool may give a hint as to whether there are bleeding lesions in the gastrointestinal tract. Repeated positive tests can suggest the presence of a tumor in the large bowel, but a definite diagnosis will require a direct investigation of the colon (barium enema or colonoscopy). Occult blood test should be viewed as a mass screening procedure [24]. Recently, various studies showed a reduction in the expected mortality and an increase in survival as a consequence of mass screening for occult blood in the stool [25, 26]. However, we should not forget that mass screening with Haemoccult is expensive, requires a close collaboration between patients and physicians, and yields many false-positive and false-negative results [27].

With a few exceptions (α-fetoprotein, prostate specific antigen), serum markers have generally been disappointing for the early diagnosis of cancer [28]. The carcinoembryonic antigen (CEA) is an oncofetal protein produced by most colorectal carcinomas [29]; although the diagnostic sensitivity and specificity of CEA is very low, this marker found a definitive clinical application as an indicator of early recurrence in the follow-up of patients operated on for colorectal cancer [30]. Moreover, according to some observations, preoperative CEA serum levels might also be related to the clinical outcome, but not without controversies [28].

Diagnosis of Colorectal Cancer: Old Methods and Recent Imaging Techniques

At the beginning of the new millennium, sigmoidoscopy and especially pancolonoscopy represent the standard procedures for the diagnosis of benign and malignant lesions of the large bowel. Colonoscopy allows the direct inspection of the entire colorectal mucosa, while flexible sigmoidoscopy visualizes a more limited region (rectum, sigmoid and descending colon). Although 2/3 of colorectal tumors are located in the distal large bowel, a trend towards a more frequent occurrence of proximal lesions has been reported [31, 32]; moreover, in hereditary non-polyposis colorectal cancer (HNPCC) and related syndromes, neoplasms are more often located in the right colon [33, 34]. Thus, there is well-founded evidence that sigmoidoscopy can miss a relevant fraction of colorectal lesions; consequently, most endoscopists tend to avoid sigmoidoscopy and perform colonoscopy whenever possible [35, 36]. Endoscopy can detect precancerous lesions that do not bleed – such as adenomatous and other types of polyps – and tumors that are not bleeding at the time of examination. Even more important, during endoscopy colorectal lesions can be removed or, when this is not possible, biopsies can be taken for histological examination; this is an aspect of paramount importance, which should not be overlooked when discussing the advantages of the new imaging techniques (see below).

Colonoscopy, however, is an unpleasant experience, even with sedation, and many patients are reluctant to undergo repeated investigations (for example, in the surveillance of adenomatous polyps) owing to abdominal discomfort, pain or bowel preparation [37]. Indeed, a clean colon is a prerequisite for optimal endoscopy, and this requires several enemas or the ingestion of a variety of cathartic compounds [38]. Sometimes colonoscopy can be difficult (i.e. the caecum is not reached within 15–20 min); the most frequent cause of difficulty is recurrent looping of the colonoscope in a long or mobile colon [39]. Technical difficulties occur appreciably more frequently in women; the reason for this can be attributed – at least in part – to an inherently longer colon in the female sex [40].

Digital rectal exploration and rigid rectosigmoidoscopy have at present a limited role in the diagnosis of colorectal malignancies, since they can detect only lesions located in the most distal portions of the large bowel. These techniques, however, can be useful for the surgeon in planning the type of operation.

Imaging Studies in Primary Cancer

Barium enema remains an excellent investigation for the diagnosis of colorectal cancer, especially in symptomatic patients. Since radiographs rely on a detailed definition of the colonic wall, double-contrast barium enema has been shown to be more sensitive (91%) than single-contrast examination (70%–80%), and it is at present the technique of choice [41]. It should be noted, however, that it is often difficult to visualize low rectal cancers on a radiograph; consequently, given the suspicion of cancer, the anorectal region should be examined with digital palpation or rigid sigmoidoscopy. For an optimal investigation of the large bowel, this is covered with barium and then inflated with air; the inflation can cause considerable discomfort to the patient. Putting together patient discomfort, radiation exposure, moderate sensitivity (when compared to colonoscopy) and possibility (with endoscopy) to remove polyps, we are not surprised if colonoscopy has gradually replaced barium enema as first choice investigation for colorectal tumors [42].

Virtual colonoscopy (computed tomography colonography) is a new imaging method which takes advantage of computed tomography (CT) or magnetic resonance imaging to obtain three-dimensional images of the whole colon [43, 44]. The technique combines rapid helical scanning with computer technology capable of rendering clear images of the various large-bowel segments. With a conventional workstation and a dynamic display of images, the radiologist may perform virtual examinations of the colon, simulating the way endoscopists explore the large bowel during standard colonoscopy. After bowel preparation, the patient is placed in a lateral or supine position, and through a small enema tube the colon is distended with air or carbon dioxide, without causing excessive discomfort to the patient. Glucagon can be given before performing helical imaging of the abdomen to avoid smooth-muscle spasm and to reduce pain further. A single acquisition of images usually requires three or four 20-s breath holds, and total scanning can be completed within a few minutes. After data acquisition, the examination is reviewed by a radiologist with a workstation and suitable software, in order to produce three- and two-dimensional images of the large bowel. It is worth noting that the radiation dose necessary for virtual colonoscopy is lower than that used for conventional CT, owing to the contrast between the air filling the colon and the density of soft tissues [45].

In a recent prospective study [43], virtual and conventional colonoscopy showed a similar efficacy in detecting polyps 6 mm or more in diameter in patients at increased risk for colorectal malignancies. However, in other investigations, polyps of 10 mm or more were missed by virtual colonoscopy, especially when located in the proximal colon or in the case of flat lesions [46, 47], which are difficult to detect even during routine endoscopy [48]. When compared with barium enema, virtual colonoscopy does not require coating the colon with barium, can produce a large number of different projections of a given colorectal segment, is more rapid and better tolerated by the patient [45].

In conclusion, computed tomography colonography is a new and promising imaging method which allows a rapid and detailed investigation of the entire large bowel. The technique, however, has a sensitivity and specificity inferior to conventional colonoscopy [49]; cannot be used to remove tissue; is available in relatively few centers; and, being rather expensive, can hardly be used as a screening procedure for the early detection of colorectal tumors.

Hydrocolonic sonography is a transabdominal ultrasound examination which is executed after retrograde instillation of water into the colon, thus improving the conditions for ultrasonic imaging and evaluation of the entire large bowel [50]. After preparation of the colon and intravenous injection of vagolytic compounds (such as scopolamine) for bowel relaxation, 1 to 2 liters of water are instilled through a rectal tube. Continuous transabdominal colonic ultrasonography is carried out beginning at the time of water instillation. The technique is less expensive than colonoscopy, less invasive, does not require sedation and seems to be well tolerated [51]. Initial observations showed that the instillation of water allowed sonographic imaging from the rectosigmoid junction to the caecum in 97% of the investigated patients [52]. Moreover, 28 of 29 carcinomas were correctly diagnosed (with conventional ultrasound only 9 carcinomas were identified), and 38 of 42 polyps larger than 7 mm could be detected. Subsequent studies, however, did not confirm these encouraging observations; thus, Chui et al. [53], in a series of 52 patients with a total of 26 polyps and 3 carcinomas, were unable to detect most of these lesions by hydrocolonic ultrasonography. The success of the technique might depend closely on the bowel preparation and cleaning, since adherent feces are difficult to differentiate from colonic lesions; in addition, colonic haustrations may mimic polyps, and some areas of the large bowel (such as the rectum, because of the overlying bladder and bones) are difficult to examine.

Endoluminal ultrasound was introduced in 1956, when the first endorectal ultrasound was carried out [54]; the technique, however, gained ample diffusion only after 1980, when the equipment designed for urological investigations was adapted for introduction into the rectum. At present, the main use of endosonography is in the preoperative staging of rectal cancer and, in particular, in determining the depth of tumor penetration and the lymph node status. This kind of information can be valuable for the surgeon for choosing the most appropriate approach to that particular situation [55]. In the few studies that addressed this problem, the endosonographic evaluation of depth of invasion and pararectal lymph node metastasis seemed superior to that of CT [56, 57]. The accuracy of endorectal ultrasound, however, is limited by several factors, including the degree of inflammation around the tumor, the possibility of microscopic tumor spread, an inaccurate definition of normal structures, and the lack of sufficient expertise by the operator. McClave et al. [58] recently showed that errors in interpretation still account for most mistakes made in endosonography for staging colorectal carcinoma. The authors advocated specific attention to instrumentation and a better preparation of radiologists in order to maximize the accuracy of ultrasound interpretation.

Radioimmunodetection of malignant tumors can be obtained by taking whole-body gamma scans in patients who have been injected intravenously with antibodies labeled with a gamma-emitting radionuclide. The antigens most commonly used in clinical studies are CEA and TAG-72 [59, 60]; though most investigators employed intact murine monoclonal antibodies, there is growing interest in the use of antibody fragments or single-chain antibodies [61, 62]. The choice of radionuclides considered for radioimmunodetection include ^{99}technetium, ^{111}indium and ^{123}iodine. In the detection of primary tumors, the technique cannot be compared with endoscopy and barium enema, while there are studies of immunodetection in the initial staging of colorectal cancer patient [63]. The available literature suggests that cancer detection with radionuclides is safe, and that the sensitivity of detection is high in selected patients, ranging from 60% to more that 90% [64]. For colorectal neoplasms, the limit of detection is of the order of 1-2 cm, and there is evidence that occult disease undiagnosed with other diagnostic procedures can be identified with radionuclides [65]. However, is not clear whether the localization of occult lesions by radioimmunodetection may improve the management and prognosis of these patients. Finally, the technique has been used more frequently, and with more success, for recurrent colorectal cancer.

Intraoperative ultrasound can be used to supplement surgical inspection and palpation, in particular of the liver. The technique can be carried out with specialized intraoperative ultrasound units or with probes used on standard diagnostic ultrasound scanner units. After manual palpation, the liver can be investigated by placing the ultrasound probe directly over the various segments and the areas of interest; an experienced radiologist may complete the investigation within 5-10 min. Intraoperative ultrasound is particularly useful for detecting liver metastasis and, thus, for determining the feasibility and the extent of liver resection [66]. In fact, some metastatic lesions can be overlooked on preoperative imaging studies, and deep intrahepatic lesions - especially when less that 2 cm in diameter - can be missed during manual examination [67]. Although this technique has not (yet) achieved a wide diffusion, some investigators consider intraoperative ultrasound as the modality of choice for hepatic surgery [68].

Imaging Studies in the Diagnosis of Recurrent or Metastatic Disease

Locoregional recurrence and distant metastasis (especially to the liver and lung) represent frequent events in colorectal cancer, and one of the major frustrations for physicians after an apparently curative resection. Cancer of the rectum can recur in 3%-30% of cases (while these rates are lower for colonic neoplasms), and most recurrences develop within 2-3 years after surgery [69]. It follows that colorectal cancer patients - and especially those with Dukes' C lesions - should be closely followed up for at least 3 years after surgical treatment [70].

Serum level of CEA, lower endoscopy, standard ultrasound and CAT scanning (Fig. 4.1) are the standard procedures commonly employed for the early detection of recurrent or metastatic colorectal cancer. In recent years, however, new techniques have been developed which seem to offer additional advantages in the follow-up of these patients.

Magnetic resonance imaging (MRI) creates images by evaluating nuclei for the absorption or emission of electromagnetic energy when a patient is placed in a magnetic field and a radiofrequency pulse is applied. A small number of protons in the tissues absorb the energy and change their initial orientation; on returning to their natural state, the hydrogen nuclei release a signal that is received and processed through a computer algorithm, and an image is reconstructed [71]. Since the various tissues and organs of the human body have different properties in regard to proton density, they can absorb and emit energy at characteristic times which are different and can be detected. According to most studies, CAT scanning and MRI seem to possess the same limitations in evaluat-

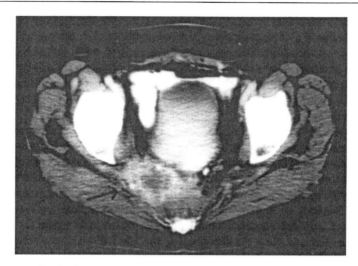

Fig. 4.1. Example of pelvic computed tomography (CT). Local recurrence of rectal cancer mainly located in the presacral region and in the ischiorectal space. *Arrow* shows the tumor mass, which has a non-homogeneous density with a necrotic center

ing liver metastasis and the depth of tumor invasion through the bowel wall and the surrounding tissues. In particular, both techniques can fall short in distinguishing between benign fibrotic changes and true neoplastic recurrence [72, 73]. However, MRI has a higher tissue contrast resolution than CAT and does not involve the use of ionizing radiation. On the other hand, MRI is more expensive, requires a longer time, and cannot be used in certain patients (such as those with cardiac pacemakers or ocular foreign bodies) (Fig. 4.2).

Radioimmunodetection has already been discussed in the diagnosis of primary tumors, but its application in patients with suspected recurrences has been more rewarding. One of the main objectives of this technique is to detect recurrent disease which has not been diagnosed by more conventional approaches, such as CAT scanning and ultrasound. In some investigations, radioimmunoscintigraphy showed a sensitivity and specificity of the order of 80%; even more importantly, immunodetection was superior to other techniques in identifying recurrences [74, 75]. Another objective is to distinguish neoplastic tissue from benign fibrotic reactions in the site of previous surgery, an aspect for which there is no definitive answer, and that remains intriguing despite the availability of sophisticated techniques, such as CAT or MRI [72].

Endoluminal ultrasound has also been employed to evaluate local recurrences of rectosigmoid cancer following apparently curative resection. The available literature suggests that the technique may be useful in the detection of asymptomatic recurrence [76]. However, when endoluminal ultrasound was compared with conventional approaches, CAT scanning showed a higher sensitivity and specificity in identifying recurrent tumors [77]. Thus, more studies are needed to ascertain whether endorectal ultrasound should become a routine procedure in the follow-up of patients with malignancies of the rectosigmoid tract.

Imaging Studies in the Diagnosis of Recurrent or Metastatic Disease 87

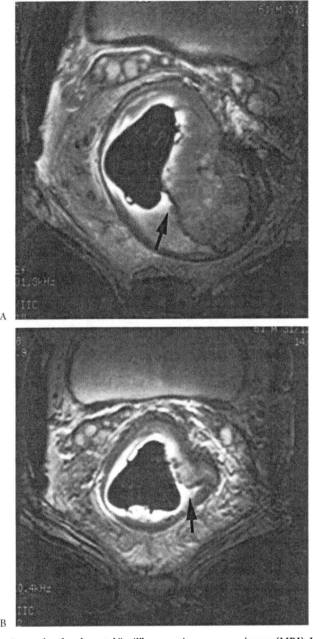

Fig. 4.2 A, B. Example of endorectal "coil" magnetic resonance image (MRI). Large vegetating mass of the left rectal wall with reduction of the lumen (**A**) and retraction of the wall (*arrow*). The same patient after preoperative chemoradiotherapy (**B**): a marked reduction of the previously described mass is evident, with widening of the rectal lumen, while retraction of the wall is still evident

Positron-emission tomography (PET) is a new imaging technique which uses a positron-emitting isotope incorporated into a biochemical process occurring in organs and tissues of the body. When the isotope decays, a positron is emitted, collides with an electron, and causes both particles to be annihilated; this results in the release of two 511-keV photons that radiate outward in opposite directions. The scanner is designed to detect these photons and to determine their point of origin; determining the point of origin creates images similar to CAT scans [78]. However, images are actually the result of a functional, metabolic process; consequently, the anatomic details are not as well delineated as with CAT or MRI. On the other hand, the metabolic origin of these images may provide information on the functional status of a given organ or tissue, which cannot be obtained with more conventional techniques [79]. The most common compound used for PET imaging is fluorodeoxyglucose (FDG), which allows the direct assessment of the cellular glucose metabolism [80]. FDG given to patients is trapped into cells in amounts that reflect their glucose metabolism; the uptake depends on several factors, including blood flow, energy demand, plasma glucose and insulin levels. Tumor imaging with FDG and PET is based on the assumptions that there is an enhanced rate of glucose metabolism in malignancies and that high-grade tumors require more glucose for their metabolic activity than low-grade neoplasms [81]. PET has been used in staging several malignant tumors; as far as colorectal neoplasms are concerned, the main application of FDG-PET was the discrimination between fibrosis and local recurrence of cancer following apparently curative surgery. As we have already discussed, none of the standard procedures (ultrasound, CAT scanning and MRI) can provide a definitive answer to this frequent and challenging clinical problem [72–75]. There are various studies indicating that PET is highly effective in discriminating between recurrent colorectal cancer and reactive fibrosis, with a sensitivity and specificity undoubtedly better than those seen with CAT scanning or MRI [82, 83, 54]. However, false-positive results have been reported also with FDG-PET and can be due to abdominal abscesses, proctitis or other inflammations [84, 85]; it follows that a clear definition of the clinical status of the patient is essential for an accurate interpretation of PET scan images. A recent investigation, carried out in a relevant number of patients, showed that FDG-PET was more sensitive than CAT for the detection of recurrent or metastatic colorectal cancer, and that in approximately 25% of cases PET altered the clinical management in a beneficial manner [86]. Moreover, Johnson et al. [87] confirmed that PET scanning is more sensitive than CT scanning and more likely to give the correct results when metastatic disease is present.

Conclusions

In conclusion, clinical symptoms are of little help in managing patients affected by colorectal malignancies, since they appear in the late phases of the disease and can be identical to symptoms occurring in irritable bowel syndrome, constipation or hemorrhoids. It follows that the objective of an early diagnosis can be reached through the detection of the disease in its asymptomatic phase, which may last several years.

Despite the availability of new and promising imaging techniques, colonoscopy maintains a preminent role in the diagnosis of primary colorectal tumors, because it explores the whole large bowel and allows us to take samples for analysis and, in some cases, to remove the neoplasm. CT and the newly developed PET represent our best choices for diagnosing tumor recurrences.

References

1. Gatta G, Capocaccia R, Sant M et al. Understanding variations in survival for colorectal cancer in Europe: a EUROCARE high resolution study. Gut 2000; 47:533-8.
2. Gatta G, Faivre J, Capocaccia R et al. Survival of colorectal cancer patients in Europe during the period 1978-89. Eur J Cancer 1998; 34:2176-83.
3. Herrera L, Luna P, Villarreal JR et al. Perspectives in colorectal cancer. J Surg Oncol 1991; 2:92-103.
4. Boland R, Sato J, Appelman HD et al. Microallelotyping defines the sequence and tempo of allelic losses at tumour suppressor gene loci during colorectal cancer progression. Nature Med 1995; 1:902-9.
5. Kane MJ. Adjuvant systemic treatment for carcinoma of the colon and rectum. Semin Oncol 1991; 18:421-42.
6. Kemeny N, Huang Y, Cohen AM et al. Hepatic arterial infusion of chemotherapy after resection of hepatic metastases from colorectal cancer. N Engl J Med 1999; 341:2039-48.
7. Heald RJ, Moran BJ, Ryall RDH et al. Rectal cancer. The Basingstoke experience of total mesorectal excision, 1978-97. Arch Surg 1998; 133:894-9.
8. Khalili TM, Fleshner PR, Hiatt JR et al. Colorectal cancer. Comparison of laparoscopic with open approaches. Dis Colon Rectum 1998; 41:832-8.
9. Winawer SJ, Zauber AG, O'Brien MJ et al. Randomized comparison of surveillance intervals after colonoscopic removal of newly diagnosed adenomatous polyps. N Engl J Med 1993; 328:901-6.
10. Winawer SJ, Zauber AG, Nah Ho M et al. Prevention of colorectal cancer by colonoscopic polypectomy. N Engl J Med 1993; 329:1977-81.
11. Gerard A, Bleiberg H. Delay in diagnosis of colorectal cancer. Eur J Cancer Clin Oncol 1987; 23:1089-90.
12. Crerand S, Feeley TM, Waldron RP et al. Colorectal carcinoma over 30 years at one hospital: no evidence for a shift to the right. Int J Colorect Dis 1991; 6:184-7.
13. Copeland EM, Miller LD, Jones RS. Prognostic factors in carcinoma of the colon and rectum. Am J Surg 1968; 166:875-9.
14. Ponz de Leon M, Sacchetti C, Sassatelli R et al. Cancer of the large bowel: Dukes' staging, duration of symptoms, multiple tumours and other relevant clinical features derived from a population-based registry. Ital J Gastroenterol 1988; 20:175-9.
15. Jones R, Lydeard S. Prevalence of symptoms of dyspepsia in the community. BMJ 1989; 298:30-2.
16. Thiis-Evensen E, Hoff GS, Sauar J et al. Population-based surveillance by colonoscopy: effect on the incidence of colorectal cancer. Scand J Gastroenterol 1999; 34:414-20.
17. Irvin TT, Greaney MG. Duration of symptoms and prognosis of carcinoma of the colon and rectum. Surg Gynecol Obstet 1977; 144:883-6.
18. Holliday HW, Hardcastle JD. Delay in diagnosis and treatment of symptomatic colorectal cancer. Lancet 1979; 1:309-11.

19. Robinson E, Mohilever J, Zidan J et al. Colorectal cancer: incidence, delay in diagnosis and stage of disease. Eur J Cancer Clin Oncol 1986; 22:157-61.
20. Curless R, French J, Williams GV et al. Comparison of gastrointestinal symptoms in colorectal carcinoma patients and community controls with respect to age. Gut 1994; 35:1267-70.
21. Winawer SJ, Zauber AG, O'Brien MJ et al. The National Polyp Study: design, methods, and characteristics of patients with newly diagnosed polyps. Cancer 1992; 70:1236-45.
22. O'Brien MJ, Winawe SJ, Zauber AG et al. The National Polyp Study: patient and polyp characteristics associated with high-grade dysplasia in colorectal adenomas. Gastroenterology 1990; 98:371-9.
23. Weisburger JH. Causes, relevant mechanisms, and prevention of large bowel cancer. Semin Oncol 1991; 18:316-36.
24. Faivre J, Tazi MA, El Mrini T et al. Faecal occult blood screening and reduction of colorectal cancer mortality: a case-control study. Br J Cancer 1999; 79:680-3.
25. Kronborg O, Wahrendorf J. Colorectal cancer screening: methods, benefits and costs. Colorectal cancer screening: methods, benefits and costs. Eur J Cancer 1994; 30:877-9.
26. Allison JE, Tekawa IS, Ransom LJ et al. A comparison of fecal occult-blood tests for colorectal-cancer screening. N Engl J Med 1996; 334:155-9.
27. Robinson MHE, Hardcastle JD, Moss SM et al. The risks of screening: data from the Nottingham randomised controlled trial of faecal occult blood screening for colorectal cancer. Gut 1999; 45:588-92.
28. Torosian MH. The clinical usefulness and limitations of tumor markers. Surg Gynecol Obstet 1988; 166:567-79.
29. Minton JP, Martin EW. The use of serial CEA determinations to predict recurrence of colon cancer and when to do a second-look operation. Cancer 1978; 42:1422-7.
30. Wanebo H, Stearns M, Schwartz M. Use of CEA as indicator of early recurrence and as guide to selected second-look procedure in patients with colorectal cancer. Ann Surg 1978; 188:481-93.
31. Sariego J, Byrd ME, Kerstein M et al. Changing patterns in colorectal carcinoma: a 25-year experience. Am Surg 1992; 58:686-91.
32. Nazarian HK, Giuliano AE, Hiatt JR. Colorectal carcinoma: analysis of management in two medical eras. J Surg Oncol 1993; 52:46-9.
33. Lynch HT, Watson P, Kriegler M et al. Differential diagnosis of hereditary nonpolyposis colorectal cancer (Lynch syndrome I and Lynch syndrome II). Dis Colon Rectum 1988; 31:372-7.
34. Vasen HFA, den Hartog Jager FCA, Menko FH et al. Screening for hereditary non-polyposis colorectal cancer: a study of 22 kindreds in the Netherlands. Am J Med 1989; 86:27881.
35. Rex DK, Smith JJ, Ulbright TM et al. Distal colonic hyperplastic polyps do not predict proximal adenomas in asymptomatic average-risk subjects. Gastroenterology 1992; 102:317-9.
36. Thiis-Evensen E, Hoff GS, Sauar J et al. Flexible sigmoidoscopy or colonoscopy as a screening modality for colorectal adenomas in older age groups? Findings in a cohort of the normal population aged 63-72 years. Gut 1999; 45:834-9.
37. Schutz SM, Lee JG, Schmitt CM et al. Clues to patient dissatisfaction with conscious sedation for colonoscopy. Am J Gastroenterol 1994; 89:1476-9.
38. Lazzaroni M, Bianchi Porro G. Preparation, premedication, and surveillance. Endoscopy 1996; 28:6-12.
39. Saunders BP, Macrae F, Williams CB. What makes colonoscopy difficult? Gut 1993; 34(1).
40. Saunders BP, Fukumoto M, Halligan S et al. Why is colonoscopy more difficult in women? Gastrointest Endosc 1996; 43:124-6.
41. Ott DJ, Chen YM, Gelfand DW et al. Single-contrast vs double-contrast barium enema in the detection of colonic polyps. Am J Roentgenol 1986; 146:993-6.

References 91

42. Neugut AI, Forde KA. Screening colonoscopy: has the time come? Am J Gastroent 1988; 83:295-7.
43. Fenlon HM, Nunes DP, Schroy PC et al. A comparison of virtual and conventional colonoscopy for the detection of colorectal polyps. N Engl J Med 1999; 341:1496-503.
44. Schenenberger AW, Bauerfeind P, Krestin GP et al. Virtual colonoscopy with magnetic resonance imaging: in vitro evaluation of a new concept. Gastroenterology 1997; 112:1863-70.
45. Johnson CD, Ahlquist DA. Computed tomography colonography (virtual colonoscopy): a new method for colorectal screening. Gut 1999; 44:301-5.
46. Hara AK, Johnson CD, Reed IE et al. Detection of colorectal polyps with CT colography: initial assessment of sensitivity and specificity. Radiology. 1997; 205:59-65.
47. Rex DK, Vining D, Kopecky KK. An initial experience with screening for colon polyps using spiral CT with and without CT colography. Gastrointest Endosc 1999; 50:309-13.
48. Lanspa SJ, Rouse J, Smyrk T et al. Epidemiologic characteristics of the flat adenoma of Muto. A prospective study. Dis Colon Rectum 1992; 35:543-6.
49. Hara AK, Johnson CD, Reed JE et al. Reducing data size and radiation dose for CTC (CT colography). Am J Roentgenol 1997; 168:1181-4.
50. Limberg B. Diagnosis of large bowel tumours by colonic sonography. Lancet 1990; 335:144-6.
51. Limberg B. Diagnosis of acute ulcerative colitis and colonic Crohn's disease by colonic sonography. J Clin Ultrasound 1989; 17:25-31.
52. Limberg B. Diagnosis and staging of colonic tumors by conventional abdominal sonography as compared with hydrocolonic sonography. N Engl J Med 1992; 327:65-9.
53. Chui DW, Gooding GAW, McQuaid KR et al. Hydrocolonic ultrasonography in the detection of colonic polyps and tumors. N Engl J Med 1994; 331:1685-8.
54. Tempero M, Brand R, Holdeman K et al. New imaging techniques in colorectal cancer. Semin Oncol 1995; 22:448-71.
55. Katsura Y, Yamada K, Ishizawa T et al. Endorectal ultrasonography for the assessment of wall invasion and lymph node metastasis in rectal cancer. Dis Colon Rectum 1992; 35:362-8.
56. Katsura Y, Ishizawa T. Yoshinaka H et al. Diagnosis of mural invasion and lymph node metastasis of rectal cancer by endorectal ultrasonography. J Jpn Soc Colo-proctl 1990; 43:388-95.
57. Hildebreandt U, Klein T, Feifel G et al. Endosonography of pararectal lymph nodes: in vitro and in vivo evaluation. Dis Colon Rectum 1990; 33:863-8.
58. McClave SA, Jones WF, Woolfolk GM et al. Mistakes on EUS staging of colorectal carcinoma: error in interpretation or deception from innate pathologic features? Gastrointest Endosc 2000:51:682-9.
59. Goldenberg DM, Goldenberg H, Sharkey RM et al. Clinical studies of cancer radioimmunodetection with carcino-embryonic antigen monoclonal antibody fragments labeled with ^{123}I or ^{99m}Tc. Cancer Res 1990; 50:909-121.
60. Gero EJ, Colcher D, Ferroni P et al. The CA 72-4 radioimmunoassay for the detection of the TAG-72 carcinoma associated antigen in serum of patients. J Clin Lab Analysis 1989; 3:360-9.
61. Bischof Delaloye A, Delaloye B, Buchegger F et al. Clinical value of immunoscintigraphy in colorectal carcinoma patients: a prospective study. J Nucl Med 1989; 30:1646-56.
62. Colcher D, Bird R, Roselli M et al. In vivo tumor targeting of a recombinant single-chain antigen-binding protein. J Natl Cancer Inst 1990; 82:1191-7.
63. Lind P, Leichner P, Arian Schad K et al. Anticarcinoembryonic antigen immunoscintigraphy (Technetium 99m-monoclonal antibody BW 431/26) and serum CEA levels in patients with suspected primary and recurrent colorectal carcinoma. J Nucl Med 1991; 32:1319-25.

64. Abdel Nabi HH, Schwartz AN, Higano CS et al. Colorectal carcinoma: detection with indium-111 anticarcinoembryonic-antigen monoclonal antibody ZCE-025. Radiology 1987; 164:617-21.
65. Doerr RJ, Abdel Nabi H, Krag D et al. Indium 111 ZCE-025 immunoscintigraphy in occult recurrent colorectal cancer with elevated carcinoembryonic antigen level. Arch Surg 1990; 125:226-9.
66. Bismuth H, Castaing D, Garden OJ. The use of operative ultrasound in surgery of primary liver tumors. World J Surg 1987; 11:610-4.
67. Clarke MP, Kane RA, Steele G Jr et al. Prospective comparison of preoperative imaging and intraoperative ultrasonography in the detection of liver tumors. Surgery 1989; 106:849-55.
68. Jakimowicz JJ. Intraoperative ultrasonography during minimal access surgery. J R Coll Surg 1993; 38:231-8.
69. Beynon J, Mortensen NJ McC, Foy DMA et al. The detection and evaluation of locally recurrent rectal cancer with rectal endosonography. Dis Colon Rectum 1989; 32: 509-17.
70. Huguler M, Houry S. Treatment of local recurrence of rectal cancer. Am J Surg 1998; 175:288-92.
71. Balter S. An introduction to the physics of magnetic resonance imagining. Radiographics 1987; 7:371-83.
72. Blum L, Kressel HY, de Roos A et al. MR imaging differentiation of fibrosis versus recurrent colorectal carcinoma in the pelvis quantitative assessment. Radiology 1988; 169: 167.
73. Beets-Tan RGH, Beets GL, Vligen RFA et al. Accuracy of magnetic resonance imaging in prediction of tumour-free resection margin in rectal cancer surgery. Lancet 2001; 357:497-504.
74. Moffat FL, Vargas-Cuba RD, Serafini AN et al. Radioimmunodetection of colorectal carcinoma using technetium-99m-labeled Fab' fragments of IMMU-4 anti-carcinoembryonic antigen monoclonal antibody. Cancer 1994; 73:836-45.
75. Patt YZ, Podoloff DA, Curley S et al. Monoclonal antibody (MoAb) imaging in patients with colorectal cancer with rising serum CFA: experience with ZCE-025 and IMMU-4 MoAb and proposed directions for future clinical trials. Cancer 1993; 71: 4293-7.
76. Mascagni D, Corbellini L, Urciuoli P et al. Endoluminal ultrasound for early detection of local recurrence of rectal cancer. Br J Surg 1989; 76:1176-80.
77. Romano G, Esercizio L, Santangelo M et al. Impact of computed tomography vs. intrarectal ultrasound on the diagnosis, resecability and prognosis of locally recurrent rectal cancer. Dis Colon Rectum 1993; 36:261-5.0.
78. Moh CK, Schiepers C, Seltzer MA et al. PET in oncology: will it replace the other modalities? Semin Nucl Med 1997; 27:94-106.
79. Gupta N, Bradfield H. Role of positron emission tomography scanning in evaluating gastrointestinal neoplasms. Semin Nucl Med 1996; 26:65-73.
80. Phelps ME, Huang SC, Hoffman EJ et al. Tomographic measurements of local cerebral glucose metabolism in humans with (F-18)-2-fluoro-2-deoxy-D-glucose: validation of method. Ann Neurol 1979; 6:371-88.
81. Strauss LG, Conti PS. The application of PET in clinical oncology. J Nucl Med 1991; 32:623-48.
82. Staib L, Schirrmeister H, Reske SN et al. Is 18F-fluorodeoxyglucose positron emission tomography in recurrent colorectal cancer a contribution to surgical decision making? Am J Surg 2000; 180:1-5.
83. Ito M, Takashi K, Tadokoro M et al. Recurrent rectal cancer and scar: differentiation with PET and MR imaging. Radiology 1992; 182:549-52.
84. Tahara T, Ichiya Y, Kuwabara Y et al. High (18F)-fluorodeoxyglucose uptake in abdominal abscesses: a PET study. J Comput Assist Tomogr 1989; 13:829-31.

85. Holdeman KP, McIntosh DG, Smith ML et al. PET imaging of ovarian cancer prior to second look laparotomy. J Nucl Med 1994; 35:117.
86. Whiteford MH, Whiteford HM, Yee LF et al. Usefulness of FDG-PET scan in the assessment of suspected metastatic or recurrent adenocarcinoma of the colon and rectum. Dis Colon Rectum 2000; 53:759-70.
87. Johnson K, Bakhsh A, Young D et al. Correlating computed tomography and positron emission tomography scan with operative findings in metastatic colorectal cancer. Dis Colon Rectum 2001; 44:354-7.

5 Colorectal Cancer Screening and Surveillance

Introduction

Colorectal cancer is the most preventable neoplasm of the digestive organs and one of the most preventable of all [1]. This is mainly due to the existence of well-defined premalignant lesions – the adenomatous polyps – which take years to transform into carcinoma [2], thus allowing their early detection and removal through endoscopy [3]. Colorectal tumors occur extremely frequently in Western society, with crude incidence rates of the order of 40–70 new cases/100,000 inhabitants/year and a lifetime probability for an individual of developing this malignancy of 4%–6% [4, 5]. In other words, approximately 150,000 new colorectal cancer cases are diagnosed annually in the USA, and 30,000 in countries such as Italy or Britain [6]. There is evidence, however, that the survival of patients with colorectal cancer is gradually increasing [7], a result which can be attributed to many factors, including better screening procedures.

Although colorectal cancer screening is an old problem, which has been debated for years [8], the general impression is that we are moving from a long "incubation" phase of controlled and uncontrolled studies to the time in which we are called to apply this accumulated knowledge to the general population or at least to high-risk individuals [9]. Indeed, several medical societies – including the American Cancer Society – advocate screening for colorectal neoplasms [10], and an interdisciplinary panel of health care professionals came to the conclusion that all screening strategies were found to have a net benefit [11].

Screening for colorectal tumors involves the use of appropriate tests in order to identify individuals likely to have malignant or premalignant (adenomatous polyps) lesions in their bowel. At present, either lower endoscopy (colonoscopy and sigmoidoscopy) or fecal occult blood tests have been found to be effective in reducing the incidence and mortality of colorectal neoplasms and appear to be suitable tools for screening the general population [12]. Some persons, however, are at higher risk for colorectal cancer and may require a closer examination of the large bowel [13, 14]; this approach is referred to as *surveillance*.

Colorectal Cancer Screening in the General Population

Colorectal cancer screening is probably unwarranted in many Asian and African countries, where the disease is relatively rare, with incidence rates as low as 5 new cases/100,000 inhabitants/year [15, 16]. In Western society, the disease has the dimension of an epidemic, and "it is a cruel irony that billions of dollars are spent treating patients with colorectal cancer when the disease is almost entirely preventable" [17]. Moreover, there is evidence that colorectal cancer detected by screening is usually found at an earlier stage, and that patients in whom cancer is diagnosed at these stages have a more favorable outcome [18]. One more reason for promoting screening is that the main causes associated with an increased risk for colorectal malignancies are closely related to our diet and lifestyle [19], two factors that can hardly be modified in a society in which people are becoming progressively more wealthy, sedentary and overweight [20].

Despite the evidence, mass screening remains a difficult objective to achieve. Probably the guidelines on colorectal cancer are still imprecise or may appear redundant; for example, what should general physicians suggest to their patients? Search of fecal occult blood starting at age 45 for all individuals? Flexible sigmoidoscopy or, even better, colonoscopy for all their patients irrespective of their risk? And why not combine a Haemoccult test with endoscopy when approaching 50? A more scrupulous physician will attempt to stratify his/her patients according to different risk levels, in order to subject various subgroups to different screening procedures.

Patients may resist mass screening for colorectal neoplasia, probably because they do not feel like a "patient" but are invited to behave like one. Many individuals – at least in some countries – continue to adopt a "fatalistic attitude" towards diseases (especially cancer) and, in their irrational thinking, believe that certain diseases happen to others but not to themselves. In addition, dealing with feces or undergoing lower endoscopy is undoubtedly unpleasant, especially compared with measuring blood pressure or taking a blood sample for glucose or cholesterol levels. Selecting a high-risk group might have more success, but this is not always the case. In a recent study [21], 223 individuals were identified as at risk for hereditary colorectal cancer by their position in the family tree; of these, only 86 (38.6%) underwent colonoscopy, after recommendation by the interviewer. In a similar investigation [22], a higher compliance (63%) was obtained in a different population (Finnish), but once again the response rate was lower than expected.

Despite these limitations, evidence has been accumulated – in the last 10 years – indicating that mortality for colorectal neoplasms can be reduced through mass screening in the general population, using either a search for fecal occult blood or lower endoscopy (sigmoidoscopy or colonoscopy).

Role of Fecal Occult Blood Testing

The best investigated of several fecal occult blood test methods is the guaiac impregnated slide test, where the peroxidase activity of hemoglobin is the basis for a true positive result. Although the method is widely diffused, there are many important causes of false-positive and false-negative results [23]. The former occur more often from other, non-neoplastic sources of bleeding in the gastrointestinal tract (inflammation, diverticula, hemorrhoids, etc.) or from foods containing peroxidase-like activity. False-negative tests are due to intermittently bleeding or non-bleeding tumors. According to the most common tests, bleeding from the gastrointestinal tract must exceed physiological bleeding 5 to 10 times for a positive test [24]. New methods have been developed for detecting blood in the stools, such as tests based on the porphyrin-like moiety of hemoglobin or on the assay of human hemoglobin [25, 26]. Although these new tests may be more useful than the conventional guaiac assay, they have not yet been investigated in large-scale clinical trials, especially regarding their cost/benefit aspects [27].

Five case-control studies [28-32] and three randomized controlled trials [33-35] showed a reduction in the mortality for colorectal cancer by fecal occult blood test screening. In addition, a meta-analysis of six controlled Haemoccult screening studies found a net 16% reduction in mortality for colorectal malignancies [36]. Since screening may also detect large and bleeding adenomas – the natural precursor of carcinoma – this approach, if pursued for years, might also lead to a reduction in the colorectal cancer incidence rate. In one of these studies [33], 46,551 subjects between the ages of 50 and 80 years were invited to participate; individuals were followed for 13 years, and in this period nearly half of them (i.e. 46.2% of those screened annually and 59.7% of those screened biannually) completed the tests required by the protocol; on average, 6 samples were submitted for each patient. Almost 10% of samples were positive, and 80% of patients with positive tests underwent colonoscopy. In the screening group, cumulative mortality for colorectal cancer during this follow-up period was 5.88/1,000 for individuals screened annually versus 8.83/1,000 in the control group, which means a highly significant 33% reduction of mortality among screened subjects. Most of the lesions detected through screening were Dukes' A or B neoplasms, i.e. those associated with a more favorable clinical outcome, a factor which explains the lower mortality rate in the screened group.

Yet, despite the undoubted evidence of success, fecal occult blood tests have not gained widespread diffusion among the medical community, and there is some resistance – in most countries – to performing mass screening. Though the test is simple, safe, acceptable and relatively inexpensive, lack of accuracy remains the main problem. It has recently been shown that after 5-10 years, patients' compliance with the screening program falls to below 50%, and that too many patients leave the project long before its completion [23]. The high rate of false-positive tests leads many individuals to undergo colonoscopy which in many cases may appear unnecessary or redundant. Even more important, a false-negative test may induce a false sense of security in patients with colorectal lesions, which postpones the execution of more appropriate diagnostic procedures. In this respect, physicians play a crucial role in explaining to patients the advantages but also the many limitations of the test, that does exclude the presence of polyps or cancer, unlike colonoscopy, but may at most raise a suspicion, and that only in a minority of cases. Moreover, the test cannot be proposed to patients at major risk for colorectal cancer development – such as individuals with a strong family history of cancer or patients with inflammatory bowel diseases – in whom colonoscopic surveillance is mandatory [37].

In conclusion, despite the many supporters of fecal occult blood test screening – because of its efficacy in reducing colorectal cancer mortality [38] – many physicians remain skeptical and suggest different screening procedures.

Role of Sigmoidoscopy

Flexible sigmoidoscopy allows the visualization of the lower portions of the large bowel, i.e. rectum, sigmoid and descending colon. Owing to the limited value of the fecal occult blood test, this technique has been proposed as a mass-screening procedure for colorectal tumors. The American Cancer Society recommends periodic sigmoidoscopy beginning at the age of 50 years and repeated at 3- to 5-year intervals for screening of all average-risk subjects [39]; however, only 15%–30% of eligible persons undergo such testing [40].

Sigmoidoscopy has several advantages over a fecal occult blood test; being an endoscopic investigation, it allows direct visualization and removal of polypoid lesions, with specificity and sensitivity for the detection of distal tumors of the order of 95% or more [41]. The main benefits of sigmoidoscopy, in screening for colorectal tumors, are the detection and removal of non-malignant precursor lesions – thus preventing colorectal cancer development – and the detection of early lesions (Dukes' A and B), which are usually associated with a more favorable clinical outcome. Sigmoidoscopy, however, is an invasive technique which may be embarrassing for many patients, especially when their risk of cancer is relatively low. Moreover, flexible sigmoidoscopy does not provide information on lesions of the proximal colon, where more than 30% of colorectal tumors are localized, and with an increasing frequency [42]; indeed, some authors commented that sigmoidoscopy is "as clinically logic as performing mammography of one breast to screen women for breast cancer" [43] since it explores only a limited portion of the large bowel. Finally, one might argue that sigmoidoscopy actually produces frequent false-positive results when taking into account the very low malignant potential of small (less than 0.5 cm) and hyperplastic polyps [44].

Despite these limitations, two case-control studies showed that the risk of death from colorectal malignancies was reduced by 70%–80% for those individuals who had at least one sigmoidoscopic investigation within the previous 10 years compared with subjects who were not examined [45, 46]. In one of these studies, colorectal cancer developed in 8.8% of patients who reported undergoing at least one sigmoidoscopy (within the previous 10 years) versus 24.2% among individuals who were not investigated ($p < 0.0001$) [45]. In another investigation [47], 1,618 patients were followed up for 14 years (on average) after polypectomy by rigid sigmoidoscopy. For those individuals in whom polyps had completely been removed, the risk of subsequent colorectal cancer was nearly one-half that of the general population; the observed findings lend further support to the possible role of sigmoidoscopy in reducing the incidence and, presumably, mortality of colorectal neoplasms through the removal of precursor lesions. This contention has recently been confirmed by a prospective investigation in which endoscopic screening was able to reduce the incidence of colorectal cancer in a normal Norwegian population [47a].

Role of Colonoscopy and Barium Enema

Periodic examination of the whole colon by colonoscopy appears to be the most effective tool for mass screening for colorectal cancer. The best evidence supporting this approach comes from the National Polyp Study [48, 49]. The investigation included 1,418 patients who had undergone a colonoscopy at the beginning of the study; of these, 1,210 were followed with colonoscopies at regular intervals until the end of the study (average follow-up 5.9 years). At the time of enrolment, 494 patients (35%) had adenomas larger than 1 cm, and 137 (10%) had adenomatous lesions with high-grade dysplasia. Five completely asymptomatic colorectal malignancies (Dukes' A or B carcinoma) were detected at follow-up endoscopy in five different patients. The numbers of colorectal neoplasms expected on the basis of reference groups [50, 51] were 48.3, 43.4 and 20.7, corresponding to a reduction in the incidence of cancer of 76%–90%. The authors concluded that the incidence rates of colorectal malignancies can be significantly reduced by colonoscopic surveillance and polypectomy; this provides further evidence in favor of the adenoma-carcinoma sequence and supports the current practice of removing adenomatous lesions in the colon.

The main problems associated with colonoscopy screening are cost, discomfort for the patients and risk of major complications (such as bowel perforation), which are estimated at 2/1,000 procedures [52]. Moreover, colonoscopy is more difficult to learn and to perform than flexible sigmoidoscopy. For all these reasons, some authors consider colonoscopy unsuitable for general screening, but the investigation of choice for testing high-risk patients [53]. In a recent investigation, Sonnenberg et al. [54] compared the cost-effectiveness of fecal occult blood testing, sigmoidoscopy and colonoscopy; they concluded that colonoscopy represents a cost-effective means of screening for colorectal neoplasms, since it reduces mortality rates at relatively low incremental costs. Compared with colonoscopy, an annual Haemoccult test costs less but saves fewer life-years.

Single contrast barium enema is inadequate for detecting polyps, but the results improve remarkably with the double-contrast technique, the accuracy of which in screening for colorectal lesions larger than 1 cm is of the order of 90%–95% [55]. Colonoscopy is undoubtedly more sensitive for polyps smaller than 1 cm; moreover, the main limitation of barium enema remains the impossibility to carry out biopsies or polypectomy (Table 5.1).

Table 5.1. Colorectal cancer screening in the general population: options

Investigation	Frequency	Age (years)	Reference
Fecal occult blood test	Annual	50	[28–35]
Sigmoidoscopy	3–5 year interval	50	[39, 40]
Sigmoidoscopy	"Once only"	50	[45, 46, 47]
Colonoscopy	Every 5 years	45–60	[48, 49]

New Screening Procedures Based on Molecular Analysis

A novel approach to the early detection of colorectal neoplasms is the use of sensitive molecular methods based on polymerase chain reaction (PCR) and other modern technologies [56]. Thus, Sidranski and collaborators [57] showed that *k-ras* gene mutations could be detected in the colonoscopy effluent of patients with colorectal cancer, while with similar techniques other authors found p53 mutations in approximately 30% of these patients [58]. In fact, colorectal tumorigenesis is characterized by the accumulation of mutations in many cancer-related genes [59]; since cells from neoplastic tissues shed rapidly into the colonic lumen, these mutations can be detected in the cellular debris of feces. This concept represents the basis for a potentially more accurate colorectal cancer screening approach, which might overcome the many limitations of fecal occult blood testing. In a recent investigation [60], the stools from 40 individuals were examined for *k-ras*, p53 and APC genes: mutations were found in 16 of 21 patients with colorectal cancer (76%), and in 7 of 9 subjects with adenomas of various size (78%), but in none of the controls. Rather interestingly, the fecal occult blood tests were negative in all patients with adenomas. Although these techniques are exciting, and further refinement of the methods is under way, at present two main points should be taken into consideration. First, not all colorectal tumors, but only a fraction of them, show mutations in the above-mentioned genes, and in turn, these genes appear frequently mutated in non-neoplastic clinical conditions, such as ulcerative or Crohn's colitis [61]. Second, no study has so far demonstrated any reduction in the incidence or mortality of colorectal cancer with the use of these molecular screening procedures.

Screening in Individuals with Familial Colorectal Cancer

Together with breast neoplasms, colorectal cancer is probably the most "familial" of all human tumors. By recording an accurate family history of patients with colorectal malignancies, it is easy to see how these tumors tend to aggregate in families, affecting first- and second-degree relatives of the proband [19]. In most series, some 10%–20% of colorectal cancer patients show a more or less marked site-specific familiality [62–64]. In other words, first-degree relatives of patients with colorectal cancer have a 2–3-fold increased risk for site-specific malignancies compared with the general population [65]. Moreover, close relatives of individuals with adenomas have an increased risk of colon cancer [66], and first-degree relatives of patients with colon cancer tend to have an increased risk of adenomatous polyps compared with controls [67]. The number of affected relatives and the age of onset of the neoplasms are also related to the severity of risk. Thus, if two or more close relatives had colon cancer, the risk of these tumors for other family members is higher than if only one first-degree relative was affected; the risk is four times higher if the diagnosis of cancer in the first-degree relative was reached before the age of 45 [68].

Understanding the Nature of the Familial Risk

The nature of the commonly observed familial risk remains unknown; however, since no Mendelian pattern of inheritance may explain cancer aggregation in these families, the most likely explanation seems to be a multifactorial origin, which implicates a close interaction between genes and environmental factors. Familial colorectal malignancies pose a series of relevant problems. At variance with truly hereditary cases – which represent less than 5% of all patients [69] – familial cases are extremely more common, and their prevention or early detection might save thousand of lives, especially in Western countries, where these lesions are more frequent [19]. Moreover, the identification of familial cases can be difficult, owing to the poor attention frequently given to the family history and to the small size of most modern families. Finally, due to our limited knowledge, screening recommendations or appropriate guidelines for individuals with a familial risk of cancer are lacking or should be considered empirical.

A recent study, however, offered some clues towards a better understanding of familial colorectal cancer; indeed, a few genetic alterations have been described that seem to be implicated in this mild to moderate level of cancer predisposition. Laken et al. [70] reported a constitutional mutation in the APC gene (I1307 K) that does not alter the function of the encoded protein but generates an impermutable microsatellite (a short poly-A), thus causing an increased predisposition to cancer. Although this alteration was described in Ashkenazi Jews, it is likely that the mutation contributes to a large fraction of colorectal tumors also in other ethnic groups [71]. Similarly, mutations of the MSH6 gene (a DNA mismatch repair gene, implicated in the pathogenesis of HNPCC) have recently been detected in 7.1% of patients with a family history of colorectal cancer [72]. This suggests that mutations of the MSH6 gene could be responsible for a fraction of familial colorectal malignancies that occur at somewhat older ages and do not meet the clinical criteria usually employed for defining hereditary colorectal cancer [69].

In a recent editorial, R. L. White [73] proposed the new concept of "strongly" or "weakly" predisposing alleles. The former include APC mutations which lead to FAP, alterations of mutator genes (MSH2, MLH1, PMS1–2) that are responsible for HNPCC, or mutations of BRCA1 and 2 genes, associated with hereditary breast cancer. The I1307 K APC mutation and MSH6 alterations might be examples of weakly predisposing alleles, which might be much more common than the strongly predisposing mutations and may account for a relevant fraction of those cancers at present labeled as familial.

Screening Recommendations for Individuals with Familial Risk

Despite the lack of solid guidelines, the presence of a more or less marked family history of colorectal cancer suggests a more aggressive screening procedure than for the general population. In a recent editorial, R. W. Burt [74] reports the suggestions of a multidisciplinary panel of experts who recommended that individuals with close relatives affected by colorectal cancer should undergo the same screening procedures outlined for average risk, except that it should begin at the age of 40 years. This means annual fecal occult blood testing, sigmoidoscopy every 5 years, and colonoscopy or barium enema (as an option) every 5–10 years.

According to the American Cancer Society, pancolonoscopy should be recommended when colorectal cancer, or adenomatous polyps, are detected in a first-degree relative younger than 60 years, or when two or more first-degree relatives of any age are affected by colorectal cancer. The screening should begin at age 40, or 10 years before the youngest case within a given family, and should be repeated every 3–5 years [75].

Many endoscopists would favor the ample use of colonoscopy – with little or no emphasis on fecal occult blood tests or sigmoidoscopy – for individuals with a family history of colorectal cancer [62, 76].

Surveillance After Endoscopic Polypectomy

Some of the patients who have undergone removal of one or more colorectal adenomas are at increased risk for the development of subsequent benign or malignant lesions and may benefit from endoscopic surveillance [77]. Unfortunately, we do not know in which individuals polyps will recur and in which individuals polyps appear only once in their lifetime. Some clues can be inferred from polyp size and histology; thus, there are studies suggesting that persons with only a single small polyp detected at sigmoidoscopy have no increased subsequent risk of developing cancer when compared with the risk of the general population [78, 79]. Polyps with a diameter of 5 mm or less are defined as "diminutive" [80]. In a recent study, the large majority of these diminutive polyps were hyperplastic (37%) or adenomatous (41%), and only 0.26% of 1,964 resected and examined lesions showed severe dysplasia [81]. The available evidence suggests that small adenomas grow slowly – over the course of years – into large and dysplastic adenomas, and that large adenomas take 5–10 years to develop into infiltrating carcinoma [62, 82]. It follows that when accurate methods – such as colonoscopy – are available, surveillance does not have to be carried out frequently. Indeed, the main objective of surveillance is not just to find and resect small adenomas – the large majority of which will not progress to larger lesions – but to remove recurrent polyps before they grow to a clinically important size, when they are likely to undergo malignant changes.

Until a few years ago, surveillance was much more "aggressive", with annual colonoscopic investigations and removal of all lesions. The present approach is towards larger intervals and individualization of follow-up. At the initial endoscopy, the entire colon should be explored and cleaned of polyps. After removal of large (>1 cm), multiple, villous or dysplastic adenomas, the first surveillance colonoscopy should be carried out after 3 years [83]. For lesions smaller than 1 cm, that are tubular or hyperplastic and with mild or no dysplasia, most endoscopists would recommend surveillance, with sigmoidoscopy or colonoscopy after 3–5 years [84], while for others the follow-up surveillance should be individualized [77]. After normal results of one 3-year control, further surveillance should take into account the patients' age and anxiety, concomitant diseases, discomfort of endoscopy, and cost-benefit ratio. Surveillance should be discontinued when its benefits are no longer evident for a given patient.

The first evidence of success of endoscopic removal of polyps was found by Gilbertsen in 1974 [85]; after a 25-year study of periodic sigmoidoscopy and polyp resection in a group of more than 18,000 patients, the author was able to demonstrate a significant reduction in the expected number of infiltrating carcinomas. Although the investigation was criticized owing to the lack of a control group and the large fraction of patients lost to follow-up, it remains the first experimental evidence that periodic screening might lower the mortality rate for colorectal carcinoma. Further evidence favoring endoscopic polypectomy was obtained through the National Polyp Study [48, 49, 86]: individuals who underwent regular endoscopic controls at 3-year intervals showed a subsequent frequency of colorectal carcinoma which was only 10%–20% of that predicted for the control populations. However, since the follow-up was relatively short in this study, confirmatory investigations with longer follow-up times might be helpful.

Surveillance After Surgery for Colorectal Cancer

In 20%–30% of all cases, colorectal cancer is diagnosed at an advanced stage, with little or no possibility of radical intervention [87]. In most cases however (70%–80%), apparently curative surgery can be carried out (Dukes' A, B and C carcinoma), and in these patients the prospect of cure is much more favorable. Colorectal malignancies, however, tend to recur either at the site of previous surgery (local recurrence, especially for rectal cancer) or with a metastatic spread to the liver, lung and, more rarely, other organs. In addition, metachronous lesions in the remaining large bowel tracts are particularly frequent [88, 89].

The main objective of postoperative surveillance is to detect recurrent or metastatic disease as early as possible and to prevent the development of new infiltrating lesions in the large bowel. Although these purposes are sound, their scientific basis well-grounded, and the technological advancements available to implement this approach, there is no evidence that a close postoperative surveillance may reduce the mortality rate for colorectal neoplasms, simply because curative treatment for recurrent or metastatic disease is rarely possible [90]. Moreover, two recent studies showed the lack of consensus regarding the optimal strategy for cancer surveillance after surgery, as well as the enormous economic impact of such programs [91, 92].

Despite all of these uncertainties and the lack of controlled trials, most surgeons and oncologists recommend some sort of surveillance after curative resection for cancer of the large bowel. PET scanning is useful for an early detection of local recurrences [93, 94]. Abdominal ultrasound, liver enzymes and chest X-ray are recommended for the diagnosis of distant metastasis, especially in the liver and lungs [95]. Colonoscopy is usually carried out during the perioperative period to clear the colon of all resectable lesions and to exclude the presence of synchronous malignancies. Repeated colonoscopies are executed at various intervals after the resection, depending on the type of patient (and lesion) and the personal belief of the endoscopist; in many European centers, colonoscopy is performed at the 1-year follow-up and then repeated every 3–5 years [96]. It should be stressed that most recurrences (both local and distant) occur within the first 2 years after surgery and that surveillance should be concentrated during that time. In a recent study, Golandiuk et al. [97] evaluated the pattern of recurrence in a large series of patients who underwent curative resection for large-bowel cancer; the median time to recurrence for all patients was 16.7 months. Metachronous colorectal lesions may occur at any time, so colonoscopy screening should be continued for many years.

Surveillance in Patients with Inflammatory Bowel Disease

Patients with ulcerative colitis have an increased risk of colorectal cancer [98]. The incidence of cancer increases progressively with extension and duration of the disease and has been estimated to be of the order of 0.5% per year after 8–10 years of disease [77]. Cancer may develop from polyps or other visible lesions but, more frequently, it appears to originate in colonic epithelium that has undergone dysplastic changes. Dysplastic alterations may precede or be associated with carcinoma, and their identification during routine biopsies forms the basis of surveillance in these patients [99]. Morson et al. were the first, in the late 1960s [100], to draw attention to the predictive value of dysplasia in the large bowel; the introduction of colonoscopy, in the 1970s, had a profound effect on the management of these patients.

According to the most recent guidelines, all patients with ulcerative colitis should undergo colonoscopy at various intervals of time, to control the extent and activity of the disease [101]. At 8–10 years after the diagnosis of pancolitis, surveillance should become more frequent: the current recommendation is endoscopic controls at 1–2 year intervals. During colonoscopy, a full examination should be executed, with inspection of the entire mucosa (from rectum to caecum), and taking random biopsies at 10-cm intervals along the colon [102]. The endoscopist should examine with particular attention elevated mass-like lesions (Dysplasia Associated Lesions or Masses, DALM), since these areas are at particular risk of harboring dysplasia or carcinoma [103]. For the same reason, further biopsies should be taken from irregular plaques, polyps or pseudopolyps, unusual ulcers or strictures [101, 103, 104].

Despite the well-grounded scientific approach and the availability of appropriate techniques, evidence of the efficacy of surveillance in ulcerative colitis is still lacking. Various studies have shown that surveillance led to the detection of early-stage carcinoma in only a minority of patients, resulting in a high cost-to-benefit ratio; indeed, a significant number of screened individuals developed advanced lesions despite surveillance [105, 106]. This can be due to the long period of observation in order to demonstrate an effect on cancer stage and survival, to the frequent low compliance, and to the fact that not all patients are ready to accept colectomy with ileoanal anastomosis (one of the current surgical approaches) if severe dysplasia is detected in one or more lesions. Other studies favored surveillance [107, 108]. In the experience of Choi et al. [107], for instance, data of an 18-year surveillance program were collected prospectively, and carcinomas were detected at an early stage (Dukes' A and B) in 15 of 19 patients (79%).

The risk of carcinoma among patients affected by Crohn's colitis is, again, related to the extent and duration of active disease [109]. The relation between cancer risk and dysplasia has not been investigated in detail as for ulcerative colitis; consequently, no specific indications are available to guide practice [77]. Despite this lack of information, most endoscopists recommend periodic colonoscopic surveillance after 10 years of disease for patients with extensive colitis. Particular attention should be given to newly developed symptoms and to the occurrence of strictures that might be caused by infiltrating carcinomas.

To summarize, cancer surveillance in long-standing ulcerative colitis and Crohn's colitis was introduced without the evidence of controlled studies, and it remains of unproven value in terms of cost-effectiveness. However, coupling common sense with the available scientific evidence, most endoscopists recommend surveillance for these patients; this approach, at least in some studies, has led to a more frequent detection of early-stage lesions and to a significant improvement of survival [110].

Surveillance in Hereditary Cancer Syndromes

Among hereditary colorectal cancer syndromes, familial adenomatous polyposis (FAP) and hereditary non-polyposis colorectal cancer (HNPCC or Lynch syndrome) have been extensively investigated, especially recently, and will be discussed for the surveillance of high-risk individuals. Surveillance in other, rarer hereditary cancer syndromes – such as Turcot syndrome, Cowden disease, Peutz-Jeghers disease, juvenile familial polyposis, etc. [111] – follows, in general terms, the same guidelines as for FAP and HNPCC (see also chapter 12).

Although usually executed in specialized laboratories, genetic tests are now available for the diagnosis of FAP, HNPCC and other related polyposis syndromes [112, 113]. Genetic testing – commonly carried out using DNA from peripheral mononuclear cells – can be applied for two main purposes: (1) to test individuals at risk in a given family owing to their position in the genealogical tree; (2) to confirm the clinical diagnosis in a subject suspected of having FAP or HNPCC. In daily practice, an individual (the proband) with relevant symptoms and signs suggestive of an inherited syndrome is examined first. If a mutation in one of the genes associated with the disease is found, then other family members are tested; when the genetic test is negative in the proband, there is no reason to screen other family members, unless there is the suspicion of a phenocopy in the proband (i.e. a sporadic case occurring, by chance, in a familial setting). When a mutation is not found, this does not allow us to exclude the syndrome, since the available analytic techniques do not identify all relevant mutations and other genes can be implicated in the pathogenesis of the disease (especially for HNPCC). Genetic counseling – defined as the provision of genetic education coupled with psychosocial counseling [114] – is a fundamental part of genetic testing. Counseling should be provided by a clinician with a large experience of family cancer syndromes and should include education on the disease, recommendations on management and surveillance, details on the genetic nature of the syndrome, possible consequences of genetic testing, suggestions on diet and lifestyle, and informed consent.

Familial Adenomatous Polyposis

FAP arises from constitutional mutations of the APC gene (stands for adenomatous polyposis coli) and is inherited in an autosomal dominant fashion [115]. According to the Knudson hypothesis [116], when the corresponding normal allele is lost or mutated, the complete inactivation of APC is followed by the appearance of typical signs and symptoms. FAP is characterized by the presence of hundreds or thousands of polyps of various dimensions scattered in the colorectal tracts and usually appearing during adolescence; if the colon is not removed, colorectal carcinoma almost invariably develops by the age of 30–45 years [117]. Extracolonic manifestations are frequent and include gastric polyps, duodenal periampullary adenomas, desmoid tumors, osteomas. odontomas, epidermoid cysts, retinal spots and, more rarely, other lesions. Many of these changes correlate with location of mutations in the APC gene [118].

All individuals with clinical features of FAP and their first-degree relatives should be offered genetic counseling and genetic testing, beginning at the age of 10–14 years. APC gene mutations can be detected in 80%–90% of families with the present technology [119]; once the mutation is found in the index case, other family members can be studied, and surveillance can be directed to those who test positive for the mutation. These individuals should be examined with colonoscopy annually or biannually until adenomas appear; the optimal timing for colectomy depends on several factors (size, distribution and degree of dysplasia of polyps), but in most cases is between the ages of 16 and 20 years [117]. When a mutation is not found, then all family members at risk should undergo endoscopic screening. Upper endoscopy is also recommended for affected and high-risk individuals, at regular intervals of time, for the surveillance of premalignant gastric and especially duodenal lesions [120]. Though prospective controlled studies are lacking, there is evidence from cancer registries indicating that mortality from colorectal cancer can be reduced with an appropriate surveillance of FAP families [121].

Hereditary Non-polyposis Colorectal Cancer

HNPCC poses more problems than FAP, since there are no specific phenotypic manifestations of the disease, and the accurate examination of the family tree represents the basis for a proper diagnosis [122]. HNPCC is an autosomal dominant disease characterized by an early appearance of tumors (more often of the right colon), common occurrence of synchronous or metachronous neoplasms of the large bowel, and frequent association with malignancies of other organs, in particular endometrium, stomach, ovary and urogenital tract [123]. A large fraction (30%–70%) of HNPCC arises from inherited mutations in any of the several known mismatch repair genes, whose function is to maintain DNA integrity during cell replication. Two of these genes – hMSH2 and hMLH1 – account for more than 90% of the constitutional mutations detected in HNPCC families [124]. Inactivation of mismatch repair genes induces a certain type of DNA mutation – called replication errors – which accumulate throughout the genome of involved tumors. These alterations are most easily identified in short DNA segments called "microsatellites" (since many of them are outside the coding region of the genes) which consist of sequences of repeating DNA bases (mono-, di- or polynucleotides) [125]. In the presence of multiple microsatellite errors, the tumor exhibits the "microsatellite instability" (MSI) phenotype; as expected, almost all colorectal malignancies in HNPCC show the MSI phenotype, compared with only 10%–15% of sporadic tumors [126].

In approaching HNPCC surveillance, the first step is to design an accurate genealogical tree, extended to second- and third-degree relatives. Whenever two or three relatives on one side of the family have colorectal cancer (or HNPCC-related neoplasms) – especially when this is located in the right colon and develops before the age of 50 years – the syndrome should be taken into consideration. In families that satisfy the clinical criteria for HNPCC [124], MSI testing should be executed on colon cancer tissue (fresh or paraffin embedded) from one of the affected individuals. If the tumor is unstable (MSI), then the probability that the given family has HNPCC is much greater. The subsequent step is to perform genetic testing on constitutional DNA, in order to find mutations in one of the mismatch repair genes.

Those individuals in a HNPCC family who are positive for mutations need close colonoscopic surveillance at least every 2 years, starting at the age of 20–25 years or 5 years earlier than the youngest individual with cancer in the

Table 5.2. Colorectal cancer surveillance in individuals at risk: recommendations

Clinical condition	Investigation	Frequency	Age	Reference
Familial colorectal cancer	Colonoscopy	5–10 year intervals	40–45	[74, 77]
Endoscopic polypectomy	Colonoscopy	3 year intervals	After polypectomy	[84, 86]
Surgery for colorectal cancer	Colonoscopy	1, 3, 5 years	After surgery	[96, 97]
Inflammatory bowel disease	Colonoscopy	1–2 year intervals	After 10 years of disease	[101, 102]
Hereditary non-polyposis colorectal cancer (HNPCC)	Colonoscopy	2–3 year intervals	20–25 years	[122, 129, 130]
Familial adenomatous polyposis (FAP)	Colonoscopy	1–2 year intervals	14–16 years	[117, 119, 120]

family [122]. Owing to the frequency of endometrial carcinoma, pelvic evaluation (gynecological examination and ultrasound) beginning at 18 years of age is recommended for women. The same approach (colonoscopic surveillance) is also indicated: (1) in families with a strong clinical suspicion of HNPCC (on the basis of clinical findings) but who do not fulfil the standard criteria for HNPCC [127]; (2) in HNPCC – or suspected HNPCC [128] – families who do not show positive results on genetic tests. A surveillance strategy in HNPCC families showed some efficacy in reducing the burden of colorectal cancer. In a large series of HNPCC families, Jarvinen et al. [129] reported the occurrence of fewer colorectal malignancies and fewer cancer-related deaths among HNPCC family members who accepted endoscopic screening every 3 years compared with those who declined this surveillance program. The same authors [130] reassessed their families after completion of a 15-year follow-up and confirmed the excellent results of surveillance: colorectal cancer developed in 8 screened subjects (6%) compared with 19 control subjects (16%, $p < 0.014$; a reduction in cancer rate of 62%). Moreover, all colorectal malignancies in the study group were localized (Dukes' A or B), causing no deaths, compared with 9 cancer-related deaths among controls (Table 5.2).

Conclusion: Media, Society and Colorectal Cancer Screening

As we entered the last decade of the twentieth century, the benefits of colorectal cancer screening were uncertain. The key questions were: can screening the general population reduce colorectal cancer mortality? Can society afford the cost of screening programs? Entering the new millennium, the available literature and the results of many controlled studies seem to suggest that screening asymptomatic individuals can lower the incidence and mortality of colorectal malignancies [131], and that the cost of screening per added years of life does not exceed that of other well-accepted prevention programs, as in the case of hypertension or coronary artery disease [132]. We might, of course, discuss whether a fecal occult blood test is more convenient or feasible when compared with other procedures, such as sigmoidoscopy or colonoscopy; but there is no doubt that the currently available techniques might all be effective in reducing the incidence and mortality of colorectal cancer if applied in large-scale projects. In a recent study, Slusser et al. [133] evaluated the efficacy of a television-advertised screening program for colorectal cancer using a fecal occult blood test. The results showed that this approach was effective in recruiting a large number of participants; moreover, patients diagnosed with colorectal cancer through the television program tended to have early stage disease and improved 5-year survival.

March 2000 was called the "Month of Colorectal Cancer Awareness" by some American cancer foundations [74]. On that occasion, President Clinton gave a speech strongly in favor of colorectal cancer screening, as shown in this sentence: "I encourage health care providers, advocacy groups, policymakers, and concerned citizens across the country to help raise public awareness of the risk and methods of colorectal cancer, and to use the power of our knowledge to defeat this silent disease...".

With these auspices, and this high patronage, the forthcoming century appears more than promising in this field of research.

References

1. Rosen L, Abel ME, Gordon PH et al. The American Society of Colon and Rectal Surgeons Standards Task Force. Practice parameters for the detection of colorectal neoplasms – supporting documentation. Dis Colon Rectum 1992; 35:391–4.
2. Hardy RG, Meltzer SJ, Jankowski JA. ABC of colorectal cancer. Molecular basis for risk factors. BMJ 2000; 321:886–9.
3. Reinus JF. Guidelines for clinical practice. Dig Dis Sci 1994; 39:2282–4.
4. Johansen C, Mellemgaard A, Skov T et al. Colorectal cancer in Denmark 1943–1988. Int J Colorect Dis 1993; 8:42–7.
5. Troisi RJ, Freedman AW, Devesa SS. Incidence of colorectal carcinoma in the U.S. An update of trends by gender, race, age, subsite, and stage, 1975–1994. Cancer 1999; 85: 1670–6.
6. Franceschi S, Levi F, La Vecchia C et al. Comparison of cancer mortality trends in major European areas, 1960–89. Eur J Cancer Prev 1994; 3:145–206.
7. Gatta G, Faivre J, Capocaccia R et al. Survival of colorectal cancer patients in Europe during the period 1978–89. Eur J Cancer 1998; 34:2176–83.
8. Chamberlain J. Is screening for colorectal cancer worthwhile? Br J Cancer 1990; 62: 1–3.
9. Bhattacharya I, Sack EM. Screening colonoscopy: the cost of common sense. Lancet 1996; 347:1744–5.
10. Simmang CL, Senatore P. Practice parameters for detection of colorectal neoplasms. Dis Colon Rectum 1999; 42:1123–9.
11. Winawer SJ, Fletcher RH, Miller L et al. Colorectal cancer screening: clinical guidelines and rationale. Gastroenterology 1997; 112:594–642.

12. Toribara NW, Sleisenger MH. Screening for colorectal cancer. N Engl J Med 1995; 332: 861-7.
13. Lynch HT, Smyrk T. Hereditary Nonpolyposis Colorectal Cancer (Lynch syndrome). An updated review. Cancer 1996; 78:1149-67.
14. Lynch HT, Tinley ST, Lynch J et al. Familial Adenomatous Polyposis. Discovery of a family and its management in a cancer genetics clinic. Cancer 1997; 80: 6154-20.
15. Naaeder SB, Archampong EQ. Cancer of the colon and rectum in Ghana: a 5-year prospective study. Br J Surg 1994; 81:456-9.
16. Al-Jaberi TM, Ammari F, Gharieybeh K et al. Colorectal adenocarcinoma in defined Jordanian population from 1990 to 1995. Dis Colon Rectum 1997; 49:1089-94.
17. Kronborg O. Screening for early colorectal cancer. World J Surg 2000; 24:1069-74.
18. Weinberg DS, Strom BL. Screening for colon cancer: a review of current and future strategies. Semin Oncol 1995; 22:433-47.
19. Ponz de Leon M, Roncucci L. The cause of colorectal cancer. Digest Liver Dis 2000; 32: 426-39.
20. Hu FB, Stampfer MJ, Manson JE et al. Trends in the incidence of coronary heart disease and changes in diet and lifestyle in women. N Engl J Med 2000; 343:530-7.
21. Ponz de Leon M, Della Casa G, Benatti P et al. Frequency and type of colorectal tumors in asymptomatic high-risk individuals in families with Hereditary Nonpolyposis Colorectal Cancer. Cancer Epidemiol Biomarkers Prev 1998; 7:639-41.
22. Järvinen HJ, Mecklin JP, Sistonen P. Screening reduces colorectal cancer rate in families with hereditary nonpolyposis colorectal cancer. Gastroenterology 1995; 108: 1405-11.
23. Delcò F, Sonnenberg A. Limitations of the faecal occult blood test in screening for colorectal cancer. Ital J Gastroenterol Hepatol 1999; 31:119-26.
24. Gnauck R, Macrae FA, Fleisher M. How to perform the fecal occult blood test. CA Cancer J Clin 1984; 34:134-47.
25. Ahlquist DA, McGill DB, Schwartz S. Fecal blood levels in health and disease: a study using Hemoquant. N Engl J Med 1985; 312:1422-8.
26. St John DJB, Young GP, Alexeyeff M. Most large and medium colorectal adenomas can be detected by immunochemical occult blood tests. Gastroenterology 1990; 98: 312 A.
27. Allison JE, Tekawa IS, Ransom LJ et al. A comparison of fecal occult-blood tests for colorectal-cancer screening. N Engl J Med 1996; 334:155-9.
28. Selby JV, Friedman GD, Quesenberry CP et al. Effect of fecal occult blood testing on mortality from colorectal cancer; a case-control study. Ann Intern Med 1993; 118: 1294-7.
29. Saito H, Soma Y, Koeda J et al. Reduction in risk of mortality from colorectal cancer by fecal occult blood. Int J Cancer 1995; 61:465-9.
30. Wahrendorf J, Robra BP, Wiebelt H et al. Effectiveness of colorectal cancer screening: results from a population-based case-control evaluation in Saarland, Germany. Eur J Cancer Prev 1993; 2:221-7.
31. Lazovich DA, Weiss NS, Stevens NG et al. A case-control study to evaluate efficacy of screening faecal occult blood. J Med Screen 1995; 2:84-9.
32. Zappa M, Castiglione G, Grazzini G et al. Effect of faecal occult blood testing on colorectal cancer mortality: results of a population-based case-control study in the district of Florence, Italy. Int J Cancer 1997; 73:208-10.
33. Mandel JS, Bond JH, Church TR et al. Reducing mortality from colorectal cancer by screening for fecal occult blood. N Engl J Med 1993; 328:1365-71.
34. Hardcastle JD, Chamberlain JO, Robinson MHE et al. Randomised controlled trial of faecal occult blood screening for colorectal cancer. Lancet 1996; 348:1472-7.
35. Kronborg O, Fenger C, Olsen J et al. Randomised study of screening for colorectal cancer with faecal-occult-blood test, Haemoccult. Lancet 1996; 348:1467-71.

36. Towler B, Irwing L, Glasziou P et al. A systematic review of the effects of screening for colorectal cancer using the faecal occult blood test, Haemoccult. BMJ 1998; 317: 559–65.
37. Syngal S, Weeks JC, Schrag D et al. Benefits of colonoscopic surveillance and prophylactic colectomy in patients with Hereditary Nonpolyposis Colorectal Cancer mutations. Ann Intern Med 1998; 129:787–96.
38. Faivre J, Tazi MA, El-Mrini T et al. Faecal occult blood screening and reduction of colorectal cancer mortality: a case-control study. Br J Cancer 1999; 79:680–3.
39. Lieberman D. Endoscopic colon screening: is less more? Gastroenterology 1996; 111: 1385–9.
40. Woo B, Cook EF, Weisberg M et al. Screening procedures in the asymptomatic adult. Comparison of physicians' recommendations, patients' desires, published guidelines and actual practice. JAMA 1985; 254:1480–4.
41. Williams CB, Macrae FA, Bartram CI. A prospective study of diagnostic methods in adenoma follow-up. Endoscopy 1982; 14:74–8.
42. Beart RW, Melton J, Maruta M et al. Trends in right and left-sided colon cancer. Dis Colon Rectum 1983; 26:393–8.
43. Podolsky DK. Going the distance – The case for true colorectal cancer screening. N Engl J Med 2000; 343:207–8.
44. Ponz de Leon M, Di Gregorio C. Pathology of colorectal cancer. Dig Liver Dis 2000 2001; 33:372–88.
45. Selby JV, Friedman GD, Quesenberry Jr. CP et al. A case-control study of screening sigmoidoscopy and mortality from colorectal cancer. N Engl J Med 1992; 326: 653–7.
46. Newcomb PA, Norfleet RG, Storer BE et al. Screening sigmoidoscopy and colorectal cancer mortality. J Natl Cancer Inst 1992; 84:1572–5.
47. Atkin WS, Morson BC, Cuzick J. Long-term risk of colorectal cancer after excision of rectosigmoid adenomas. N Engl J Med 1992; 326:658–62.
47a. Thiis-Evensen E, Hoff GS, Sauar F et al. Population-based surveillance by colonoscopy; effect on the incidence of colorectal cancer. Scan J Gastroenterol 1999; 34:414–20.
48. Winawer SJ, Zauber AG, Ho MN et al. Prevention of colorectal cancer by colonoscopic polypectomy. N Engl J Med 1993; 329:1977–81.
49. Winawer SJ, Zauber AG, Ho MN et al. Randomized comparison of surveillance intervals after colonoscopic removal of newly diagnosed adenomatous polyps. N Engl J Med 1993; 328:901–6.
50. O'Brien MJ, Winawer SJ, Zauber AG et al. The National Polyp Study: patient and polyp characteristics associated with high-grade dysplasia in colorectal adenomas. Gastroenterology 1990; 98:371–9.
51. Gloeckler-Ries LA, Cuzick J. Long-term risk of colorectal cancer after excision of rectosigmoid adenomas. N Engl J Med 1992; 326:658–62.
52. Rankin GB. Indications, contraindications and complications of colonoscopy, in Sivak MV Jr. (ed): "Gastrointestinal Endoscopy". Philadelphia, PA, Saunders, 1997, pp 873–8.
53. Scholefield JH. ABC of colorectal cancer. Screening. BMJ 2000; 321:1004–6.
54. Sonnenberg A, Delcò F, Inadomi JM. Cost-effectiveness of colonoscopy in screening for colorectal cancer. Ann Int Med 2000; 133:573–84.
55. Fork FT. Reliability of routine double contrast examination of the large bowel: a prospective study of 2,590 patients. Gut 1983; 24:672–7.
56. Hecht JR. Genetics, epidemiology, prevention, and early detection of colorectal cancer. Curr Opin Gastroenterol 1997; 13:5–10.
57. Sidransky D, Tokino T, Hamilton SR et al. Identification of ras oncogene mutations in the stool of patients with curable colorectal tumors. Science 1992; 256:102–4.
58. Villa E. Molecular screening: why haven't we started yet? Am J Gastroenterol 1997; 92: 2144–6.

59. Ponz de Leon M, Percesepe A. Pathogenesis of colorectal cancer. Dig Liver Dis 2000; 32:807-21.
60. Ahlquist DA, Harrington JJ, Shuber AP. Detection of altered DNA in stool: feasibility for colorectal neoplasia screening. (Abstr.) Gastroenterology 1999; 116:A369.
61. Lyda MH, Noffsinger A, Belli J et al. Multifocal neoplasia involving the colon and appendix in ulcerative colitis: pathological and molecular features. Gastroenterology 1998; 115:1566-73.
62. Ponz de Leon M, Antonioli A, Ascari A et al. Incidence and familial occurrence of colorectal cancer and polyps in a health-care district of Northern Italy. Cancer 1987; 62: 2848-59.
63. Duncan JL, Kyle J. Family incidence of carcinoma of the colon and rectum in north-east Scotland. Gut 1982; 23:169-71.
64. Maire P, Morichau-Beauchant M, Drucker J et al. Familial occurrence of cancer of the colon and rectum: results of a 3-year survey. Gastroenterol Clin Biol 1984; 8: 22-7.
65. Ponz de Leon M, Sassatelli R, Sacchetti C et al. Familial aggregation of tumors in the three-year experience of a population-based colorectal cancer registry. Cancer Res 1989; 49:4344-8.
66. Bonelli L, Martines S, Conio M et al. Family history of colorectal cancer as a risk factor for benign and malignant tumours of the large bowel. A case-control study. Int J Cancer 1988; 41:513-7.
67. Cannon-Albright LA, Skolnick MH, Bishop DT et al. Common inheritance of susceptibility to colonic adenomatous polyps and associated colorectal cancers. N Engl J Med 1988; 319:533-7.
68. St John JB, McDermott FT, Hopper JL et al. Cancer risk in relatives of patients with common colorectal cancer. Ann Intern Med 1993; 118:785-90.
69. Giardiello FM, Brensinger JD, Petersen GM. AGA technical review on Hereditary Colorectal Cancer and Genetic Testing. Gastroenterology 2001; 121:198-213.
70. Laken SJ, Petersen GM, Gruber SB et al. Familial colorectal cancer in Ashkenazim due to a hypermutable tract in APC. Nature Genet 1997; 17:79-83.
71. Lothe RA, Hektoen M, Johnsen H et al. The APC gene I1307 K variant is rare in Norwegian patients with familial and sporadic colorectal or breast cancer. Cancer Res 1998; 58:2923-4.
72. Kolodner RD, Tytell JD, Schmeits JL et al. Germ-line MSH6 mutations in colorectal cancer families. Cancer Res 1999; 59:5068-74.
73. White RL. Excess risk of colon cancer associated with a polymorphism of the APC gene? Cancer Res 1998; 58:4038-9.
74. Burt RW. Colon cancer screening. Gastroenterology 2000; 119:837-53.
75. Winawer SJ, Fletcher RH, Miller L et al. Colorectal cancer screening clinical guidelines and rationale. Gastroenterology 1997; 112:594-42.
76. Pariente A, Milan C, Lafon J et al. Colonoscopic screening in first-degree relatives of patients with "Sporadic" colorectal cancer: a case-control study. Gastroenterology 1998; 115:7-12.
77. Bond JH. Colorectal surveillance for neoplasia: an overview. Gastrointest Endosc 1999; 49:S35-S40.
78. Spencer RJ, Melton LJ III, Ready RL et al. Treatment of small colorectal polyps: a population-based study of risk of subsequent carcinoma. Mayo Clin Proc 1984; 59:305-10.
79. Atkin WS, Morson BC, Cuzick J. Long-term risk of colorectal cancer after excision of rectosigmoid adenomas. N Engl J Med 1992; 326:658-62.
80. Kim EC, Lance P. Colorectal polyps and their relationship to cancer. Gastroenterol Clin North Am 1997; 26:1-17.
81. Weston AP, Campbell DR. Diminuitive colonic polyps: histopathology, spatial distribution, concomitant significant lesions and treatment complications. Am J Gastroenterol 1995; 90:24-8.

82. Stryker SJ, Wolff BG, Culp CE et al. Natural history of untreated colonic polyps. Gastroenterology 1987; 93:1009-13.
83. Winawer SJ, Zauber AG, O'Brien MJ et al. Randomized comparison of surveillance intervals after colonoscopic removal of newly diagnosed adenomatous polyps. N Engl J Med 1993; 328:901-6.
84. Pennazio M, Arrigoni A, Risio M et al. Small rectosigmoid polyps as markers of proximal neoplasm. Dis Colon Rectum 1993; 36:1121-5.
85. Gilbertsen CA. Proctosigmoidoscopy, polypectomy and rectal cancer. Cancer 1974; 34:936-9.
86. Winawer SJ, Stewart ET, Zauber AG et al. A comparison of colonoscopy and double-contrast barium enema for surveillance after polypectomy. N Engl J Med 2000; 342: 1766-72.
87. Ponz de Leon M, Sassatelli R, Scalmati A et al. Descriptive epidemiology of colorectal cancer in Italy: the 6-year experience of a specialized registry. Eur J Cancer 1993; 29: 367-71.
88. Fante R, Roncucci L, Di Gregorio C et al. Frequency and clinical features of multiple tumors of the large bowel in the general population and in patients with hereditary colorectal carcinoma. Cancer 1996; 77:2013-21.
89. Fajobi O, Yiu CY, Sen-Gupta SB et al. Metachronous colorectal cancers. Br J Surg 1998; 85:897-901.
90. Schoemaker D, Black R, Giles L et al. Annual colonoscopy, chest radiography, and computed tomography of the liver did not prolong survival in patients with colorectal cancer. Gastroenterology 1998; 114:7-14.
91. Edelman MJ, Meyers FJ, Siegel D. The utility of follow up testing after curative cancer therapy. J Gen Intern Med 1997; 12:318-31.
92. Virgo KS, Vernava AM, Longo WE et al. Cost of patient follow up after potentially curative colorectal cancer treatment. JAMA 1995; 273:1837-41.
93. The Standard Task Force of the American Society of Colon and Rectal Surgeons. Practice parameters for the detection of colorectal neoplasms. Dis Colon Rectum 1992; 35: 389-94.
94. Lamki LM. Positron Emission Tomography in oncology. Cancer 1996; 78:2039-42.
95. Bruinvels DJ, Stiggelbout AM, Kievit J et al. Follow up of patients with colorectal cancer: a meta-analysis. Ann Surg 1994; 219:174-82.
96. Kjeldsen BJ, Kronborg O, Fenger C et al. A prospective randomized study of follow-up after radical surgery for colorectal cancer. Br J Surg 1997; 84:666-9.
97. Galandiuk S, Wieand HS, Moertel CG et al. Patterns of recurrence after curative resection of carcinoma of the colon and rectum. Surg Gynecol Obstet. 1992; 174:27-32.
98. Levin B. Colorectal cancer screening. Cancer 1993; 72(Suppl): 1056-60.
99. Lennard-Jones JE. Prevention of cancer mortality in inflammatory bowel disease. In: Young C, Rozen P, Levin B, editors. "Prevention and early detection of colorectal cancer." WB Saunders, Philadelphia, 1996; 217-38.
100. Morson BC, Pang LSC. Rectal biopsy as an aid to cancer control in ulcerative colitis. Gut 1967; 8:423-34.
101. Brostrom O, Lofberg E, Ost A et al. Cancer surveillance of patients with long standing ulcerative colitis: a clinical, endoscopical and histological study. Gut 1986; 27:1408-13.
102. Riddell RH. Screening strategies in gastrointestinal cancer. Scand J Gastroenterol 1990; 175(suppl):177-84.
103. Blackstone MO, Riddell RH, Rogers G et al. Dysplasia-associated lesion or moss (DALM) detected by colonoscopy in long-standing ulcerative colitis: an indication for colectomy. Gastroenterology 1981; 80:366-74.
104. Eaden JA, Mayberry JF. Colorectal cancer complicating ulcerative colitis: a review. Am J Gastroenterol 2000; 95:2710-9.
105. Lofberg R, Brostrom O, Karlen P et al. Colonoscopic surveillance in long-standing total ulcerative colitis - A 15 year follow-up study. Gastroenterology 1990; 99:1021-31.

106. Collins RH, Feldman M, Fordtran JS. Colon cancer, dysplasia and surveillance in patients with ulcerative colitis: a critical review. N Engl J Med 1987; 316:1654-8.
107. Choi PM, Nugent FW, Schoetz Dj et al. Colonoscopic surveillance reduces mortality from colorectal cancer in ulcerative colitis. Gastroenterology 1993; 105:418-24.
108. Lashner BA, Kane SV, Hanauer SB. Colon cancer surveillance in chronic ulcerative colitis: historical cohort study. Am J Gastroenterol 1990; 85:1083-7.
109. Ekbom A, Helmick C, Zack M et al. Ulcerative colitis and colorectal cancer. N Engl J Med 1990; 323:1228-33.
110. Giardiello FM, Bayless TM. Colorectal cancer and ulcerative colitis. Radiology 1996; 199:28-30.
111. Giardiello FM, Offerhaus JGA. Phenotype and cancer risk of various polyposis syndromes. Eur J Cancer 1995; 31 A:1085-7.
112. Chung DC, Rustgi AK. DNA mismatch repair and cancer. Gastroenterology 1995; 109:1685-99.
113. Ficari F, Cama A, Valanzano R et al. APC gene mutations and colorectal adenomatosis in familial adenomatous polyposis. Br J Cancer 2000; 82:348-53.
114. Kessler S. Psychological aspects of genetic counseling. IX. Teaching and counseling. J Genet Counsel 1997; 6:287-95.
115. Guillem JG, Smith AJ, Culle J et al. Gastrointestinal polyposis syndromes. Curr Prob Surg 1999; 36:219-323.
116. Knudson Jr AG. Hereditary cancer, oncogenes, and antioncogenes. Cancer Res 1985; 45:1437-43.
117. Ponz de Leon M, Benatti P, Percesepe A et al. Clinical features and genotype phenotype correlations in 41 Italian families with Adenomatosis Coli. Ital J Gastroenterol Hepatol 1999; 31:850-60.
118. Gebert JF, Dupon C, Kadmon M et al. Combined molecular and clinical approaches for the identification of families with Familial Adenomatous Polyposis Coli. Ann Surg 1999; 229:350-61.
119. Laken SJ, Papadopoulos N, Petersen GM et al. Analysis of masked mutations in familial adenomatous polyposis. Proc Natl Acad Sci 1999; 96:2322-6.
120. Wallace MH, Phillips RKS. Upper gastrointestinal disease in patients with familial adenomatous polyposis. Br J Surg 1998; 85:742-50.
121. Berk T, Stern HS. Screening, management, and surveillance for families with familial adenomatous polyposis. Gastroenterol Clin N Am 1993; 3:725-36.
122. Marra G, Boland CR. Hereditary Nonpolyposis Colorectal Cancer: the syndrome, the genes and historical perspectives. J Natl Cancer Inst. 1995; 87:1114-25.
123. Evans DGR, Walsh S, Jeancock J et al. Incidence of hereditary non-polyposis colorectal cancer in a population-based study of 1137 consecutive cases of colorectal cancer. Br J Surg 1997; 84:1281-5.
124. Peltomaki P, Vasen HFA, the International Collaborative Group on Hereditary Nonpolyposis Colorectal Cancer. Mutations predisposing to Hereditary Nonpolyposis Colorectal Cancer: database and results of a collaborative study. Gastroenterology 1997; 113:1146-58.
125. Frayling JM. Microsatellite instability. Gut 1999; 45:1-4.
126. Konishi M, Kikuchi-Yanoshita R, Tanaka K et al. Molecular nature of colon tumors in Hereditary Nonpolyposis Colon Cancer, familial polyposis, and sporadic colon cancer. Gastroenterology 1996; 111:307-17.
127. Vasen HFA, Watson P, Mecklin J-P et al. New clinical criteria for Hereditary Nonpolyposis Colorectal Cancer (HNPCC, Lynch syndrome) proposed by the International Collaborative Group on HNPCC. Gastroenterology 1999; 116:1453-6.
128. Park JG, Vasen HFA, Park KJ et al. Suspected Hereditary Nonpolyposis Colorectal Cancer. International Collaborative Group on Hereditary Nonpolyposis Colorectal Cancer (ICG-HNPCC) criteria and results of genetic diagnosis. Dis Colon Rectum 1999; 42:710-6.

129. Jarvinen HJ, Mecklin JP, Sistonen P. Screening reduces colorectal cancer rate in families with hereditary nonpolyposis colorectal cancer. Gastroenterology 1995; 108:1401–5.
130. Järvinen HJ, Aarnio M, Mustonen H et al. Controlled 15-year trial on screening for colorectal cancer in families with Hereditary Nonpolyposis Colorectal Cancer. Gastroenterology 2000; 118:829–34.
131. Mandel JS, Church TR, Bond JH et al. The effect of fecal occult-blood screening on the incidence of colorectal cancer. N Engl J Med 2000; 343:1603–7.
132. Lieberman D, Sleisenger MH. Is it time to recommend screening for colorectal cancer? Lancet 1996; 348:1463–4.
133. Slusser SO, Liberski SM, McGarrity TJ. Survival of patients diagnosed with colorectal cancer through a television-advertised screening program. Am J Gastroenterol 1996; 91:1563–6.

6 Prevention and Chemoprevention of Colorectal Neoplasms

Introduction

It is almost a paradigm in the medical community to state that "Prevention is better than cure". This has been proven in cardiovascular diseases [1] and in many metabolic conditions [2], and it is expected to be true for many neoplasms, especially those closely related to strong environmental causative agents, such as lung and liver tumors [3, 4]. However, we should not forget that for most human malignancies there are several factors which contribute to cancer development, and that it is often difficult, if not impossible, to find a single causative agent fully responsible for the disease.

When considering colorectal tumors, it is widely accepted that they develop due to a close interaction between genetic factors, environmental agents and precancerous lesions [5]. Genetic factors are well defined only in certain inherited conditions, such as familial adenomatous polyposis (FAP) or hereditary non-polyposis colorectal cancer (HNPCC or Lynch syndrome) [6, 7], but remain elusive in the large majority of colorectal malignancies; in addition, there is no chance of intervention – at least at present – for modifying our genetic background. Environmental factors are even more elusive, and the many case-control or cohort studies have only contributed to render the issue complex and controversial, especially when considering dietary factors [8, 9]. The adenoma-carcinoma sequence [10] is a mainstay in colorectal tumorigenesis; for this reason, most of the efforts in colorectal cancer prevention involve the removal of polyps [11]. This approach, however, requires colonoscopy and can hardly be proposed to the general population.

A new alternative strategy is chemoprevention, which can be defined as the use of natural or synthetic compounds in order to block, reverse or prevent the development of cancer [12]. Although the approach can be considered still in its infancy, various human and animal investigations suggest that certain compounds can prevent colorectal cancer progression [13]. Chemoprevention seems particularly attractive in some high-risk groups, such as mutation carriers in FAP or HNPCC families [14] or patients with long-standing inflammatory bowel diseases.

The main purpose of the present chapter is to critically analyze the ways by which we can try to prevent the development of colorectal malignancies. As recently pointed out [15], the term "prevention" should be used when there is evidence of complete protection from cancer; for colorectal (as well as breast and many other) malignancies, "risk reduction" is undoubtedly more appropriate for describing the objectives of the available interventions. For the purpose of the present chapter, however, the two terms will be used with the same meaning. Moreover, primary prevention will refer to the removal or inhibition of exogenous risk factors (such as diet and lifestyle), while secondary prevention will refer to interventions on premalignant lesions (i.e. removal of adenomatous polyps).

Can We Prevent Colorectal Cancer with an Appropriate Diet?

The answer to this question is not simple. Various dietary factors, including excess calories, high meat consumption, high saturated fat content, and a low intake of bran, fruit, vegetables, calcium, selenium and several vitamins have been implicated in the pathogenesis of colorectal cancer [8, 9]. Animal studies have been instructive and consistent in indicating that dietary factors can influence all stages of colorectal tumorigenesis, from crypt cell replication to aberrant crypt and adenoma formation, and eventually to malignant changes [16, 17]. Thus, low-fat and caloric-restricted diets in rats are associated with a reduced rate of chemically induced colorectal tumors [18]. Moreover, migrant studies showed that when individuals born in countries with a low incidence of colorectal cancer (and used to a low consumption of meat and animal fat) move to Western countries, where the consumption of these products is much higher, they acquire an increased risk for these tumors [19]. Finally, several case-control studies have suggested that among the individual dietary components, the consumption of red meat and of saturated fat seems to be related to an increased risk for colorectal cancer [20]. Similarly, there is a general consensus that diets rich in fruit and vegetables protect against colorectal cancer; this effect can be attributed either to their content of fiber or to the presence of various micronutrients [21, 22].

Despite the many investigations, the role of the main dietary components in colorectal cancer development remains ill-defined. Thus, in a recent analysis of 19 controlled studies, J.D. Potter concluded that the evidence that saturated fat and meat could be related to the risk of the disease was not entirely convincing [8]. Similarly, some epidemiologic studies supported the hypothesis that fiber can protect against colorectal cancer [23, 24], while others did not [25]. In a recent prospective investigation involving 2,079 individuals followed for approximately 4 years, a diet low in fat and rich in fiber, fruit and vegetables did not influence the risk of recurrent adenomas of the large bowel [26]. Similar inconsistent results were reported for calcium [27, 28], several antioxidant vitamins (carotene, vitamins A, E and C) [29, 30], selenium and folate [31].

Thus, can colorectal cancer be prevented by a more appropriate diet? The available evidence does not suggest that changes in the diet might have a great impact on colorectal cancer prevention, for two main reasons. First, the scientific evidence linking an improvement of our diet to a reduced risk of colorectal cancer is poor despite the numerous studies carried out over the last 20 years; in the absence of definite proof, it is difficult to propose rigid guidelines to average-risk individuals, despite the benefits that these changes might have for cardiovascular diseases. Second, even if the evidence were strong, changes in diet might be difficult to implement; indeed, the trend in Western countries is towards a larger consumption of rich, expensive and sophisticated foods, in parallel with the general increase in welfare. The incidence of obesity is on the rise in the USA as well as in many European countries [32], and the consumption of fiber, whole grain, fruit and vegetables remains low [33]. Even when the relative intake of these foods is moderate to high, this is usually in addition to a typical Western diet; we cannot exclude that in populations where fruit and vegetables are the most important dietary components, this confers a protection against colorectal cancer development [34]. These considerations, however, do not imply that physicians should not encourage their patients to lose weight and to increase their consumption of fiber, fruit and vegetables.

Can We Prevent Colorectal Cancer by Modifying Our Lifestyle?

There are several studies indicating that physical activity – both occupational and recreational – may protect against colonic cancer, whereas this effect is virtually inconsistent for rectal neoplasms [35–38]. In a longitudinal investigation, 17,000 individuals were followed for 25 years: those who expended more than 2,500 kcal/week in added physical activity had half the risk of developing colorectal malignancies than those who expended less than 1,000 kcal/week [39]. As expected, physical activity may also affect the rate of adenoma recurrence [40]. The relationship between level of physical activity and risk of colonic neoplasia is fairly consistent: 10 of 11 case-control studies showed an inverse relationship between these two variables [8]. The reasons and mechanisms by which occupational or leisure activity reduces the susceptibility to large-bowel malignancies remain unclear.

Obesity is closely associated with physical activity in several ways; there are studies indicating that obese individuals are at increased risk for colorectal cancer and polyps [41, 42]. However, other investigations failed to find an association between body mass index and risk of colorectal cancer [43]. It has been proposed that moderate physical activity together with a lean body mass might induce a "metabolic environment" (low insulin levels, low glucose and triacylglycerol levels and, probably, low circulating levels of hormones and growth factors) which is less favorable for cancer development, especially for neoplasms of the large bowel and breast. The hypothesis, still largely unproven, is nevertheless provocative, since it might lead to consider colorectal (and other) malignancies among the many metabolic disorders induced by energy imbalance [8, 44].

Colorectal tumors are usually not included in the long (and growing) list of tobacco-related malignancies. There are studies, however, indicating a significantly increased risk of adenoma or cancer in heavy smokers [45, 46], though the data have not been confirmed by other investigators [47]. Similar inconsistent results have been reported concerning the association between the consumption of alcoholic beverages and the risk of colorectal cancer [8, 48].

In summary, the relationship between Western lifestyle and colorectal cancer risk – although intuitively attractive and acceptable – remains to be proven in scientific terms. At present, the strongest evidence is that favoring a protective effect of physical activity against these common neoplasms. Thus, can we prevent colorectal cancer by modifying our lifestyle? Western society at the beginning of the twenty-first century does not offer many chances of effective prevention. Nearly 70% of the active population in a typical well-developed country works in the service trades; for most of these subjects, this means spending 6–8 h per day looking at the monitor of a computer and using their hands only for digitating numbers and letters. To this we should add an average 5 h of television (per day) that recent surveys attribute to each individual. Jobs requiring intense physical activity are not requested, and workmen are gradually being substituted by machines. There is no doubt that our life has become more comfortable and sedentary, and that this trend will continue. The many individuals struggling for fitness and against overweight by jogging, trekking or other leisure activity do not represent a countertendency of our society. In my opinion, therefore, the prevention of colorectal neoplasms by modification of our lifestyle remains improbable, though the benefits of physical activity remain undisputed.

Secondary Prevention: Is the Removal of Adenomas Effective?

The elucidation of the adenoma-carcinoma sequence [10] opened the way for a new type of prevention – usually defined as "secondary" – consisting of the systematic removal of all premalignant lesions from the large bowel, particularly adenomatous polyps. The National Polyp Study has recently shown that this approach, when pursued for years, may induce a significant reduction in the incidence and mortality rates for colorectal cancer [11, 49]. This favorable effect can be attributed either to the systematic removal of all newly detected adenomas or to the earlier detection of malignant lesions.

In theory, therefore, removal of adenomas would appear to be an effective way to prevent the development of colorectal cancer. However, when we move to clinical practice, there are several considerations that should be taken into account. Thus, adenomatous polyps are extremely frequent in the general population, with autopsy series indicating the presence of these lesions in up to 30%–40% of individuals [50]; moreover, polyps are usually asymptomatic, a factor that limits their detection to subjects who spontaneously undergo colonoscopic investigation or seek medical advice owing to symptoms, such as rectal bleeding or abdominal discomfort, which have no relation to the polyps. The prevention of colorectal cancer through endoscopic surveillance of the general population would require thousands and thousands of endoscopies, with a cost/benefit ratio unsustainable for any National Health Service [51]. For example, one of the two endoscopic units of the Health Care District of Modena (Italy, 263,000 residents) recorded 1,688 lower endoscopies (mostly colonoscopies) in 1995 [52]; with a population at average risk (> 50 years) of more than 100,000 individuals, this would have required almost 20,000 examinations per year in order to provide an accurate surveillance, assuming one colonoscopy for each individual at risk every 5 years. As alternative approaches, once-only sigmoidoscopy or sigmoidoscopy "every 10 years" has been proposed [53, 54] for the prevention and, thus, the reduction of mortality due to colorectal cancer. Though undoubtedly more feasible and cost-effective, these "simplified" screening procedures fall short in evaluating only the distal portion of the large bowel; in fact, various studies [55, 56] indicate a gradual increase in the prevalence of lesions located in the right colon (approximately 40% of the total), which are beyond the range of a common sigmoidoscope.

In addition, colonoscopy is an unpleasant experience, and many average-risk individuals do not accept this procedure in the absence of symptoms, only for screening purposes. In a recent investigation dealing with subjects at risk for HNPCC (thus, in theory, with a strong motivation for surveillance), only 86 of 223 (38.6%) individuals accepted undergoing colonoscopy when recommended to do so by the interviewers [57].

In summary, although theoretically feasible, secondary prevention through the removal of adenomas can hardly be applicable in the general population. Perhaps a more realistic strategy might consist in the stratification of the general population according to different levels of risk (for example, subjects with a more or less evident familiality for colorectal neoplasms, obese or extremely sedentary individuals, and so on), and thereafter to concentrate our efforts in the close surveillance of these groups.

Colorectal Cancer Prevention Under Special Conditions

There are well-defined clinical conditions in which prevention appears more feasible and effective – at least in theory – in reducing the prevalence of the disease.

In FAP, patients inherit a constitutional mutation in one of the alleles of the APC gene [58]. Adenomas and other extracolonic changes are not present at birth, but develop during the second and third decades of life, due to the inactivation of the wild-type allele. When this occurs, adenomas begin to appear in the gastrointestinal tract, being usually denser and larger in the rectosigmoid region. In time, one of these adenomatous lesions may change into an infiltrating neoplasm, in most cases during the third or fourth decade of life [58]. This slow progression to cancer gives time for an appropriate prevention, which mainly consists in the identification of the syndrome and in the execution of a prophylactic proctocolectomy [60]. Molecular analysis of the APC gene allows the detection of the deleterious mutation in most investigated families [61]; carriers of mutations should undergo close endoscopic surveillance until the development of "full-blown" polyposis; individuals who test negative can be reassured. It has recently been shown [62] that the administration of sulindac (200–400 mg/day) may induce a certain regression – though not a complete disappearance – of adenomas in FAP patients. This effect, however, the intimate mechanism of which remains unclear, has not been translated into clinical practice, especially after the occurrence of rectal cancer in FAP patients treated with sulindac [63]. Despite the limitations of the medical approach, prevention of cancer is feasible in most FAP families, through a combination of molecular, endoscopic and surgical procedures. In a recent investigation, Heiskanen et al. [64] concluded that survival in FAP patients was significantly improved by close surveillance and surgery.

Individuals with HNPCC (or Lynch syndrome) inherit – in most cases – a constitutional mutation in one of several genes responsible for repairing DNA mismatches [7, 65]. When a somatic mutation inactivates the corresponding wild-type allele, the affected cell – in the colorectal mucosa or other target organs – tends to accumulate other mutations at a very high rate, and this eventually leads to cancer development. In the "full-blown" syndrome, early onset colorectal malignancies, often localized in the proximal colon, aggregate in families with striking "verticality", in accordance with a fully penetrant autosomal dominant transmission [66]. The tumor spectrum of HNPCC includes neoplasms of the endometrium, ovary, urothelium, brain and stomach [67]. To date, there is no medical approach that can reduce the risk of cancer in this genetically determined syndrome, though some chemopreventive agents (see below) are under evaluation [68]. The prevention of HNPCC is based on the identification of affected families and close endoscopic surveillance of individuals at risk, with systematic removal of all precancerous lesions [69]. Molecular testing of MSH2 and MLH1 – the two genes more frequently involved in HNPCC – allows the identification of deleterious mutations in approximately 50% of the investigated families [70]; mutation carriers require colonoscopic screening starting at age 20–25, whereas individuals who test negative should be screened the same as the general population. Recent studies showed that systematic surveillance of high-risk subjects in HNPCC families leads to a significant reduction in the incidence and mortality of colorectal malignancies [71, 72].

Various studies showed that patients with ulcerative or Crohn colitis (IBD) are at increased risk for colorectal tumors [73]. The risk is closely related to the duration and extent of the disease; except for the conventional treatment, there is no medical intervention which is effective in reducing the risk of cancer in IBD. Thus, the current approach for cancer prevention requires colonoscopic surveillance at regular intervals of time (especially after 10 years of disease), with multiple biopsies, in order to detect severe dysplasia or early carcinoma [74]. Despite the soundness of lower endoscopy for monitoring the risk of cancer in IBD, there is no convincing evidence of efficacy. This can be attributed to the long period of observation required, to frequent low compliance, and to the reluctance of patients to accept radical approaches – such as colectomy and ileoanal anastomosis – when severe dysplasia is detected [75].

Chemoprevention of Colorectal Cancer

Chemoprevention can be defined as the use of natural compounds or drugs to block, reverse or prevent the development of benign or malignant tumors [76]. It is rather straightforward that the best strategy for cancer control is the removal of the causative agents; this may be relatively simple for tumors such as lung cancer or hepatocellular carcinoma, where precise aetiological factors (tobacco smoking, hepatitis B and C viruses) have been identified. In contrast, this approach can be disappointing for neoplasms such as breast or colorectal carcinoma, the causes of which are less well defined or cannot easily be removed, because they are strictly related to the Western diet and lifestyle [8, 9, 35, 36, 41]. In these cases, a "second line" of prevention based on the administration of chemical compounds (chemoprevention) may assume considerable importance.

General Concepts of Chemoprevention

Chemoprevention is one of the most recent strategies in cancer research [77], which means that many years of basic and clinical investigations will be required to assess the real value of this novel approach. In chemoprevention studies, at least three fundamental aspects should be considered: choice of an appropriate synthetic or natural compound; choice of a valuable intermediate or definitive end-point; and definition of the population to be investigated.

The main features of a candidate compound for chemoprevention are a well-documented biological basis of activity, an almost absolute absence of toxic effects, a cost that an individual or the society can afford, and a simple way of administration. Although none of the compounds commonly used for chemoprevention meet all these requirements, this should not discourage the design and the execution of further clinical studies. Lack of toxicity is particularly relevant, since we should not forget that chemopreventive agents are given to unaffected normal individuals, with the purpose of prevention and not for cure. In addition, chemoprevention usually lasts several years, an aspect that makes safety and low cost critical points in this novel strategy. Approximately 2,000 synthetic or natural compounds seem to possess chemopreventive activity [78]; some of them presumably block or reverse the initiation of tumors, others their promotion or progression; in addition, many of these compounds may influence more than one phase of carcinogenesis. The main classes of drugs used in the chemoprevention of colorectal tumors can be summarized in the following groups: (1) vitamins, provitamins and vitamin-like compounds (vitamins A, C, E, D, β-carotene, folate, retinoids in general); (2) non-steroidal anti-inflammatory drugs (in particular, aspirin and sulindac); (3) minerals (calcium or selenium); (4) bile acids (ursodeoxycholic acid); (5) antioxidants (the above-mentioned vitamins, acetylcysteine); (6) miscellaneous (flavonoids, difluoromethylornithine, others) (Table 6.1).

The choice of the end-point is a crucial aspect in chemoprevention. The ideal end-point is the reduction of the incidence or mortality for a specific tumor;

Table 6.1. Main drugs used in the chemoprevention of colorectal neoplasms in humans (*Cox* cyclooxygenase, *UDCA* ursodeoxycholic acid)

Compounds	Effect	Dose	End-point	Reference
Sulindac	Inhibition of Cox1 and 2	200–400 mg	Polyp disappearance	[87, 88]
Aspirin	Inhibition of Cox1 and 2	300–500 mg	Cancer prevention	[93, 94]
Celecoxib	Inhibition of Cox2	100–400 mg	Polyp disappearance	[97]
Vitamin A	Antiproliferation effect, differentiation, antioxidant	30,000 IU	Polyp recurrence	[100]
β-carotene	Antiproliferation effect, differentiation, antioxidant	25 mg	Polyp recurrence	[101]
Vitamin E	Antiproliferation effect, differentiation, antioxidant	70–400 mg	Polyp recurrence	[100, 101]
Vitamin C	Antiproliferation effect, differentiation, antioxidant	1000 mg	Polyp recurrence	[100, 101]
Calcium	Antiproliferative effect	1–3 g	Polyp recurrence	[104, 106, 107]
Vitamin D	Cell differentiation	–	Cancer prevention	[110]
UDCA acid	Reduced concentration of DCA	150–450 mg	Cancer prevention	[118]
Folate	DNA methylation	400 µg	Cancer prevention	[124]

however, when this is the objective of the investigation, a very large number of individuals would have to be recruited, and their follow-up extended for many years. These factors render impractical the choice of these "definitive" end-points and favor the use of so-called "intermediate" (or "surrogate") end-points: short-term changes of premalignant lesions (i.e. adenoma, dysplasia) or cellular-molecular markers (cell proliferation, expression of oncogenes, instability of microsatellites and others). An ideal biomarker for use in cancer chemoprevention should have – at least in part – the following characteristics: (1) variability of expression during carcinogenesis; (2) detectable early in tumorigenesis; (3) expressed differently in normal and in high-risk sites or populations; (4) subject to modulation by a certain class of chemopreventive agents; (5) easily detectable in body fluids or tissues; and, finally, (6) a low rate of spontaneous changes [76, 79]. Although the search for the ideal intermediate biomarker is still in progress, Table 6.2 shows the main surrogate end-point markers which have been employed so far.

The third main aspect in chemopreventive studies is the choice of an appropriate target population. Of course an investigator may choose to explore the

Table 6.2. Main intermediate end-point markers used in colorectal cancer chemoprevention

Colorectal polyps (mostly adenomas)
Dysplastic changes in adenomas or flat mucosa
Aneuploidy
Presence or number of micronuclei
Cell proliferation (H^3thymidine, bromodeoxyuridine)
Oncogene expression
Tumor-related gene expression
Microsatellite instability

---

possible chemopreventive effect of a given compound in individuals from the general population, i.e. without any specific risk for cancer. As already mentioned, this approach implies the recruitment of a very large number of subjects and the use of sensitive and reliable end-point biomarkers. As an alternative and more practical approach, high-risk subjects can be selected. In the case of colorectal tumorigenesis, examples of high-risk groups include: individuals with adenomatous polyps of the large bowel; patients previously operated on for colorectal malignancies (and, thus, at risk of local recurrence and/or metachronous tumors); first-degree relatives of colorectal cancer patients; subjects affected by inflammatory bowel diseases; and family members at risk in HNPCC or FAP families [80]. A special group of individuals at risk is represented by carriers of constitutional mutations of the APC gene or of other cancer-related genes, such as the DNA mismatch repair genes. These apparently healthy individuals carry a risk of colorectal cancer that approaches 100% for fully penetrant mutations and justifies the use of chemopreventive agents in order to reduce the risk of tumor development [81–83].

Main Compounds Used in the Chemoprevention of Colorectal Tumors

There is evidence that the use of *non-steroidal anti-inflammatory drugs* (NSAID) is somehow associated with a certain protection against colorectal cancer and adenomatous polyps [84]. NSAIDs block both cyclooxygenase 1 and cyclooxygenase 2, catalytic enzymes involved in prostaglandin synthesis, the expression of which is markedly elevated in colorectal tumors [85]. An example of their effect can be observed in experimental colonic carcinogenesis of rodents [86]: when these animals are treated with sulindac, the number of intestinal tumors is markedly reduced [87]. The intimate mechanisms whereby the blockade of cyclooxygenase leads to an inhibition of colorectal tumorigenesis are not completely understood, though there are reasons to believe that they may involve an increase in apoptosis [88] and an effect on angiogenesis [89]. The effect of sulindac can also be observed in humans; there are various clinical studies showing that in patients with FAP the administration of this drug – at the dose of 200–400 mg/day – is associated with a significant reduction in the number and size of colonic adenomas [84, 90]. Two points, however, should be stressed: first, in no patient has complete disappearance of polyps been reported; second, in occasional reports [91], colorectal cancer developed during treatment with sulindac. Both these observations limited the clinical use of sulindac in FAP patients; at present, the drug is mostly used for preventing polyp recurrence in the rectal stump after subtotal colectomy and ileorectal anastomosis [92]. Apart from sulindac, the other anti-inflammatory compound extensively evaluated for colorectal cancer prevention in humans remains aspirin. Several case-control investigations have shown a significant reduction in the risk of colorectal tumors (both adenomas and carcinomas) among subjects who were regular users of aspirin [93, 94]. However, in the only prospective, randomized study performed so far, the administration of 325 mg of aspirin every other day was not associated with any reduction in the incidence of colorectal cancer or polyp, even after 12 years of follow-up [95]. Thus, although the use of conventional NSAIDs in colorectal cancer prevention is rather attractive – because they have been licensed for many years and their mechanism of action is clearly understood – we have at present few reasons for recommending these drugs to the general population or even to high-risk groups. In addition, the minimum effective dose of NSAIDs and the duration of treatment have not been established; both these factors are of relevance, on account of the risk of peptic ulcer and gastric erosions associated with the use of the commonly available NSAIDs [96]. In this respect, the newly developed cyclooxygenase 2 inhibitors are of interest, since their selectivity might prevent the upper gastrointestinal damage of conventional NSAIDs; preliminary studies with celecoxib in FAP are encouraging, either for the effect on polyp regression or for the lack of relevant adverse effects [97].

Antioxidant vitamins and provitamins – in particular, β-carotene, retinol, retinoic acid, ascorbic acid and tocophenol – show some promise as chemopreventive agents in colorectal tumorigenesis. These agents exhibit an antiproliferative effect [98] and can induce differentiation and apoptosis in myeloid cells [99]. Clinical studies, however, have so far been controversial and difficult to reconcile. Thus, the association of vitamin C (1 g/day), retinol (30,000 IU/day) and vitamin E (70 mg/day) appeared to be protective against polyp recurrence in a study of 255 patients with adenomas removed at endoscopy [100]. However, in a larger study involving 864 patients, a similar association (but with β-carotene instead of retinol) was ineffective in reducing polyp recurrence [101]. Similar negative results were obtained in other investigations in which various antioxidant vitamins were combined for the purpose of inhibiting colorectal tumorigenesis in different clinical settings [102, 103]. To summarize, the evidence for supporting the use of antioxidant vitamins in colorectal cancer chemoprevention is rather weak; difficulties in designing and interpreting clinical studies can be attributed to different combinations of vitamins and provitamins and to the lack of consensus on the appropriate dose to be used.

A high intake of calcium might be associated with a reduced incidence of colorectal neoplasms [104]. It has been suggested that calcium reduces the risk of colorectal carcinoma by forming insoluble soaps with ionized fatty acids and secondary bile acids (especially deoxycholic acid) in the gut lumen, potentially decreasing the proliferative stimulus of these substances on the colonic mucosa [105]. This effect might be particularly important in the early stages of tumor development, represented by the formation and growth of colorectal adenomas. Some human case-control and cohort studies showed an inverse relationship between calcium intake and the risk of colon cancer, but the association was statistically weak [106, 107]. Similar inconsistent results were observed in prospective, randomized investigations in which daily supplements of calcium were given to patients at risk for colorectal neoplasia [108, 109].

According to some investigations, individuals with a low intake of *vitamin D* seem to be at increased risk for colon cancer [110]. Moreover, animal studies showed a protective effect of 1,25-dihydroxy vitamin D in chemically induced rat colon carcinogenesis [111], and vitamin D receptor expression has been demonstrated in colorectal neoplasms of humans [112]. Vitamin D plays a fundamental role in the process of cell differentiation, presumably through the activation of protein kinase C [113]. Taken together, these observations make the possible use of vitamin D in colorectal cancer chemoprevention particularly attractive. However, human investigations have so far been inconclusive and showed, if at all, a weak and statistically insignificant protective effect of vitamin D against colon cancer [114, 115].

Among the various bile acids, *ursodeoxycholic acid* (the 7-β-epimer of chenodeoxycholic acid) showed some promise in chemoprevention. When given to humans at a dose of 150–450 mg/day, ursodeoxycholic acid reduces the synthesis of the other bile acids, thus decreasing the concentration of the secondary bile acid deoxycholic acid, which is a promoter of colorectal tumorigenesis [116, 117]. Although experimental evidence in an animal model may indicate that ursodeoxycholic acid administration inhibits colorectal tumor development, no definitive evidence of inhibitory activity has been reported in human studies [118].

Folic acid and its metabolites are critical components of DNA synthesis and methylation. DNA hypomethylation is rather frequent in colorectal tumors, and lack of folate reduces the availability of methyl groups for DNA methylation, which is strictly related to gene silencing [119]. It is not surprising, therefore, that folate has been suggested as a possible chemopreventive agent. Moreover, folate is a micronutrient abundant in vegetables and fruit, and various studies – unfortunately not without controversies – have suggested the existence of an inverse relationship between vegetables and fruit consumption and risk of colorectal malignancies [8, 26]. Various epidemiological investigations showed a lower incidence of colorectal cancer among individuals with the highest intake of folate [120, 121], while subjects used to diets low in folate had an increased risk of colorectal adenomas and carcinomas [122, 123]. In a recent prospective investigation [124], folate supplementation showed some protection against colorectal cancer development, especially among individuals taking daily doses (400 µg or more) of folate; risk reduction, however, became significant only after 15 years of folate consumption, a factor which might limit the use of this natural compound in chemoprevention.

Other drugs whose administration has been proposed – or is under evaluation – for colorectal cancer chemoprevention include *N-acetylcysteine* (an antioxidant compound, commonly used as an expectorant in chronic obstructive lung diseases) [125], *histamine H_2 antagonist* (which showed some effect in preventing growth in animal models of colorectal tumors) [126], and *estrogens*, which may exert a direct antiproliferative effect on colorectal mucosal cells [117] and may inhibit the production of insulin-like growth factor I [128].

Conclusions

Primary colorectal cancer prevention remains difficult, owing to the inherent difficulties in modifying diet and lifestyle in Western countries in the twenty-first century (diet and lifestyle which have been associated with – and related to – better health and a significant increase of life expectancy). Secondary prevention might offer a better prospect of success; however, sigmoidoscopy or colonoscopy can hardly be proposed to the general population. This approach remains extremely valuable and effective for cancer prevention in special groups of individuals, such as patients – or gene carriers – in hereditary colorectal cancer syndromes and patients with long-standing inflammatory bowel diseases. Chemoprevention is still at the beginning of a long story; such studies, however, require several years to be carried out in human beings and owing to the many variables implicated (dose, time of administration, type of association, etc.), their interpretation has so far been rather controversial. The final impression is that despite the real advancements in our knowledge about colorectal cancer prevention, the practical application of these new concepts remains difficult, at least in the short term.

References

1. Hu FB, Stampfer MJ, Manson JAE et al. Trends in the incidence of coronary heart disease and changes in diet and lifestyle in women. N Engl J Med 2000; 343:530–7.
2. Byers T. Body weight and mortality. N Engl J Med 1995; 333:723–4.
3. Loeb LA, Ernster VL, Warner KE et al. Smoking and lung cancer: an overview. Cancer Res 1984; 44:5940–58.
4. Schafer DF, Sorrell MF. Hepatocellular carcinoma. Lancet 1999; 353:1253–7.
5. Ponz de Leon M. Familial and Hereditary tumors. Springer Verlag, Heidelberg 1994; 1–347.
6. Wallis Y, Macdonald F. The genetics of inherited colon cancer. J Clin Pathol 1996; 49: M65-M73.
7. Marra G, Boland CR. Hereditary nonpolyposis colorectal cancer: the syndrome, the genes, and historical perspectives. J Natl Cancer Inst 1995; 87:1114–25.
8. Potter JD. Colorectal cancer: molecules and populations. J Natl Cancer Inst 1999; 91: 916–32.
9. Miller AB, Berrino F, Hill M et al. Diet in aetiology of cancer: a review. Eur J Cancer 1994; 30 A: 207–28.
10. Bedenne L, Faivre J, Boutron MC et al. Adenoma – Carcinoma sequence or "de novo" carcinogenesis? A study of adenomatous remnants in a population-based series of large bowel cancers. Cancer 1992; 69:883–8.

11. Winawer SJ, Zauber AG, Ho MN et al. Prevention of colorectal cancer by colonoscopic polypectomy. N Engl J Med 1993; 329:1977-81.
12. Halama M. Chemoprevention of cancer. Acta Oncol 1998; 37:227-30.
13. Lippman S, Benner S, Hong W. Cancer chemoprevention. J Clin Oncol 1994; 12: 851-73.
14. Blackburn GL, Giardiello FM. Developing strategies for intervention/prevention trials of individuals at risk of hereditary colon cancer. Monogr Natl Cancer Inst 1995; 17: 107-10.
15. Chlebowski RT. Reducing the risk of breast cancer. N Engl J Med 2000; 343:191-8.
16. McLellan EA, Bird RP. Aberrant crypts: potential preneoplastic lesions in the murine colon. Cancer Res 1988; 48:6187-92.
17. Clinton SK, Imrey PB, Mangian HJ et al. The combined effects of dietary fat, protein, and energy intake on azoxymethane-induced intestinal and renal carcinogenesis. Cancer Res 1992; 52:857-65.
18. Reddy BS, Wang CX, Maruyama H. Effect of restricted caloric intake on azoxymethane-induced colon tumor incidence in male F344 rats. Cancer Res 1987; 47:1226-8.
19. Haenszel W, Kurihara M. Studies of Japanese migrants. I. Mortality from cancer and other diseases among Japanese in the United States. J Natl Cancer Inst 1968; 40:43-68.
20. Manousos O, Day NE, Trichopoulos D et al. Diet and colorectal cancer: a case-control study in Greece. Int J Cancer 1983; 32:1-5.
21. Wilmink ABM. Overview of the epidemiology of colorectal cancer. Dis Colon Rectum 1997; 40:483-93.
22. Weisburger JH. Causes, relevant mechanisms, and prevention of large bowel cancer. Semin Oncol 1991; 18:316-36.
23. MacLennan R, McCrae F, Bain C et al. Randomized trial of intake of fat, fiber, and beta carotene to prevent colorectal adenomas. J Natl Cancer Inst. 1995; 87:1760-6.
24. The Surgeon General's Report on Nutrition and Health, Washington, DC, 1988. US Dept of Health and Human Services publication n°. 88-50210.
25. Walker AR, Walker BF, Walker AJ. Faecal pH, dietary fibre intake, and proneness to colorectal cancer in four South African populations. Br J Cancer 1986; 53:489-95.
26. Schatzkin A, Lanza E, Corle D et al. Lack of effect of a low-fat, high-fiber diet on the recurrence of colorectal adenomas. N Engl J Med 2000; 342:1149-55.
27. Garland C, Shekell RB, Barrett-Connor E et al. Dietary vitamin D and calcium and risk of colorectal cancer: a 19-year prospective study in men. Lancet 1985; 1:307-9.
28. Heilbrun LK, Hankin JH, Nomura AM et al. Colon cancer and dietary fat, phosphorus, and calcium in Hawaiian-Japanese men. Am J Clin Nutr 1986; 43:306-9.
29. Miller HW. The emerging role of retinoids and retinoic acid metabolism blocking agents in the treatment of cancer. Cancer 1998; 83:1471-82.
30. Knekt P. Role of vitamin E in the prophylaxis of cancer. Ann Med 1991; 23:3-12.
31. Slattery ML, Schaffer D, Edwards SL et al. Are dietary factors involved in DNA methylation associated with colon cancer? Nutr Cancer 1997; 28:52-62.
32. Manson JE, Willett WC, Stampfer MJ et al. Body weight and mortality among women. N Engl J Med 1995; 333:677-85.
33. Shike M. Diet and lifestyle in the prevention of colorectal cancer: an overview. Am J Med 1999; 106:11S-15S.
34. Michels KB, Giovannucci E, Joshipura KJ et al. Prospective study of fruit and vegetable consumption and incidence of colon and rectal cancers. J Natl Cancer Inst 2000; 92:1740-52.
35. Garabrant DH, Peters JM, Mack TM et al. Job activity and colon cancer risk. Am J Epidemiol 1984; 119:1005-14.
36. Gerhardsson M, Norell SE, Kiviranta H et al. Sedentary jobs and colon cancer. Am J Epidemiol 1986; 123:775-80.
37. Fraser G, Pearce N. Occupational physical activity and risk of cancer of the colon and the rectum in New Zealand males. Cancer Causes Control 1993; 4:45-50.

38. Giovannucci E, Ascherio A, Rimm EB et al. Physical activity, obesity, and risk for colon cancer and adenoma in men. Ann Int Med 1995; 122:327-34.
39. Lee IM, Paffenbarger RS Jr, Hsieh C. Physical activity and risk of developing colorectal cancer among college alumni. J Natl Cancer Inst 1991; 83:1324-9.
40. Kono S, Shinchi K, Ikeda N et al. Physical activity, dietary habits and adenomatous polyps of the sigmoid colon: a study of self-defense officials in Japan. J Clin Epidemiol. 1991; 44:1255-61.
41. Singh PN, Fraser GE. Dietary risk factors for colon cancer in a low-risk population. Am J Epidemiol 1998; 148:761-74.
42. Palmer S. Diet, nutrition, and cancer: the future of dietary policy. Cancer Res 1983; 43:2509s-14 s.
43. Shike M. Body weight and colorectal cancer. Am J Clin Nutr 1996; 63:422-4.
44. Schoen RE, Tangen CM, Kuller LH et al. Increased blood glucose and insulin, body size, and incident colorectal cancer. J Natl Cancer Inst 1999; 91:1147-54.
45. Monnet E, Allemand H, Farina H et al. Cigarette smoking and the risk of colorectal carcinoma in men. Scand J Gastroentrol 1991; 26:758-62.
46. Hoff G, Vatn MH, Larsen S. Relationship between tobacco smoking and colorectal polyps. Scand J Gastroenterol 1987; 22:13-6.
47. Sandler RS, Lyles CM, McAuliffe C et al. Cigarette smoking, alcohol, and the risk of colorectal adenomas. Gastroenterology 1993; 104:1445-51.
48. Ponz de Leon M, Roncucci L. The cause of colorectal cancer. Digest Liver Dis 2000; 32:426-39.
49. Winawer SJ, Fletcher RH, Miller L et al. Colorectal cancer screening: clinical guidelines and rationale. Gastroenterology 1997; 112:594-642.
50. Offerhaus GJA, Giardiello FM, Tersmette KWF et al. Ethnic differences in the anatomical location of colorectal adenomatous polyps. Int J Cancer 1991; 49:641-4.
51. Lieberman D. Cost-effectiveness of colon cancer screening. Am J Gastroenterol 1991; 86:1789-94.
52. Ponz de Leon M, Benatti P, Percesepe A et al. Epidemiology of cancer of the large bowel – The 12-year experience of a specialized Registry in Northern Italy. Ital J Gastroenterol Hepatol 1999; 31:10-8.
53. Selby JV, Friedman GD, Quesenberry CP Jr et al. A case-control study of screening sigmoidoscopy and mortality from colorectal cancer. N Engl J Med 1992; 326:653-7.
54. Atkin WS, Cuzick J, Northover JMA et al. Prevention of colorectal cancer by once-only sigmoidoscopy. Lancet 1993; 341:736-40.
55. Nazarian HK, Giuliano AE, Hiatt JR. Colorectal carcinoma: analysis of management in two medical eras. J Surg Oncol 1993; 52:46-9.
56. Podolsky DK. Going the distance – The case for true colorectal-cancer screening. N Engl J Med 2000; 343:207-8.
57. Ponz de Leon M, Della Casa G, Benatti P et al. Frequency and type of colorectal tumors in asymptomatic high-risk individuals in families with Hereditary Nonpolyposis Colorectal Cancer. Cancer Epidemiol Biomarkers Prev 1998; 7:639-41.
58. Boland CR, Sinicrope FA, Brenner DE et al. Colorectal cancer prevention and treatment. Gastroenterology 2000; 118:S115-S128.
59. Ponz de Leon M, Sassatelli R, Zanghieri G et al. Hereditary adenomatosis of the colon and rectum: clinical features of eight families from Northern Italy. Am J Gastroenterol 1989; 84:906-16.
60. Ambroze WL, Dozois RR, Pemberton JH et al. Familial adenomatous polyposis: results following ileal pouch-anal anastomosis and ileorectostomy. Dis Colon Rectum 1992; 35:12-5.
61. Laken SJ, Papadopoulos N, Petersen GM et al. Analysis of masked mutations in familial adenomatous polyposis. Proc Natl Acad Sci 1999; 96:2322-6.
62. Giardiello FM, Offerhaus JA, Tersmette AC et al. Sulindac induced regression of colorectal adenomas in familial adenomatous polyposis: evaluation of predictive factors. Gut 1996; 38:578-81.

63. Niv Y, Fraser GM. Adenocarcinoma in the rectal segment in familial polyposis coli is not prevented by Sulindac therapy. Gastroenterology 1994; 107:854-7.
64. Heiskanen I, Luostarinen T, Järvinen HJ. Impact of screening examinations on survival in familial adenomatous polyposis. Scand J Gastroenterol 2000; 35:1284-7.
65. Wheeler JMD, Bodmer WF, Mortensen NJMcC. DNA mismatch repair genes and colorectal cancer. Gut 2000; 47:148-53.
66. Lynch HT, Smyrk T. Hereditary nonpolyposis colorectal cancer (Lynch syndrome). An updated review. Cancer 1996; 78:1149-67.
67. Benatti P, Sassatelli R, Roncucci L et al. Tumour spectrum in hereditary non-polyposis colorectal cancer (HNPCC) and in families with "suspected HNPCC". A population-based study in Northern Italy. Int J Cancer 1993; 54:371-7.
68. Hawk E, Lubet R, Limburg P. Chemoprevention in Hereditary Colorectal Cancer syndromes. Cancer 1999; 86:1731-43.
69. Järvinen HJ, Aarnio M, Mustonen H et al. Controlled 15-year trial on screening for colorectal cancer in families with Hereditary Nonpolyposis Colorectal Cancer. Gastroentrology 2000; 118:829-34.
70. Liu B, Parsons R, Papadopoulos N et al. Analysis of mismatch repair genes in hereditary non-polyposis colorectal cancer patients. Nature Med 1996; 2:169-74.
71. Hall NR, Bishop DT, Stephenson BM et al. Hereditary susceptibility to colorectal cancer. Relatives of early onset cases are particularly at risk. Dis Colon Rectum 1996; 39: 739-43.
72. Lynch HT, Smyrk T, Lynch J. An update on HNPCC (Lynch syndrome). Cancer Genet Cytogenet 1997; 93:84-99.
73. Eaden JA, Mayberry JF. Colorectal cancer complicating ulcerative colitis: a review. Am J Gastroenterol 2000; 95:2710-9.
74. Karlén P, Kornfeld D, Broström O et al. Is colonoscopic surveillance reducing colorectal cancer mortality in ulcerative colitis? A population based case control study. Gut 1998; 42:711-4.
75. Choi PM, Nugent FW, Schoetz DJ et al. Colonoscopic surveillance reduces mortality from colorectal cancer in ulcerative colitis. Gastroenterology 1993; 105:418-24.
76. Shureiqi I, Reddy P, Brenner DE. Chemoprevention: general perspective. Critical Reviews in Oncology/Hematology 2000; 33:157-67.
77. Wattenberg LW. Chemoprevention of cancer. Cancer Res 1985; 45:1-8.
78. Bertram JS, Kolonel LN, Meyskens FL. Rationale and strategies for chemoprevention of cancer in humans. Cancer Res 1987; 47:3012-31.
79. Krishnan K, Ruffin MT, Brenner DE. Chemoprevention for colorectal cancer. Critical Reviews in Oncology/Hematology 2000; 33:199-219.
80. Ponz de Leon M, Roncucci L. Chemoprevention of colorectal tumors: role of lactulose and of other agents. Scand J Gastroenterol 1997; 32:72-5.
81. Wu JS, Paul P, McGannon EA et al. APC genotype, polyp number, and surgical options in familial adenomatous polyposis. Ann Surg 1998; 227:57-62.
82. Yuan Y, Han HJ, Zheng S, Park JG. Germline mutations of hMLH1 and hMSH2 genes in patients with suspected hereditary nonpolyposis colorectal cancer and sporadic early-onset colorectal cancer. Dis Colon Rectum 1998; 41:434-40.
83. Miyaki M, Konishi M, Tanaka K et al. Germline mutation on MSH6 as the cause of hereditary nonpolyposis colorectal cancer. Nature Genet 1997; 17:271-2.
84. Jänne PA, Mayer RJ. Chemoprevention of colorectal cancer. N Engl J Med 2000; 342:1960-8.
85. Eberhart CE, Coffey RJ, Radhika A et al. Up-regulation of cyclooxygenase 2 gene expresso in human colorectal adenomas and adenocarcinomas. Gastroenterology 1994; 107:1183-8.
86. Williams CS, Luongo C, Radhika A et al. Elevated cyclooxygenase-2 levels in Min mouse adenomas. Gastroenterology 1996; 111:1134-40.

87. Boolbol SK, Dannenberg AJ, Chadburn A et al. Cyclooxygenase-2 overexpression and tumor formation are blocked by sulindac in a murine model of familial adenomatous polyposis. Cancer Res 1996; 56:2556–60.
88. Sheng H, Shao J, Morrow JD et al. Modulation of apoptosis and Bcl-2 expression by prostaglandin E2 in human colon cancer cells. Cancer Res 1998; 58:362–6.
89. Tsujii M, Kawano S, Tsujii S et al. Cyclooxygenase regulates angiogenesis induced by colon cancer cells. Cell 1998; 93:705–16.
90. Waddell WR, Loughry RW. Sulindac for polyposis of the colon. Am J Surg 1989; 157:175–9.
91. Lynch HT, Thorson AG, Smyrk T. Rectal cancer after prolonged sulindac chemoprevention. Cancer 1995; 75:936–8.
92. Labayle D, Fisher D, Vielh P et al. Sulindac causes regression of rectal polyps in familial adenomatous polyposis. Gastroenterology 1991; 101:635–9.
93. Thun MJ, Namboodiri MM, Heath CW Jr. Aspirin use and reduced risk of fatal colon cancer. N Engl J Med 1991; 325:1593–6.
94. Giovannucci E, Rimm EB, Stampfer MJ et al. Aspirin use and the risk for colorectal cancer and adenoma in male health professionals. Ann Intern Med 1994; 121:241–6.
95. Sturmer T, Glynn RJ, Lee IM et al. Aspirin use and colorectal cancer; post-trial follow-up data from the Physicians' Health Study. Ann Intern Med 1998; 128:713–20.
96. Langman MJS, Weil J, Wainwright P et al. Risks of bleeding peptic ulcer associated with individual non-steroidal anti-inflammatory drugs. Lancet 1994; 343:1075–8.
97. Steinbach G, Lynch PM, Phillips RKS et al. The effect of celecoxib, a cyclooxygenase-2 inhibitor, in familial adenomatous polyposis. N Engl J Med 2000; 342:1946–52.
98. Paganelli GM, Biasco G, Brandi G et al. Effect of vitamin A, C and E supplementation on rectal cell proliferation in patients with colorectal adenomas. J Natl Cancer Inst 1992; 84:47–51.
99. Castaigne S. All trans retinoic acid as a differentiation therapy for acute promyelocytic leukaemia. Blood 1988; 76:567–72.
100. Roncucci L, Di Donato P, Carati L et al. Antioxidant vitamins or lactulose for the prevention of the recurrence of colorectal adenomas. Dis Colon Rectum 1993; 36:227–34.
101. Greenberg ER, Baron JA, Tosteson TD et al. A clinical trial of antioxidant vitamins to prevent colorectal adenoma. N Engl J Med 1994; 331:141–7.
102. De Cosse JJ, Miller HH, Lesser ML. Effect of wheat fibre and vitamins C and E on rectal polyps in patients with familial adenomatous polyposis. J Natl Cancer Inst 1989; 81:1290–7.
103. McKeown-Eyssen G, Holloway C, Jazmaji V et al. A randomised trial of vitamins C and E in the prevention of recurrence of colorectal polyps. Cancer Res 1988; 48:4701–5.
104. Sorenson AW, Slattery ML, Ford MH. Calcium and colon cancer: a review. Nutr Cancer 1988; 11:135–45.
105. Newmark HL, Wargovich MJ, Bruce WR. Colon cancer and dietary fat, phosphate, and calcium: a hypothesis. J Natl Cancer Inst 1984; 72:1323–5.
106. Martinez ME, Willett WC. Calcium, vitamin D, and colorectal cancer: a review of the epidemiologic evidence. Cancer Epidemiol Biomarkers Prev 1998; 7:163–8.
107. Hyman J, Baron JA, Dain BJ et al. Dietary and supplemental calcium and the recurrence of colorectal adenomas. Cancer Epidemiol Biomarkers Prev 1998; 7:291–5.
108. Baron JA, Beach M, Mandel JS et al. Calcium supplements for the prevention of colorectal adenomas. N Engl J Med 1999; 340:101–7.
109. Lipkin M, Newmark H. Effect of added dietary calcium on colonic epithelial-cell proliferation in subjects at high risk for familial colonic cancer. N Engl J Med 1985; 313:1381–4.
110. Garland CF, Comstock GW, Garland FC et al. Serum 25-hydrosyvitamin D and colon cancer: eight year prospective study. Lancet 1989; 2:1176–8.
111. Belleli A, Shany S, Levy J et al. A protective role of 1,25 dihydroxy vitamin D3 in chemically induced rat colon carcinogenesis. Carcinogenesis 1992; 13:2293.

112. Kane KF, Langman MJS, Williams GR. 1,25 hydroxy vitamins D3 and retinoid X receptor expression in human colorectal neoplasms. Gut 1995; 36:255-8.
113. Slater SJ, Kelly MB, Taddeo FJ et al. Direct activation of protein kinase C by 1,25-dihydroxy vitamin D3. J Biol Chem 1995; 270:6639-43.
114. Kampman E, Giovannucci E, van't Veer P et al. Calcium vitamin D, dairy foods, and the occurrence of colorectal adenomas among men and women in two prospective studies. Am J Epidemiol 1994; 139:16-29.
115. Bostick RM, Potter JD, Sellers TA et al. Relation of calcium, vitamin D, and dairy food intake to incidence of colon cancer among older women. The Iowa Women's Health Study. Am J Epidemiol 1993; 137:1302-17.
116. Rodrigues CM, Kren BT, Steer CJ et al. The site-specific delivery of ursodeoxycholic acid to the rat colon by sulfate conjugation. Gastroenterology 1995; 109:1835-44.
117. Narisawa T, Fukaura Y, Terada K et al. Prevention of N-methylnitrosourea-induced colon tumorigenesis by ursodeoxycholic acid in F344 rats. Jpn J Cancer Res 1998; 89:1009-13.
118. Earnest DL, Holubec H, Wali RK et al. Chemoprevention of azoxymethane-induced colonic carcinogenesis by supplemental dietary ursodeoxycholic acid. Cancer Res 1994; 54:5071-4.
119. Bestor TH. Methylation meets acetylation. Nature 1998; 393:311-2.
120. Benito E, Stiggelbout A, Bosch FX et al. Nutritional factors in colorectal cancer risk: a case-control study in Majorca. Int J Cancer 1991; 49:161-7.
121. Ferraroni M, La Vecchia C, D'Avanzo B et al. Selected micronutrient intake and the risk of colorectal cancer. Br J Cancer 1994; 70:1150-5.
122. Giovannucci E, Rimm EB, Ascherio A et al. Alcohol, low-methionine - low-folate diets, and risk of colon cancer in men. J Natl Cancer Inst 1995; 87:265-73.
123. Baron JA, Sandler RS, Haile RW et al. Folate intake, alcohol consumption, cigarette smoking, and risk of colorectal adenomas. J Natl Cancer Inst 1998; 90:57-62.
124. Giovannucci E, Stampfer MJ, Colditz GA et al. Multivitaminic use, folate, and colon cancer in women in the Nurses' Health Study. Ann Intern Med 1998; 129:517-24.
125. De Flora S, Astengo M, Serra D et al. Inhibition of urethan-induced lung tumors in mice by dietary N-acetylcysteine. Cancer Lett 1986; 32:235-41.
126. Watson SA, Wilkinson LJ, Robertson JR et al. Effect of histamine on the growth of human gastro-intestinal tumours: reversal by cimetidine. Gut 1993; 34:1091-6.
127. McMichael AJ, Potter JD. Reproduction, endogenous and exogenous sex hormones and colon cancer: a review and hypothesis. J Natl Cancer Inst 1980; 65:1201-7.
128. Campagnoli C, Biglia N, Altare F et al. Differential effects of oral conjugated estrogens and transdermal estradiol on insulin-like growth factor 1, growth hormone and sex hormone binding globulin serum levels. Gynecol Endocrinol 1993; 7:251-8.

7 Treatment of Colorectal Cancer

Introduction

Despite the recent advances in medical and surgical approaches, treatment of colorectal cancer remains unsatisfactory in many patients. The main factor associated with the relatively poor prognosis for colorectal malignancies is the advanced stage of the disease at the time of diagnosis; indeed, some 20%-40% of patients show locally advanced or metastatic disease which is beyond the scope of a radical approach [1]. Even among those patients who undergo apparently curative resection, some 20% to 30% die within 5 years. Local recurrences (more frequent after the excision of rectal cancers) are responsible for the failure of treatment in 5%-30% of all cases, usually within 2-3 years from the operation; liver and lung metastases are also frequent in the follow-up of patients undergoing curative resection, especially in Dukes' C carcinoma [2-4].

These figures should not obscure the fact that colorectal tumors remain the most curable among neoplasms of the digestive organs, and that the last two decades have been distinguished by several advances in colorectal cancer treatment. Thus, fluorouracil-based chemotherapy has been accepted as a standard adjuvant therapy in Dukes' C carcinoma, and continues to be the mainstay of treatment for metastatic lesions [5]. Laparoscopic surgery appeared in the early 1990s and rapidly became widespread, though not without controversies [6]. Total mesorectal excision improved the cure rates for rectal cancer and probably reduced the variability of outcome among surgeons [7]. Finally, judicious use of radiotherapy (especially preoperative) has been followed by a reduction of local recurrences after surgery for rectal cancer [8]. The above-mentioned new approaches – together with a more frequent early diagnosis [9] – induced a significant improvement of the 5-year survival (in most series), which is at present about 50%-60% [10].

This chapter will review our present knowledge of colorectal cancer treatment, giving particular emphasis to novel or more promising approaches and to the existing controversies.

Staging Colorectal Neoplasms

Staging at diagnosis represents the single most important factor affecting survival for patients with colorectal malignancies and influencing the choice of surgical, endoscopic and/or medical treatment. The staging system proposed by Cuthbert Dukes – pathologist at St. Mark's Hospital – in 1932 [11] is still widely employed in its principles and easy to apply. According to this system, tumors are staged into three categories, depending on the degree of local infiltration and on the presence of lymph node metastases; the issue, however, became more complex owing to the modifications introduced by several authors [5, 12]. In 1986, Hutter and Sabin [13] proposed a universal staging procedure showing a close correspondence between the TNM system employed for most neoplasms and Dukes' staging. The authors followed simple physiopathologic considerations which eliminated ambiguities and confusion consequent to the numerous revisions of the Dukes' procedure. Thus, stage I tumors (corresponding to Dukes' A and to Astler-Coller A and B1) are confined within the muscular wall; in stage II (Dukes' B or Astler-Coller B2 and B3), the neoplasm spreads beyond the smooth muscle, may infiltrate perirectal (or pericolic) tissues, and even adjacent organs (bladder, uterus). In stage III tumors (Dukes' C and Astler-Coller C), metastases in the lymph nodes are present, whereas in stage IV (corresponding to the D class of Astler-Coller and other classifications) the tumor diffuses through the blood, metastasizing to the liver, lung and, less frequently, other organs [14] (Fig. 7.1).

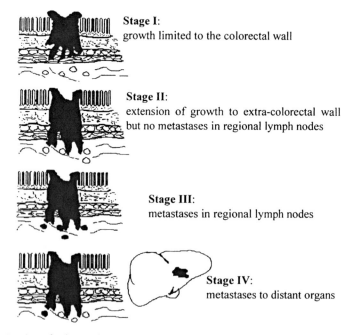

Fig. 7.1. Staging of colorectal carcinoma into four main categories [13]

More subtle staging procedures have been described with the purpose of identifying micrometastasis in the lymph nodes of patients with stage I and especially stage II colorectal carcinoma. Thus, various authors reported the use of immunohistochemical staining for cytokeratin (in haematoxylin & eosin-negative nodes) as a means for discovering occult metastases [15, 16]. These investigations found micrometastasis in 20%-30% of stage II colorectal cancers, though a clear correlation with the clinical outcome was not reported. Since cytokeratin staining is only able to distinguish cells of epithelial origin, without giving any information on their benign or malignant nature, a further advance involved the use of molecular tumor markers to identify micrometastasis. Among the many candidate oncogenes and tumor suppressor genes, *k-ras* and p53 received particular attention [17-20]. In one of these studies [20], *k-ras* mutation analysis in 20 Dukes' B patients revealed the same type of mutation in the primary tumor and in the lymph nodes in 80% of patients; moreover, none of the patients with mutation-free nodes developed local recurrences compared with 6 of 16 individuals with *k-ras*-positive lymph nodes. The authors suggested that the assessment of mutational status of *k-ras* (together with other cancer-related genes, such as p53, DCC and possibly others) might allow the definition of a "molecular fingerprint" of a given tumor, which could be used to find micrometastasis in stage I and II colorectal cancers. The fact is not without practical relevance, since chemotherapy is indicated in stage III lesions, while its benefit in stage II patients is still under investigation (see below). To summarize, "molecular staging" of colorectal malignancies is an appealing concept, but not yet ready to be introduced into clinical practice; further studies are needed to evaluate the correlation of micrometastasis with survival and to assess the possible value of adjuvant chemotherapy in patients with occult metastases.

Treatment of Resectable Colorectal Tumors

Endoscopic Treatment of Malignant Polyps

Malignant polyps can be defined as adenomas in which carcinoma develops and infiltrates across the muscularis mucosae into the submucosa. Data from cancer registries indicate that malignant polyps are relatively rare: their incidence is of the order of 2-3 cases/100,000/year, corresponding to 3%-6% of all registered large-bowel cancers [1, 21]. Due to the presence of lymphatic vessels in the submucosa, malignant polyps might in theory give rise to distant metastases; however, endoscopic polypectomy is curative in 99.7% of pedunculated polyps [22] and in 98.5% of sessile lesions [23]. Both these studies came to the conclusion that endoscopic removal of malignant polyps with "favorable prognostic criteria" did not impair the clinical outcome. Favorable criteria include resection margins free of neoplasia, lack of vascular or lymphatic invasion, and well-differentiated carcinoma at histology [24]. After excision of a polyp with malignant features, the pathologist plays a determinant role in establishing the completeness of removal and, thus, the possible need of surgery. If margins of resection do not show residual tumor, the lymphatics do not appear to have been invaded, and the neoplasm appears well differentiated, then the patient is invited for endoscopic follow-up, but the available evidence suggests that surgery is not necessary. When the margins of the resected polyp are infiltrated or there is evidence of vascular or lymphatic invasion, especially in the presence of poorly differentiated tumors, then surgical resection – with the consequent removal and examination of the mesenteric lymph nodes – appears to be the most appropriate choice [23].

Surgical Treatment of Resectable Tumors of the Colon

The current surgical approach to the treatment of colonic cancer developed in the years following World War II. The main concepts were complete excision of the tumor mass and extent of resection based on wide removal of the lymphatic drainage. While right hemicolectomy (from the caecum to half of the transverse colon) was already a well-known approach [25], Rosi [26] stressed the role of left hemicolectomy (excision of half of the transverse, descending and sigmoid colon) for lesions of the distal colon instead of segmental resection. While it is rather obvious that removal of the neoplasm and an adjacent portion of the colon remains the basis of surgical cure, there is no standard management policy as to the exact length of colonic resection (hemicolectomy versus segmental resection), extent of lymph node excision and ligation of the inferior mesenteric artery [27]. In a recent prospective, multicentre trial involving 270 consecutive patients with colonic carcinoma, left segmental resection and left hemicolectomy showed comparable results in terms of pathology findings, early postoperative abdominal and extra-abdominal complications and, most important, 5- and 10-year survival [28]. The authors concluded that left segmental resection is a "legitimate alternative" to left hemicolectomy, a finding of practical relevance also for the emergence of laparoscopic surgery (see below). It seems, therefore, that the extent of resection does not affect the prognosis.

At variance with sporadic tumors, large resections and, more often, subtotal colectomy with ileorectal anastomosis are required for patients with HNPCC (or Lynch syndrome) because of the frequent synchronous and metachronous lesions [29–31]. Similarly, in FAP the presence of hundreds or thousands of polyps scattered in the various segments of the large bowel requires subtotal colectomy with ileorectal anastomosis [32, 33] or restorative proctocolectomy with ileoanal anastomosis [34, 35]. Owing to the frequent (up to 30%) occurrence of cancer in the rectal stump [26], the latter approach has become more popular recently.

Five-year survival, after surgery for resectable colonic neoplasms is about 90% for patients with stage I lesions, 60%–80% for stage II and 30%–40% for individuals with lymph node metastasis (stage III) [37, 38].

Laparoscopic surgery was introduced for cholecystectomy in 1989 [39] and since then has been applied to several clinical conditions such as appendicectomy, hernia repair, fundoplication, diverticulitis and, from the early 1990s, colorectal cancer [40]. A recent review confirmed that laparoscopic colorectal cancer surgery is technically feasible and presents numerous advantages over conventional surgery [6]; however, the disadvantages are also evident, and some concerns still remain. Among the possible advantages of the laparoscopic approach are a reduced loss of blood during the procedure [41], less postoperative pain owing to the smaller scar [42], a shorter postoperative ileus (presumably related to less bowel manipulation with laparoscopy) [43], with a consequent shorter hospitalization (6 versus 11 days in one series) [44], a possible reduced immunosuppression [45] and a more rapid resumption of oral intake [46]. Disadvantages of the laparoscopic approach include a longer operating time (although the difference between the two procedures tends to become smaller over time), the overall cost of the equipment [6] and a number of complications usually not observed with conventional surgery, such as herniation of the small bowel into the trocar site [42], inadvertent enterotomy, injury to mesenteric vessels and transection of the inferior epigastric artery [47]. Some authors raised concerns about the extent of resection and removal of lymph nodes with laparoscopy; although definitive data on survival from prospective investigations are still lacking, the available evidence indicates that there is no significant difference between the conventional and laparoscopic approach in the extent of resection and lymphadenectomy [6, 42, 48, 49]. Probably the major concern related to colorectal cancer laparoscopy is the development of recurrent tumor at the port-site of laparoscopy, which has been reported in 1%–2% of all patients [50, 51]. The reasons for this complication (which has been observed also with stage I tumors) remain unclear, but possible explanations include contamination of the wound by tumor cells on instrument removal, exfoliation of tumor cells during laparoscopic manipulation, and the promotional effect of pneumoperitoneum on tumor cell attachment and proliferation [6, 52, 53]. Intraperitoneal heparin, preoperative antitumoral compounds and "gasless" laparoscopy have been proposed as preventive strategies [6, 54].

Surgical Treatment of Resectable Tumors of the Rectum

Surgical treatment of rectal tumors includes a large spectrum of operative procedures, ranging from radical operations to new sphincter-preserving techniques. At the beginning of the twentieth century, most patients with rectal neoplasms presented with symptoms, and operations usually required a perineal approach, in which the tumor was dissected out from inside the rectum by splitting the rectal wall [15]. This type of surgery implied complete division of the sphincter and was associated with a significant dysfunction of the anal sphincter; in addition, operative mortality was of the order of 8%–12% [56]. W.E. Miles, in 1908, and W. Mayo, in 1916, suggested total rectal excision for tumor of the rectum through the *abdominoperineal resection* [57, 58], a type of surgery that in its original application required removal of the anal canal and sphincters, wide excision of the levator muscles and ligation of the main sigmoid artery. Despite the complexity of the operation, 5-year survival exceeded 40%, a value not very different from that observed one century later [5, 57]. An alternative treatment for neoplasms of the rectum was proposed by Hartmann in 1923 [59]; the two-stage procedure involved colostomy as a first step, followed by a second operation consisting of the removal of the tumor. Though the technique does not allow a radical approach to cancer of the rectum, it is still used as palliative resection, especially for patients with obstructed or perforated lesions, in whom there are clinical contraindications to more radical operations.

Although the first *anterior resection* for cancer of the rectum was carried out in 1910 [60], the technique became popular from the 1950s, and competed against the abdominoperineal approach after the introduction of stapling devices [61, 62]. Indeed, various controlled and uncontrolled investigations showed that lower anterior resection (executed with at least 2-cm margins) and abdominoperineal resection gave comparable results in terms of 5-year survival, local recurrences, main complications, perioperative and postoperative mortality [63-67]. Of course, the main advantage of the anterior approach was the avoidance of a preternatural anus (permanent colostomy). For all these reasons, anterior resection replaced Miles operation for neoplasms located in the midrectum and in selected cases of the distal rectum, while the latter intervention remains the technique of choice for tumors located less than 2 cm from the uppermost part of the anorectal ring.

Total *mesorectal excision* was introduced by Heald [68] in 1982 with the purpose of reducing the rate of local recurrence of rectal carcinoma in the pelvis. The technique involves an anterior approach in which complete excision of the mesorectum is carried out below the levator muscle, thus removing all perirectal fat and facilitating sphincter preservation. The procedure was developed with an awareness of the importance of complete excision – under direct vision – of the envelope of lymphovascular fatty tissue surrounding the rectum and its mesorectum. The author hypothesized that local recurrence was more the result of leaving mesorectal residue than of the aggressive nature of tumors to spread beyond the limits of perimesorectal dissection. This postulate proved to be true, since in the most recent reviews on total mesorectal excision the local recurrence rate was 3% at 5 years and 4% at 10 years – among the lowest reported in the literature – with a disease-free survival of 80% at 5 years and 78% at 10 years after curative resection for rectal cancer [69-71]. Total mesorectal excision is now a well established surgical approach for reducing the local recurrence of rectal cancer and for facilitating complete pathological evaluation.

When compared with surgery for colonic lesions, the operations for rectal carcinoma are undoubtedly more complex and require more surgical skill. At least three additional problems should be mentioned: pelvic lymphadenectomy, autonomic nerve preservation, and variation among surgeons.

Radical abdominopelvic resection of lymph nodes for rectal carcinoma is based on the simple principle of removing all potentially infiltrated lymphatic tissue in order to lower the rate of locoregional recurrence, thus improving survival. The technique involves dissection of lymph nodes along the aorta, iliac vessel and obturator space. Despite the soundness of this approach, the available literature fails to document a definite improvement in local recurrence or overall survival [72-74]. Moreover, urinary dysfunction and impotence develop frequently after this type of surgery and represent major deterrents to widespread application [75].

Despite the technical advances (especially stapling devices), urinary and sexual dysfunctions remain serious problems after rectal surgery. For this reason, operative techniques have been developed that combine autonomic nerve preservation with radical resections [76, 77]. These essentially consist in the identification and consequent preservation of the bilateral hypogastric nerves (located 2 cm medial to the ureter, at the level of the sacral promontory), nervi erigentes (adherent to the mesorectum) and the inferior hypogastric plexus. With these precautions, postoperative sexual alterations have been reduced from more than 50% to 10%-30% [78].

Finally, most surgeons recognize that the frequency of postoperative complications varies widely among individual surgeons. For example, in a series of 1,400 patients with rectal cancer, local recurrence and death rates were significantly lower among individuals operated on by surgeons with more than 19 years' experience as a specialist [79]. In another investigation, the risk of local recurrence was significantly higher in patients treated by surgeons not specifically trained in colorectal surgery, or by surgeons executing less than 21 resections per year [80]. These findings clearly demonstrate that both specialization (in oncologic surgery) and the absolute number (i.e. "volume") of operations may be important factors in determining the clinical outcome.

Medical Treatment of Colorectal Tumors

In most cases, colorectal cancer is grossly completely resectable, and any residual malignant tissue is microscopic in nature. This is particularly true for patients with regional lymph node involvement (stage III), who have a 40%-50% 5-year survival rate [37, 38]. This is an ideal clinical setting for any attempt to reduce cancer mortality by adding adjuvant chemotherapy (or radiotherapy) to apparently curative surgery. Pursuing this objective, clinical efforts at adjuvant therapy began approximately 40 years ago and involved numerous trials enrolling several thousands of patients treated with cytostatic and cytotoxic compounds - often in combination - as well as non-specific immune stimulants. Despite these efforts, no definite evidence for the effectiveness of any regimen was documented, and in a meta-analysis published in 1988 [81], Buyse et al. reported that the probability of dying of colorectal cancer was 8% higher for treated than for untreated patients.

After so many years of negative results, the benefits of chemotherapy administered in an adjuvant setting for colonic neoplasms were established by an intergroup trial involving 979 stage III patients who were randomly assigned to treatment with levamisole + 5-fluorouracil, vs levamisole alone, vs no treatment [82]. In this keystone investigation, patients treated with the combination regimen had a striking 41% reduction in the recurrence rate ($p < 0.0001$) and a 33% reduction in the mortality rate ($p < 0.006$) compared with the untreated controls.

These results were confirmed by the same authors, but with a longer follow-up of patients (no less than 5 years) [83]. They concluded that the combination of levamisole + 5-fluorouracil "should be considered standard treatment for all such patients not entered into clinical trials".

Fluorouracil is a prodrug that is converted intracellularly to various metabolites that bind to the enzyme thymidylate synthase, thus inhibiting the synthesis of thymidine, DNA and RNA [84]. Levamisole is an anthelmintic compound which is supposed to have an immunostimulatory action [85]. In the above-mentioned investigations [82, 83], patients assigned to the combination therapy received levamisole 1–4 weeks after surgery at the oral dose of 50 mg three times/day for 3 days, repeated every 2 weeks for 1 year. Fluorouracil was added at a dose of 450 mg/m^2 body surface daily for 5 days through rapid intravenous injection, 3–4 weeks after surgery. Twenty-eight days after the start of chemotherapy, weekly treatment with fluorouracil was begun, at the same dose, and continued for almost 1 year. Further studies showed that 6 months of chemotherapy is as effective as 12 months [86, 87].

Side-effects due to levamisole alone were mild and infrequent (nausea, fatigue, taste change), so that reactions to fluorouracil + levamisole were those which might be expected for fluorouracil alone. These included nausea (but vomiting was rare), stomatitis, diarrhea, dermatitis, fatigue and mild alopecia [82]. Approximately half of the treated patients developed haematologic depression, usually limited to mild leukopenia; however, the only observed drug-related death was due to profound leukopenia and sepsis in a patient treated with the combination regimen [83]. An unexpected adverse reaction to fluorouracil + levamisole was the occurrence of abnormal liver function tests (elevation of alkaline phosphatase and aminotranferase levels), with biopsy-proven steatosis in some individuals; these alterations, however, were not associated with clinical symptoms and regressed after discontinuation of the therapy [88].

In the Moertel study [82], 20% of patients with stage II (Dukes' B) tumors who did not receive combination therapy had recurrences, as opposed to 14% (not significant) of those who were treated with levamisole + fluorouracil, during a follow-up of 3 years. The general impression is that for patients with stage II disease, adjuvant chemotherapy does not offer any survival benefit [89]. However, this group of patients is very heterogeneous and includes individuals with limited infiltration beyond the muscular wall as well as patients with lesions infiltrating the bladder and other contiguous organs. It is likely, therefore, that stage II tumors with prognostic indicators that suggest a high risk of recurrence (such as extent of disease, perforation and vascular invasion) might benefit from adjuvant chemotherapy much more than neoplasms without high-risk indicators [87]. Future studies should take into account various subgroups of stage II subjects with different degrees of risk for recurrent and metastatic disease.

Among the efforts directed in the past years at identifying ways of improving the efficacy of 5-fluorouracil in colorectal cancer, the most successful was the combination with folinic acid [84]. Experimental studies have shown that leucovorin (folinic acid) enhances the intracellular concentration of reduced folates, and this, in turn, stabilizes the binding of fluorouracil to thymidylate synthase, thus increasing the inhibition of DNA synthesis and improving the cytotoxic action of the drug [90]. In accordance with this contention, several studies carried out in patients with advanced colorectal tumors showed a significant improvement in the probability of response, favoring 5-fluorouracil + leucovorin over fluorouracil alone [91, 92]. In contrast to the combination with levamisole, therefore, the combination of 5-fluorouracil with folinic acid possesses a well-grounded pharmacological basis of activity. In addition, the documented benefit in advanced disease led to the logical extension of this combination treatment into adjuvant therapy. Over the last decade, several controlled phase-III investigations definitively showed an improved disease-free survival and a significant improvement in overall survival in patients with stage-III colorectal cancer treated with the combination of fluorouracil and folinic acid as an adjuvant therapy, with a 25%-30% decrease in the odds of dying of the disease (i.e. a result comparable to that obtained with 5-fluorouracil + levamisole) [93-95]. In one of these studies [93], 1,081 patients with stage II and III colonic tumors were treated either with 5-fluorouracil and leucovorin administered weekly or a combination of 5-fluorouracil, semustine and vincristine. After a median follow-up of almost 4 years, 5-fluorouracil + leucovorin adjuvant therapy was associated with an improved disease-free (73% vs 64%) and overall (84% vs 77%; $p < 0.003$) survival. According to some authors [87], the combination of fluorouracil with leucovorin should be accepted as "standard" adjuvant chemotherapy for patients with stage-III colonic cancer.

Owing to its anatomical location, carcinoma of the rectum (i.e. located within 7-10 cm from the anal verge) represents a special challenge not only to surgeons but also to adjuvant therapy. Since other pelvic organs are close to the rectum, it is difficult to achieve a wide tumor-free margin during operation. As a consequence of these difficulties, nearly half the recurrences of rectal neoplasms are located in the pelvis [96, 97]. Radiotherapy (given either preoperatively or postoperatively) has proven to be effective for palliating the symptoms and for reducing the rate of recurrence, though the treatment has rarely been associated with an increase in survival (see below). A further approach for reducing local and distal failures after rectal surgery is the administration of 5-fluorouracil-based chemotherapy with or without concomitant radiation therapy [85]. This approach is also favored by animal observations showing that fluorouracil may prime tumor cells and increase the cytotoxic effect of subsequent radiotherapy [87]. There is evidence that the administration of 5-fluorouracil by bolus injection or protracted infusion together with radiation therapy improves the local control and overall survival in patients with resectable rectal cancer [98-101]. In one of these studies [100], 227 patients with stage II or III rectal neoplasms were randomly allocated to receive no postoperative treatment, semustine-based chemotherapy, irradiation of the pelvis, or combined chemotherapy + irradiation. After a median follow-up of more than 10 years, combined therapy was better than surgery alone for both disease-free survival (65% vs 45%, $p < 0.006$) and overall survival (45% vs 26%, $p < 0.04$). Combined therapy was also superior to irradiation or chemotherapy alone, though the differences did not reach statistical significance. In a more recent European investigation [102], 144 patients with stage II or III rectal carcinoma were randomized to surgery alone or surgery combined with postoperative radiotherapy plus 5-fluorouracil bolus injection (500–750 mg) 30 min before 6 of the radiotherapy fractions. After a follow-up of 4–8 years, patients in the combined therapy group had a cumulative local recurrence rate significantly lower than that observed in the group that had surgery alone; overall 5-year survival was 64% in the adjuvant group compared with 46% in the surgery group ($p < 0.01$).

The above-mentioned as well as other observations prompted some authors [5, 103] to consider postoperative or preoperative combined radiation and chemotherapy as the "standard" of care for stage II and III rectal cancer. Other authors, however, are more cautious about the possible role of chemotherapy in rectal cancer [67, 104] and advocate further clinical evidence of benefit before this treatment modality could be considered for routine use.

Radiation Treatment of Rectal Cancer

In contrast to colonic tumors, radiotherapy is widely used in the management of carcinomas of the rectum. This treatment, however, has a limited capability to eradicate bulky primary carcinomas and can be considered as an alternative to surgery only in specific circumstances, such as palliation of symptoms in locally extensive, recurrent or metastatic disease. Endorectal irradiation is a highly effective treatment for superficial tumors of the distal rectum but as a single approach does not allow an evaluation of possible regional lymph node metastasis [105, 106]. For this reason, surgical resection combined with external beam radiation (with or without chemotherapy) became the treatment of choice for rectal carcinoma [5].

Once the definite role of external irradiation as an adjuvant treatment of resectable rectal malignancies was established, researchers tried to find the most favorable approach and, in particular, to evaluate the advantages and disadvantages of postoperative or preoperative radiotherapy; like a pendulum, in fact, the favor of radiotherapists and surgeons seems to oscillate between these two treatment modalities.

Postoperative radiation therapy is usually delivered a few weeks after surgery at recommended doses of 45–55 Gy over a period of 5–6 weeks [107]. Preoperative radiation can be given at the same fractionated doses 4–5 weeks before surgery [108], or as a short course at smaller doses (25 Gy delivered in five fractions in 1 week), followed by surgical excision within 1 week after the completion of radiotherapy [109]. Postoperative radiotherapy is carried out after an accurate pathologic staging; its main advantage is therefore the selection of patients, thus avoiding possible overtreatment and allowing treatment only for high-risk individuals (i.e. those with extensive local infiltration or lymph node metastasis) [104]. On the other hand, preoperative irradiation has several advantages, including cleaning of cancerous peripheral areas, cancer down-staging, which makes conservative surgery easier, and use of lower doses of radiation, with a consequently reduced toxicity [109]. A major disadvantage of postoperative radiotherapy is the possible small-bowel fixation in the irradiated field, which exposes the small bowel to injury and complications [110]. The disadvantages of the preoperative approach include the treatment of patients not requiring therapy – owing to low-stage primary lesions – and an increased risk of surgical complications [111]. Finally, one common limitation of most studies on adjuvant radiotherapy in rectal cancer is that while control of local recurrences is frequently achieved, overall survival is rarely affected [110, 112].

A few representative investigations deserve to be analyzed in more detail. In 1996, two studies of the Medical Research Council Rectal Cancer Working Party [112, 113] evaluated the role of surgery preceded or followed by irradiation for operable, locally advanced rectal cancer (versus surgery alone). These prospective, randomized trials included a total of 5,021 patients who were followed for a minimum of 5 years or until death. The results provided evidence that either preoperative or postoperative adjuvant irradiation was able to reduce the rate of local recurrences, approximately to a similar extent, but failed to show significant survival advantage for any of the investigated subgroups. In the Swedish Rectal Cancer Trial [109], 1,168 patients with resectable rectal cancer were randomized to preoperative radiotherapy (25 Gy, in 1 week) followed by surgery or to surgery alone. After 5 years of follow-up, local recurrences were diagnosed in 11% of patients who received the combined therapy and in 27% of individuals treated with surgery alone ($p < 0.001$). Moreover, the overall 5-year survival was 58% in the radiotherapy-plus-surgery group and 48% in the surgery alone group ($p < 0.004$). The authors concluded that a short-term regimen of preoperative radiation not only reduces the rates of local recurrence but can also increase survival in patients with resectable rectal malignancies. In keeping with these encouraging results, a recent meta-analysis of 14 randomized clinical trials published between 1975 and 1997 [114] on preoperative radiotherapy for resectable rectal cancer showed that this approach led to a significant improvement of overall and cancer-specific survival compared with surgery alone.

In conclusion, it seems that recently the pendulum has been oscillating towards preoperative irradiation + surgical excision as the standard approach for the treatment of resectable rectal cancer. However, other aspects should be taken into consideration for future research. First, total mesorectal excision without any adjuvant chemo- or radiotherapy is associated with excellent results in terms of recurrence rate and overall survival [69–71]; it is not known whether these figures can be improved by adjuvant preoperative or postoperative irradiation. Second, in order to keep the advantages and to minimize the disadvantages of both preoperative and postoperative radiotherapy, some authors suggested "sandwich" irradiation [110]; with this approach, a small preoperative dose might kill viable cells disseminated at the time of the surgical procedure, and a second postoperative dose could consolidate the results. Third, as already discussed, there is evidence that adding of 5-fluorouracil-based chemotherapy to standard surgery and radiotherapy may reduce the recurrence rate and prolong survival in patients with rectal malignancies [98–100]; it is possible that further refinements of this approach may render the choice between preoperative or postoperative irradiation less crucial. Finally, the wide diffusion of new and sophisticated diagnostic procedures (such as endorectal sonography, computed tomography and nuclear magnetic imaging) might allow a more accurate preoperative staging of these patients, with the consequent possible selection of individuals who are amenable to be treated with surgery alone or require a specific combination of radiotherapy and/or chemotherapy.

Management of Locally Recurrent Cancer

Local recurrence is a significant and persistent problem in the treatment of colorectal malignancies after apparently curative surgical excision. A recurrence can be defined as a regrowth of cancer in and around the tumor bed, including the pericolic fat, the mesentery and the suture line of the bowel anastomosis. Local recurrences are associated with profound morbidity and a severe impairment of the quality of life. The main symptoms include abdominal discomfort, pain, intestinal obstruction, bleeding, perforation and septic complications [115]. Most recurrences occur within 2-3 years of the original operation in patients who are otherwise in good clinical condition and often free from metastatic disease. The incidence of local recurrence after apparently curative resection varies between 2% and 32% and is more frequent for rectal carcinoma, presumably owing to the major complexity of pelvic surgery [116, 117]. Moreover, most recurrences of rectal cancer develop as isolated deposits, usually not associated with disseminated disease [118]; in contrast, in colonic carcinoma the majority of local recurrences occur together with metastasis in other organs [119].

As pointed out by Abulafi and Williams [120], the factors influencing local recurrence may be related to the patient, the tumor or the surgical procedure. As far as patients are concerned, there is evidence that local recurrence rates increase progressively with age [121]. Factors related to the neoplasm include stage and number of lymph nodes involved [120], mucinous histological type [122], tumor location in the rectum (i.e. neoplasms occurring within 6 cm of the anal verge are associated with an increased rate of local recurrence) [123], fixity of the tumor [124], presence of venous or perineural invasion at histology [125] and degree of tumor differentiation [126]. Among factors related to surgery, as already discussed the experience of the operator executing surgery is of major importance [79, 80]; in addition, local recurrences may be affected by the type of operation [127], the choice of mesorectal excision [68], the use of stapling devices [128] and tumor perforation during surgery [129].

The only option of cure for patients with local recurrences is the surgical removal of deposits, while chemotherapy or irradiation are of virtually no benefit. However, as underlined by Sagar and Pemberton [126], this kind of surgery may involve major procedures and "is not for the faint-hearted man". Even when a radical approach is not possible, surgery may offer good palliation and in many cases a better quality of life. A careful clinical history, together with physical examination, biochemical tests (especially carcinoembryonic antigen, CEA, serum levels during the follow-up) [130] and new imaging techniques (such as computed tomography and positron emission tomography) [131] can identify a proportion of patients with local recurrence who are candidates for a surgical attempt. The strategies depend closely on the type of recurrence. For local recurrences around the anastomosis, resection of the anastomosis – possibly with a sphincter-saving procedure – is probably the technique of choice, providing the tumor is not fixed to the surrounding structures [126]. Isolated perineal recurrences after Miles operation may be treated with local wide excision, which is more often palliative [132]. Anterior recurrences limited to the neorectum and anterior organs (such as bladder, prostate, vagina and uterus) may require exenterative procedures, with "en bloc" resection of the neoplasm and involved organs; the value of this mutilating surgery is controversial, but it does provide an option for patients in whom there is no hope of other treatments [133].

Considering that the rate of survival of patients with local recurrences is less than 4% at 5 years without surgery, with a median life expectancy of 7 months [134], and that according to some observations surgery may be curative in up to 1/3 of the patients [126], many surgeons maintain an "aggressive" attitude towards recurrence. Thus, in a retrospective study of 524 patients with colorectal neoplasms operated on by one surgeon between 1975 and 1992, local recurrences developed in 124 (23.7%) [135]. Patients in whom no intervention was possible survived an average of 28 months. Thirty patients (24.2%) underwent re-resection for cure, and half of them were alive after a mean of 80 months; moreover, those who died of the disease despite re-resection did so at an average of 53 months. The authors concluded that in those patients in whom re-resection is possible, up to 50% of them may achieve long-term survival. However, according to other studies, surgical treatment of local recurrence is possible in only 5%–10% of the patients, and over 90% of these individuals die of the disease within 3 years [136, 137].

Treatment of Advanced Colorectal Tumors

An advanced colorectal neoplasm can be defined as a tumor that at diagnosis is either metastatic (usually in the liver or lung) or so locally advanced as to preclude surgical approaches with curative intent. Data from cancer registries [138, 139] indicate that still at present about 1/3–1/4 of all colorectal malignancies become manifest in an advanced stage, and for most of them the prospects of cure are rather poor. However, in the last two decades several advances have been made in the management of these patients. Although in most cases the approach has been palliative, this nevertheless may result in an objective clinical response, improved quality of life and better survival.

Surgical Treatment of Metastatic Colorectal Cancer

The liver is the most frequent site of metastasis, and in selected patients surgical excision represents the only hope of cure. However, it should be stressed that this type of radical surgery is possible in only a minority (not exceeding 20%) of patients who have metastasis at presentation [140].

Although the first successful liver resection for metastatic colorectal cancer dates back to 1940 [141], in most recent years the technique took advantage of the definition of the segmental nature of liver anatomy, which rendered limited resection possible instead of radical lobectomy. In addition, the ability of the liver to regenerate rapidly (an event well known to mythology, as in the legend of Prometheus) allowed resections of up to 70% of the liver mass without impairing function permanently. The most important factor in determining resectability and prognosis is the number of metastatic nodules within the liver and, thus, the "metastatic burden" [142]. In the small fraction of patients in whom the liver involvement is limited to a single lobe or segment, resection is not only relatively simple but is associated with a 5-year survival of up to 35%–40% [143], while in individuals with 2 or 3 lesions survival drops to 15%–20% [144]. According to some series, even resection of multiple lesions can be followed by prolonged survival in an appreciable number of patients; thus, Doci et al. [145] reported a median survival of 28 months in 18 patients in whom 3 or more metastatic nodules were resected, and similar observations were reported by Elias and collaborators [146]. At variance with these relatively optimistic results, other investigators showed worse survival results for resections of 4 or more lesions, with virtually no patient alive at 5 years [147]. Clearly, the selection of patients and the experience of the surgeons are critical factors in this type of surgery. Another factor which may complicate or contraindicate liver resection is the presence of lung metastasis, although various investigators report the results of resecting both liver and lung metastatic lesions, with limited success [148]. Other factors which seem to have a negative impact on the prognosis after resection of liver metastases include poorly differentiated histological type of neoplasm, involvement of abdominal lymph nodes, extrahepatic sites of metastasis, surgical margins free of tumor, and bilobar liver deposits [142, 149]. The possible role of adjuvant chemotherapy after resection of liver metastases remains to be demonstrated [148].

Chemotherapy for Advanced Colorectal Cancer

Although in patients with advanced colorectal neoplasms chemotherapy is usually administered for palliation rather than for cure, several studies have shown a certain benefit of 5-fluorouracil-based treatments [150], and new promising regimes have been proposed and are under careful evaluation [151]. There is evidence from large randomized trials and from meta-analysis that 5-fluorouracil-based chemotherapy adds 5–6 months to the remaining life of these patients; in addition, treatment delays the progression of symptoms and improves symptom control and functional performance in about one-half of individuals with advanced colorectal lesions [149].

While there is consensus on the role of 5-fluorouracil-based therapy, controversies persist as to the choice of the most appropriate approach. Intravenous bolus infusion is still widely used, although there is evidence that continuous infusion of 5-fluorouracil as a single agent may be superior in terms of tumor response, but not in increasing survival [152]. Other investigations showed that modulation of 5-fluorouracil with folinic acid or methotrexate increases the tumor response compared with bolus 5-fluorouracil alone, but again, no definite improvement in survival was observed [153, 154]. Moreover, other authors failed to document any difference in tumor response between modulated bolus and infusional 5-fluorouracil [155]. In these investigations, 5-fluorouracil was given at doses of 370–600 mg/m^2 of body surface area, and leucovorin at 20–500 mg/m^2, usually for 1–5 days per week every 4–5 weeks (or weekly for 6–8 weeks). In a recent meta-analysis, Buyse et al. [156] evaluated 25 randomized trials of first-line treatment with 5-fluorouracil bolus injection versus four "experimental" treatments (5-fluorouracil + leucovorin; fluorouracil + methotrexate; fluorouracil continuous infusion; and fluorouracil hepatic artery infusion) in patients with advanced colorectal malignancies. The results showed that the experimental regimens are superior to standard bolus 5-fluorouracil in terms of tumor response and revealed a small, though significant, overall survival benefit. The advantages, however, were much more evident and impressive in terms of response rate than in terms of survival. The available evidence, therefore, suggests that modulated bolus (by folinic acid or methotrexate) as well as infusional 5-fluorouracil regimens are both effective treatments for patients with inoperable colorectal neoplasms, though we should expect only minor benefits in survival.

For at least 3 decades, fluoropyrimidine-based regimens represented the only option of treatment for advanced colorectal cancer. Recently, several interesting new drugs have shown efficacy, giving the impression to some authors that we are "moving beyond Fluorouracil for colorectal cancer" [157]. Irinotecan is a semisynthetic camptothecin derivative inhibiting DNA topoisomerase I which shows some activity against colorectal cancer cell lines "in vitro" [158]; the drug has no cross-resistance with 5-fluorouracil and, thus, functions through a novel molecular mechanism. The most relevant side-effects associated with its use are diarrhea – which may be troublesome, especially in elderly and debilitated patients – neutropenia, early cholinergic syndrome, nausea, vomiting, alopecia and fatigue [159]. In phase II studies, irinotecan showed objective antitumour activity in patients with advanced colorectal malignancies, even in those with documented resistance to 5-fluorouracil, and response rates of the order of 10%–20% [160]. These findings suggested that the development of regimens that combine irinotecan with full-dose fluorouracil and folinic acid might be beneficial as the first-line treatment of patients with colorectal neoplasms. Cunningham et al. [161] evaluated the effect of irinotecan (300–350 mg/m^2 every 3 weeks) plus supportive care versus supportive care alone in patients with metastatic colorectal cancer which had progressed despite treatment with 5-fluorouracil. With a median follow-up of 13 months, survival was significantly increased in the irinotecan group (32.6% versus 13.8% in the supportive care group); moreover, despite the expected side-effects (especially diarrhea and neutropenia), symptoms like pain, weight loss and progressive deterioration of the general status were significantly better in patients receiving irinotecan. In a recent multicentre randomized study, Douillard et al. [162] compared irinotecan

(80 mg/m²) plus 5-fluorouracil (2,300 mg/m² by 24 h infusion) and calcium folinate (500 mg/m²) versus 5-fluorouracil and calcium folinate alone. The response rate was superior in the irinotecan group (49 vs 31%, $p < 0.001$), and time to progression was significantly longer and overall survival higher (17.4 vs 14.1 months, $p = 0.031$). Moreover, Saltz et al. [163] studied 683 patients with advanced colorectal neoplasms who were randomly assigned to receive irinotecan, 5-fluorouracil and leucovorin weekly for 4 weeks every 6 weeks, 5-fluorouracil and leucovorin daily for 5 days every 4 weeks, or irinotecan alone weekly for 4 weeks every 6 weeks. Patients who were given the full regimen (irinotecan plus 5-fluorouracil and folinic acid) had a higher rate of objective response, a longer time before tumors progressed, and a longer median survival (15 months vs 13 and 12 months in the other two groups). Diarrhea and neutropenia were relevant side-effects, but were counterbalanced by the improvement of many other cancer-related symptoms, and did not preclude the administration of about 75% of the prescribed dose of irinotecan and 5-fluorouracil. Clearly, these studies indicate that irinotecan plus 5-fluorouracil/folinic acid represents a valid alternative standard front-line regimen in the treatment of patients with advanced colorectal cancer [5, 164].

Several other treatment modalities for metastatic colorectal malignancies have been suggested and are at present under active investigation. Oxaliplatin is a third-generation platinum complex with single-agent activity against colorectal cancer; moreover, this compound appears synergistic with fluorouracil both in vitro and in the active treatment of patients. This activity is of particular interest because of the inefficacy of other platinum drugs – such as cisplatin and carboplatin – in colorectal neoplasms [157]. Phase II studies [165] showed the feasibility of combining oxaliplatin with various 5-fluorouracil plus folinic acid regimens as the first-line treatment of advanced colorectal cancer. In a large controlled phase III investigation [166], 420 patients were randomized to receive a standard fluoropyrimidine-based regimen with or without oxaliplatin. Median progression-free survival was significantly longer in the oxaliplatin group (9.0 vs 6.2 months, $p < 0.003$), whereas overall survival showed only a trend in favor of oxaliplatin (16.2 vs 14.7 months, NS). These recent findings suggest that oxaliplatin and irinotecan – when either is associated with 5-fluorouracil and folinic acid – may exhibit similar activity against advanced colorectal tumors. In addition, the different mechanisms of action and non-overlapping dose-limiting toxicity profiles of irinotecan and oxaliplatin clearly suggest that these two agents might also be used in combination. This possibility has been explored in preliminary investigations [167, 168] which showed response rates ranging from 17% to 64% of the treated patients.

A combination of uracil and tegafur (UFT) showed some activity against colorectal, gastric and other neoplasms [169]; according to some authors [170], the association UFT/leucovorin might represent an acceptable alternative to intravenous 5-fluorouracil/leucovorin for the treatment of advanced colorectal neoplasms. Capecitabine is an oral fluoropyrimidine which is converted to 5-fluorouracil after gastrointestinal absorption [171]. Preliminary results indicate that this agent is superior to bolus 5-fluorouracil in terms of response rates and incidence of neutropenia [172], though the duration of response and time to disease progression were similar. Thus, capecitabine might represent a valuable option when oral regimens are required for patients with advanced disease and poor clinical condition. Eniluracil is an inhibitor of the rate-limiting enzyme in the degradation of 5-fluorouracil. This agent does not possess antitumoral activity by itself, but may improve the therapeutic activity of 5-fluorouracil [173]. In a phase II study [174], the association eniluracil plus 5-fluorouracil as the first-line treatment of advanced colorectal cancer showed a response rate of 24% without significant side-effects. Finally, bryostatin 1 [175] is a macrocyclic lactone derived from a murine intervertebrate which possesses several biological activities, including a direct cytotoxic effect in some human cancer cell lines [176], with minimal toxicity. In a phase II study including 28 patients with advanced colorectal lesions, no partial or complete tumor responses were observed [175]; the authors, however, concluded that the compound deserves further consideration, especially for evaluating the possible effect of the combination of bryostatin 1 with other cytotoxic agents.

Toxicity and Cost of Chemotherapy in Advanced Colorectal Cancer

As already discussed, the cytotoxic agents commonly used for the treatment of patients with metastatic colorectal neoplasm are not devoid of toxicity. It follows that chemotherapy should be prescribed by experienced oncologists who are familiar with the side-effects of a given regimen. However, despite these concerns, the currently used infusional treatments are well tolerated by the majority of treated subjects. The most common of these adverse effects include diarrhea, mucositis, neutropenia, nausea and vomiting, alopecia, anorexia and fatigue. Diarrhea can be treated with loperamide or other antimotility agents. Mucositis can be managed with antiseptic mouthwash and early treatment of oral candidosis. Prolonged treatment with 5-fluorouracil can induce painful erythema of the palms and soles, which may respond to treatment with pyridoxine [149].

Patients with advanced colorectal carcinoma represent approximately 1/4 of all cases [1]; in a country such as Italy or Britain this means some 6,000–8,000 new cases per year. There is evidence [149] that the overall cost of treatment in patients with advanced lesions is similar to that of no treatment, and that chemotherapy – as part of the management of the advanced disease – is cost effective. However, the burden of patients and the high cost of most of the recent available drugs pose serious problems for National Health Services in all developed and industrialized countries.

Other Treatments for Advanced Colorectal Neoplasms

Other treatments for metastatic colorectal neoplasms include loco-regional approaches (such as hepatic arterial chemotherapy or embolization) radiation therapy and liver transplantation. The general impression is that although some of these treatments achieved popularity, in most recent years the interest of investigators has been addressed towards the use of systemic combined chemotherapy, leaving a very limited role to the more invasive and cumbersome local therapies.

The hepatic arterial infusion of cytotoxic drugs (usually floxuridine) requires abdominal surgery to insert an arterial catheter and implant an expensive infusion pump [85, 148]. The rationale of this approach is based on three main observations. First, the liver is the most important and often the only site of metastatic disease; it follows that an aggressive treatment focused on this organ might yield prolonged survival for some subjects. Second, liver metastases derive their blood supply mostly from the hepatic artery (in contrast to hepatocytes, which are mainly nourished through the portal vein). Third, certain agents have a high first-pass hepatic clearance, which results in high local concentrations of drug with low systemic toxicity. The frequency of tumor shrinkage is consequently higher with hepatic arterial infusion than with systemic therapy, but injury to the liver and bile duct is common and sometimes irreversible [177]. Several randomized investigations compared arterial infusion in terms of response rates and reduction of the tumoral mass, but benefits in survival were less evident. To summarize, there is little or no evidence supporting the use of this expensive and complex approach in the palliative treatment of patients with colorectal cancer metastasized to the liver.

Hepatic artery ligation or embolization (with particles such as gel foam, polyvinyl alcohol, collagen or microspheres) have been used to treat liver metastasis from colorectal cancer, but with disappointing results, mainly due to the rapid development of collateral vessels [180, 181]. With chemoembolization, drugs (cisplatin, 5-fluorouracil) are injected in the hepatic artery together with embolization agents; this combination approach provides a prolonged exposure of tumors to the cytotoxic effect of the given compounds, with fewer systemic effects [182]. This treatment has shown some efficacy in patients with hepatocellular carcinoma [183]. In a prospective, randomized trial involving 61 patients with liver metastases from colorectal carcinoma [184], embolization and chemoembolization had virtually no effect on survival.

Radiation therapy has only a palliative role in the treatment of hepatic metastases. This treatment may improve the severe pain due to liver involvement, but results concerning tumor response and survival remain extremely poor [185]. Finally, in contrast to the promising results obtained in selected patients with hepatocellular carcinoma [186], liver transplantation has no role, at present, in the treatment of metastatic liver disease [148].

Innovative Treatments for Colorectal Cancer

Novel approaches in the treatment of colorectal cancer include the use of monoclonal antibodies directed against tumor antigens and gene therapy. Both treatment modalities should be viewed as experimental, but nonetheless represent new strategies which are attracting the attention of several investigators and deserve full consideration for future basic and applied research.

Monoclonal antibodies and radiolabelled antibodies have been used in the treatment of advanced disease [187] but with disappointing clinical effects. The results seem to be more favorable when these agents are used as adjuvant therapy. Riethmuller et al. [188] used this approach in patients with stage III colorectal carcinoma; they employed the monoclonal antibody CO17-1A (a murine IgG directed against a cell surface glycoprotein of colorectal cancer cells also expressed in normal epithelium) and obtained clinical results almost comparable to those of standard adjuvant chemotherapy. The effect of the antibody was more evident in patients with distant metastases as the first sign of relapse, whereas no favorable effect was seen for local recurrence. This can be attributed to the poorly vascularized connective scar tissue – at the site of local relapse – which partially prevented the penetration of antibodies. Behr et al. [189] treated nude mice with pulmonary micrometastases from colorectal cancer by giving a iodine (I^{131})-labeled monoclonal antibody fragment directed against carcinoembryonic antigen; untreated animals died from rapidly progressing disease within 4–8 weeks, whereas radioimmunotreated animals showed a 53%–80% cure rate. The authors concluded that in this experimental setting targeted radionuclide therapy was superior to conventional chemotherapy. In a recent study, Ward et al. [190] treated 17 patients affected by metastatic colorectal cancer with a recombinant monoclonal antibody (c30.6) directed against an antigen expressed on a high proportion of colorectal carcinomas and their metastasis. Although the results showed no complete or partial response, the authors suggested that this new chimeric antibody deserves further investigation. Clearly, more studies are needed in order to establish any possible role of monoclonal antibodies in colorectal cancer therapy.

Gene therapy is a novel approach based on the direct modification of gene expression in the somatic cells of a given patient. Cancer gene therapy involves the introduction of therapeutic genes into tumoral cells with the purpose of inhibiting tumor growth [191]. In theory, gene therapy might consist of the correction of a single gene defect which causes the neoplastic phenotype; this objective, however, remains elusive for most cancers – including colorectal neoplasms – since the malignant transformation is usually associated with a series of genetic mutations. The targets of gene therapy are oncogenes (that can be inactivated through the antisense oligonucleotide technology [192]) and especially tumor suppressor genes, which are more closely associated with the control of cell replication and differentiation. The p53 gene contributes to the regulation of the cell cycle and is implicated in the mechanisms of apoptosis [193]; inactivation of this tumor suppressor gene leads to uncontrolled replication, while restoration of wild-type p53 inhibits tumor growth. Sixteen patients with p53-mutated colorectal cancer metastases have been treated with an adenovirus encoding wild-type p53 infused through the hepatic artery. Although the procedure was well tolerated, no evidence of tumor response was seen at 1 month [194]. In other studies [195], evidence of regression was observed in some of the investigated patients, though the results remain largely preliminary. In conclusion, therefore, further studies are needed to confirm the therapeutic potential of gene therapy.

Conclusions

Surgery remains the best option of cure for patients with colorectal malignancies. If the trend towards a more frequent diagnosis of early disease continues [1, 4], the surgical approach might become curative in the large majority of these patients. Moreover, the widespread diffusion of mesorectal excision may lead to a significant reduction of local recurrence, while the recent developments of laparoscopic surgery can allow shorter hospitalization and smaller scars. Adjuvant chemotherapy has become a mainstay in treating stage III individuals and selected patients with stage II disease, though population-based evidence of a definitive survival benefit is still lacking. The treatment of recurrence and of advanced disease remains unsatisfactory; however, several new drugs and regimens are under evaluation, and novel approaches – such as monoclonal antibodies against tumor antigens and gene therapy – might expand our therapeutic armamentarium. The battle against colorectal tumors is still ongoing, but the enemy does not appears as tremendous as in the past.

References

1. Ponz de Leon M, Benatti P, Percesepe A et al. Epidemiology of cancer of the large bowel – The 12-year experience of a specialized Registry in Northern Italy. Ital J Gastroenterol Hepatol 1999; 31:10-8.
2. McArdle C. ABC of colorectal cancer. Primary treatment – does the surgeon matter? Br Med J 2000; 321:1121-3.
3. Michelassi F, Vannucci L, Ayala JJ et al. Local recurrence after curative resection of colorectal carcinoma. Surgery 1990; 108:787-93.
4. Pheils MT, Chapuis PH, Newland RC et al. Local recurrence following curative resection for carcinoma of the rectum. Dis Colon Rectum 1983; 26:98-102.
5. Boland CR, Sinicrope FA, Brenner DE et al. Colorectal cancer prevention and treatment. Gastroenterology 2000; 118:S115-S128.
6. Maxwell-Armstrong CA, Robinson MH, Scholefield JH. Laparoscopic colorectal cancer surgery. Am J Surg 2000; 179:500-7.
7. Raynolds JV, Joyce WP, Dolan J et al. Pathological evidence in support of total mesorectal excision in the management of rectal cancer. Br J Surg 1996; 83:1112-5.
8. Mohiuddin M, Marks G. Adjuvant radiation therapy for colon and rectal cancer. Semin Oncol 1991; 18:421-42.
9. Gatta G, Buiatti E, Conti E et al. Variations in the survival of adult cancer patients in Italy. Tumori 1997; 83:497-504.
10. Ponz de Leon M, Benatti P, Di Gregorio C et al. Staging and survival of colorectal cancer: are we making progress? The 14-year experience of a specialized cancer Registry. Digest Liver Dis 2000; 32:312-7.
11. Dukes CE. The classification of cancer of the rectum. J Pathol Bacteriol 1932; 35:1489-94.
12. Cooper HS, Slemmer JR. Surgical pathology of carcinoma of the colon and rectum. Semin Oncol 1991; 18:367-380.
13. Hutter RVP, Sobin LH. A universal staging system for cancer of the colon and rectum. Arch Pathol Lab Med 1986; 110:367-8.
14. Niederhuber JE. Colon and rectum cancer: pattern of spread and implications for workup. Cancer 1993; 71:4187-92.

15. Greenson JK, Isenhart CE, Rice R et al. Identification of occult micrometastases in pericolic lymph nodes of Dukes' B colorectal cancer patients using monoclonal antibodies against cytokeratin and CC49. Cancer 1994; 73:563-9.
16. Cutait R, Alves V, Lopes LC et al. Restaging of colorectal cancer based on the identification of lymph node micrometastases through immunoperoxidase staining of CEA and cytokeratins. Dis Colon Rectum 1991; 34:917-20.
17. Losi L, Benhattar J, Costa J. Stability of K-ras mutations throughout the natural history of human colorectal cancer. Eur J Cancer 1992; 28 A:1115-20.
18. Dix BR, Robbins PD, Spagnolo DV et al. Clonal analysis of colorectal tumors using K-ras and p53 gene mutations as markers. Diagn Mol Pathol 1995; 4:261-5.
19. Shibata D, Schaeffer J, Li ZH et al. Genetic heterogeneity of the c-K-ras locus in colorectal adenomas but not in adenocarcinomas. J Natl Cancer Inst 1993; 85:1058-63.
20. Thebo JS, Senagore AJ, Reinhold DS et al. Molecular staging of colorectal cancer. K-ras mutation analysis of lymph nodes upstages Dukes B patients. Dis Colon Rectum 2000; 43:155-62.
21. Chantereau MJ, Faivre J, Boutron MC et al. Epidemiology, management, and prognosis of malignant large bowel polyps within a defined population. Gut 1992; 33:259-63.
22. Eckardt VF, Fuchs M, Kanzler G et al. Follow up of patients with colonic polyps containing severe atypia and invasive carcinoma: compliance recurrence and survival. Cancer 1998; 61:2552-7.
23. Cranley JP, Peters RE, Carey WD et al. When is endoscopic polypectomy adequate therapy for colonic polyps containing invasive carcinoma? Gastroenterology 1986; 91: 419-27.
24. Anwar S, White J, Hall C et al. Sporadic colorectal polyps: management options and guidelines. Scand J Gastroenterol 1999; 34:4-11.
25. Stearns MW, Schottenfeld D. Techniques for the surgical management of colon cancer. Cancer 1971; 28:165-9.
26. Rosi PA. Hemicolectomy in the treatment of carcinoma of the left colon. Quart Bull Northwest Univ Med Sch 1949; 23:376-83.
27. Sugarbaker PH, Corlew S. Influence of surgical techniques on survival in patients with colorectal cancer. Dis Colon Rectum 1982; 25:545-7.
28. The French Association for Surgical Research. Rouffet F, Hay JM, Vacher B et al. Curative resection for left colonic carcinoma: hemicolectomy vs segmental colectomy. A prospective, controlled, multicenter trial. Dis Colon Rectum 1994; 37:651-9.
29. Mecklin JP, Svendsen LB, Peltomaki P et al. Hereditary Nonpolyposis Colorectal Cancer. Scand J Gastroenterol 1994; 29:673-7.
30. Jass JR. Current problems in diagnosis and management of Hereditary Bowel Cancer. Asian J Surgery 1995; 18(2):166-73.
31. Lynch HT, Fusaro RM, Lynch J. Hereditary cancer in adults. Cancer Detect Prev 1995; 19(3):219-33.
32. Nance FC. Management strategies for familial adenomatous polyposis. Ann Surg 1993; 217:99-100.
33. Ziv Y, Church JM, Oakley JR et al. Surgery for the teenager with familial adenomatous polyposis: ileo-rectal anastomosis or restorative proctocolectomy? Int J Colorect Dis 1995; 10:6-9.
34. Wu JS, Paul P, McGannon EA et al. APC genotype, polyp number, and surgical options in familial adenomatous polyposis. Ann Surg 1998; 227:57-62.
35. Van Duijvendijk P, Slors FM, Taat CW et al. Functional outcome after colectomy and ileorectal anastomosis compared with proctocolectomy and ileal pouch-anal anastomosis in familial adenomatous polyposis. Ann Surg 1999; 230:648-654.
36. Niv Y, Fraser GM. Adenocarcinoma in the rectal segment in familial polyposis coli is not prevented by sulindac therapy. Gastroenterology 1994; 107:854-7.
37. Wiggers T, Arends P, Schutte B et al. A multivariate analysis of pathologic prognostic indicators in large bowel cancer. Cancer 1988; 61:386-95.

38. Ponz de Leon M, Sant M, Micheli A et al. Clinical and pathologic prognostic indicators in colorectal cancer. A population-based study. Cancer 1992; 69:626-35.
39. Soper NJ, Brunt LM, Kerbl K. Laparoscopic general surgery. N Engl J Med 1994; 330: 409-19.
40. Monson JRT. Advanced techniques in abdominal surgery. Br Med J 1993; 307:1346-50.
41. Lacy AM, Garcia-Valdecasas JC, Pique JM et al. Short term outcome analysis of a randomised study comparing laparoscopic vs open colectomy for colon cancer. Surg Endosc 1995; 9:1101-5.
42. Van Ye TM, Cattey RP, Henry LG. Laparoscopically assisted colon resections compare favourably with open technique. Surg Laparosc Endosc 1994; 4:25-31.
43. Dean PA, Beart RW, Nelson H et al. Laparoscopic-assisted segmental colectomy: early Mayo Clinic experience. Mayo Clin Proc 1994; 69:834-40.
44. Gellman L, Salky B, Edye M. Laparoscopic assisted colectomy. Surg Endosc 1996; 10:1041-4.
45. Kuntz C, Wunsch A, Bay F et al. Prospective randomized study of stress and immune response after laparoscopic vs conventional colonic resection. Surg Endosc 1998; 12: 963-7.
46. Khalili TM, Fleshner PR, Hiatt JR et al. Colorectal cancer. Comparison of laparoscopic with open approaches. Dis Colon Rectum 1998; 41:832-8.
47. Lord SA, Larach SW, Ferrara A et al. Laparoscopic resections for colorectal carcinoma; a 3-year experience. Dis Colon Rectum 1996; 39:148-54.
48. Bokey EL, Moore JWE, Chapuis PH et al. Morbidity and mortality following laparoscopic-assisted right hemicolectomy for cancer. Dis Colon Rectum 1996; 39: S24-8.
49. Begos DG, Arsenault J, Ballantyne GH. Laparoscopic colon and rectal surgery at a VA hospital: analysis of the first 50 cases. Surg Endosc 1996; 10:1050-6.
50. Vukasin P, Ortega AE, Greene Fl et al. Wound recurrence following laparoscopic colon cancer resection. Results of the American Society of Colon and Rectal surgeons laparoscopic Registry. Dis Colon Rectum 1996; 39:S20-3.
51. COST Study Group. Early results of laparoscopic surgery for colorectal cancer. Retrospective analysis of 372 patients treated by Clinical Outcomes of Surgical Therapy (COST) study group. Dis Colon Rectum 1996; 39:S53-8.
52. Allardyce RA, Morreau P, Bagshaw PF. Operative factors affecting tumor cell distribution following laparoscopic colectomy in a porcine model. Dis Colon Rectum 1997; 40:939-45.
53. Paik PS, Beart RW. Laparoscopic colectomy. Surg Clin North Am 1997; 77:1-13.
54. Watson DI, Mathew G, Ellis T et al. Gasless laparoscopy may reduce the risk of port site metastases following laparoscopic tumor surgery. Arch Surg 1997; 132:166-8.
55. Lockhart-Mummery JP. Two hundred cases of cancer of the rectum treated by perineal excision. Br J Surg 1926; 14:110-24.
56. Gabriel WB. The end results of perineal excision and of radium in the treatment of cancer of the rectum. Br J Surg 1932; 20:234-48.
57. Miles WE. A method of performing abdominoperineal excision for carcinoma of the rectum and of the terminal portion of the pelvic colon. Lancet 1908; 2:1812-3.
58. Mayo WJ. The radical operation for cancer of the rectum and rectosigmoid. Trans Am Surg Assoc 1916; XXXIV:261-72.
59. Pena A, Beart RW Jr. Carcinoma of the rectum. In: Corman ML ed. Colon and rectal surgery. Philadelphia: JB Lippincott 1993:596-720.
60. Donaldson GA, Rodkey GV, Behringer GE. Resection of the rectum with anal preservation. Surg Gynecol Obstet 1966; 123:571-80.
61. Beart RW Jr, Kelly KA. Randomized prospective evaluation of the EEA stapler for colorectal anastomoses. Am J Surg 1981; 141:143-7.
62. Knight CD, Griffen FD. An improved technique for low anterior resection of the rectum using the EEA stapler. Surgery 1980; 88:710-4.

63. Williams NS, Johnston D. Survival and recurrence after sphincter saving resection and abdominoperineal resection for carcinoma of the middle third of the rectum. Br J Surg 1984; 71:278-82.
64. Lavery IC, Lopez-Kostner F, Fazio VW et al. Chances of cure are not compromised with sphincter-saving procedures for cancer of the lower third of the rectum. Surgery 1997; 122:779-84.
65. Zaheer S, Pemberton JH, Farouk R et al. Surgical treatment of adenocarcinoma of the rectum. Ann Surg 1998; 227:800-11.
66. Rosen L, Veidenheiimer MC, Coller JA et al. Mortality, morbidity, and patterns of recurrence after abdominoperineal resection for cancer of the rectum. Dis Colon Rectum 1982; 25:202-8.
67. Ruo L, Guillem JG. Major 20th-century advancements in the management of rectal cancer. Dis Colon Rectum 1999; 42:563-78.
68. Heald RJ, Husband EM, Ryall RD. The mesorectum in rectal cancer surgery – the clue to pelvic recurrence? Br J Surg 1982; 69:613-6.
69. Bonadeo FA, Vaccaro CA, Benati ML et al. Rectal cancer. Local recurrence after surgery without radiotherapy. Dis Colon Rectum 2001; 44:374-9.
70. Hainsworth PJ, Egan MJ, Cunliffe WJ. Evaluation of a policy of total mesorectal excision for rectal and rectosigmoid cancers. Br J Surg 1997; 84:652-6.
71. Heald RJ, Moran BJ, Ryall RDH et al. Rectal cancer. The Basingstoke experience of total mesorectal excision, 1978-1997. Arch Surg 1998; 133:894-9.
72. Stearns MW, Deddish MR. Five-year results of abdominopelvic lymph node dissection for carcinoma of the rectum. Dis Colon Rectum 1959; 2:169-72.
73. Glass RE, Ritchie JK, Thompson HR et al. The results of surgical treatment of cancer of the rectum by radical resection and extended abdomino-iliac lymphadenectomy. Br J Surg 1985; 72:599-601.
74. Moreira LF, Hizuta A, Iwagaki H et al. Lateral lymph node dissection for rectal carcinoma below the peritoneal reflection. Br J Surg 1994; 81:293-6.
75. Hojo K, Sawada T, Moriya Y. An analysis of survival and voiding, sexual function after wide iliopelvic lymphadenectomy in patients with carcinoma of the rectum, compared with conventional lymphadenectomy. Dis Colon Rectum 1989; 32:128-33.
76. Fazio VW, Fletcher J, Mantague D. Prospective study of the effect of resection of the rectum on male sexual function. World J Surg 1980; 4:149-52.
77. Maas CP, Moriya Y, Steup WH et al. Radical and nerve-preserving surgery for rectal cancer in The Netherlands: a prospective study on morbidity and functional outcome. Br J Surg 1998; 85:92-7.
78. Havenga K, Enker WE, McDermott K et al. Male and female sexual and urinary function after total mesorectal excision with autonomic nerve preservation for carcinoma of the rectum. J Am Coll Surg 1996; 182:495-502.
79. Holm T, Johansson H, Cedermark B et al. Influence of hospital and surgeon related factors and outcome after treatment of rectal cancer with or without pre-operative radiotherapy. Br J Surg 1997; 87:657-63.
80. Parry JM, Collins S, Mathers J et al. Influence of volume of work on the outcome of treatment for patients with colorectal cancer. Br J Surg 1998; 86:475-81.
81. Buyse M, Zeleniuch-Jacquotte A, Chalmers TC. Adjuvant therapy of colorectal cancer. Why we still don't know. JAMA 1988; 259:3571-8.
82. Moertel CG, Fleming TR, Macdonald JS et al. Levamisole and fluorouracil for adjuvant therapy of resected colon carcinoma. N Engl J Med 1990; 322:352-8.
83. Moertel CG, Fleming TR, Macdonald JS et al. Fluorouracil plus Levamisole as effective adjuvant therapy after resection of stage III colon carcinoma: a final report. Ann Intern Med 1995; 122:321-6.
84. Fuchs CS, Mayer RJ. Adjuvant chemotherapy for colon and rectal cancer. Semin Oncol 1995; 22:472-87.
85. Moertel CG. Chemotherapy for colorectal cancer. N Engl J Med 1994; 330:1136-42.

86. Midgley RS, Kerr DJ. Adjuvant treatment of colorectal cancer. Cancer Treat Rev 1997; 23:135-52.
87. Midgley RS, Kerr DJ. ABC of colorectal cancer. Adjuvant therapy. Br Med J 2000; 321; 1208-11.
88. Moertel CG, Fleming TR, Macdonald JS et al. Hepatic toxicity with fluorouracil plus levamisole adjuvant therapy. J Clin Oncol 1993; 11:2386-90.
89. Ky AJ, Sung MW, Milsom JW. Research in colon and rectal cancer, with an emphasis on surgical progress. Dis Colon Rectum 1999; 42:1369-80.
90. Grem JL, Hoth DF, Hamilton JM et al. Overview of current status and future direction of clinical trials with 5-fluorouracil in combination with folinic acid. Cancer Treat Rep 1987; 71:1249-64.
91. Poon MA, O'Connell MJ, Moertel CG et al. Biochemical modulation of fluorouracil: evidence of significant improvement of survival and quality of life in advanced colorectal carcinoma. J Clin Oncol 1989; 7:1419-26.
92. Valone FH, Friedman MA, Wittlinger PS et al. Treatment of patients with advanced colorectal carcinomas with 5-FU alone, high dose leucovorin plus 5-FU or sequential methotrexate, 5-FU, leucovorin: a randomized trial of the Northern California Oncology Group. J Clin Oncol 1989; 7:1427-36.
93. Wolmark N, Rockette H, Fisher B et al. The benefit of leucovorin-modulated fluorouracil as postoperative adjuvant therapy for primary colon cancer: results from National Surgical Adjuvant Breast and Bowel Project protocol C-03. J Clin Oncol 1993; 11:1879-87.
94. Francini G, Petrioli R, Lorenzini L et al. Folinic acid and 5-fluorouracil as adjuvant chemotherapy in colon cancer. Gastroenterology 1994; 106:899-906.
95. Midgley RS, Kerr DI. Colorectal cancer. Lancet 1999; 353:391-9.
96. Pilipsen SJ, Heilweil M, Qhan SHQ et al. Patterns of pelvic recurrence following definitive resections of rectal cancer. Cancer 1984; 53:1354-62.
97. Rich T, Gunderson LL, Lew R et al. Patterns of recurrence of rectal cancer after potentially curative surgery. Cancer 1983; 52:1317-29.
98. O'Connell M, Martenson J, Wieand H et al. Improving adjuvant therapy for rectal cancer by combining protracted-infusion fluorouracil with radiation therapy after curative surgery. N Engl J Med 1994; 331:502-7.
99. Gastrointestinal Tumor Study Group: Radiation therapy and fluorouracil with or without semustine for the treatment of patients with surgical adjuvant adenocarcinoma of the rectum. J Clin Oncol 1992; 10:549-57.
100. Gastrointestinal Tumor Study Group: Prolongation of the disease-free survival in surgically treated rectal carcinoma. N Engl J Med 1985; 312:1465-72.
101. Onaitis MW, Noone RB, Hartwig M et al. Neoadjuvant chemoradiation for rectal cancer: analysis of clinical outcomes from a 13-year institutional experience. Ann Surg 2001; 6:778-85.
102. Tveit KM, Guldvog I, Hagen S et al. Randomized controlled trial of postoperative radiotherapy and short-term time-scheduled 5-fluorouracil against surgery alone in the treatment of Dukes B and C rectal cancer. Br J Surg 1997; 84:1130-5.
103. Habr-Gama A, de Souza PMSB, Ribeiro U et al. Low rectal cancer. Impact of radiation and chemotherapy on surgical treatment. Dis Colon Rectum 1998; 41:1087-96.
104. De Vita F, Orditura M, Martinelli E et al. The New European Gold Standard treatment for rectum cancer. Tumori 2000; 86(S2):S26-S29.
105. Podgorsak EB, Evans MD. An endocavitary rectal irradiation technique. Int J Radiat Oncol Biol Phys 1987; 13:1937.
106. Sischy B. The role of endocavitary irradiation for limited lesions of the rectum. Int J Colorectal Dis 1991; 6:91.
107. Cummings BJ. Radiation treatment for rectal cancer. World J Surg 1995; 19:275-81.
108. Chari RS, Tyler DS, Anscher MS et al. Preoperative radiation and chemotherapy in the treatment of adenocarcinoma of the rectum. Ann Surg 1995; 221:778-87.

109. Swedish Rectal Cancer Trial. Improved survival with preoperative radiotherapy in resectable rectal cancer. N Engl J Med 1997; 336:980-7.
110. Sause WT, Pajak TF, Noyes RD et al. Evaluation of preoperative radiation therapy in operable colorectal cancer. Ann Surg 1994; 220:668-75.
111. Tepper JE, Cohen AM, Wood WC et al. Postoperative radiation therapy of rectal cancer. Int J Radiat Oncol Biol Phys 1987; 13:5-10.
112. Medical Research Council Rectal Cancer Working Party. Randomised trial of surgery alone versus surgery followed by radiotherapy for mobile cancer of the rectum. Lancet 1996; 348:1610-4.
113. Medical Research Council Rectal Cancer Working Party. Randomised trial of surgery alone versus radiotherapy followed by surgery for potentially operable locally advanced rectal cancer. Lancet 1996; 348:1605-9.
114. Cammà C, Giunta M, Fiorica F et al. Preoperative radiotherapy for resectable rectal cancer. A meta-analysis. JAMA 2000; 284:23-30.
115. Umpleby HC, Williamson RC. Anastomotic recurrence in large bowel cancer. Br J Surg 1987; 74:873-8.
116. Malcolm AW, Perencevich NP, Olson RM et al. Analysis of recurrence patterns following curative resection for carcinoma of the colon and rectum. Surg Gynecol Obstet 1981; 152:131-6.
117. Bentzen SM, Balslev I, Pedersen M et al. Time to loco-regional recurrence after resection of Dukes' B and C colorectal cancer with and without adjuvant postoperative radiotherapy. A multivariate regression analysis. Br J Cancer 1992; 65:102-7.
118. Cass AW, Million RR, Pfaff WW. Patterns of recurrence following surgery alone for adenocarcinoma of the colon and rectum. Cancer 1976; 62:727-30.
119. Russell AH, Tong D, Dawson LE et al. Adenocarcinoma of the proximal colon. Sites of initial dissemination and patterns of recurrence following surgery alone. Cancer 1984; 53:360-7.
120. Abulafi AM, Williams NS. Local recurrence of colorectal cancer: the problem, mechanisms, management and adjuvant therapy. Br J Surg 1994; 81:7-19.
121. Moosa AR, Ree PC, Marks JE et al. Factors influencing local recurrence after abdominoperineal resection for cancer of the rectum and rectosigmoid. Br J Surg 1975; 62:727-30.
122. Umpleby HC, Ranson DL, Williamson RC. Peculiarities of mucinous colorectal carcinoma. Br J Surg 1985; 72:715-8.
123. Stearns MW Jr, Binkley GE. The influence of location on prognosis in operable rectal cancer. Surg Gynecol Obstet 1953; 96:368-72.
124. Phillips RKS, Hittinger R, Blesovsky L et al. Local recurrence following "curative" surgery for large bowel cancer. II: The rectum and rectosigmoid. Br J Surg 1984; 71:17-20.
125. Michelassi F, Block GE, Vannucci L et al. A 5- to 21-year follow-up and analysis of 250 patients with rectal adenocarcinoma. Ann Surg 1988; 208:379-89.
126. Sagar PM, Pemberton JH. Surgical management of locally recurrent rectal cancer. Br J Surg 1996; 83:293-304.
127. Heald RJ, Ryall RD. Recurrence and survival after total mesorectal excision for rectal cancer. Lancet 1986; i:1479-82.
128. Hurst PA, Prout WG, Kelly JM et al. Local recurrence after low anterior resection using the stable gun. Br J Surg 1982; 69:275-6.
129. Patel SC, Tovee EB, Langer B. Twenty-five years' experience with radical surgical treatment of carcinoma of the extraperitoneal rectum. Surgery 1977; 82:460-5.
130. Beart RW Jr, Metzger PP, O'Connell MJ et al. Postoperative screening of patients with carcinoma of the colon. Dis Colon Rectum 1981; 24:585-8.
131. Staib L, Schirrmeister H, Reske SN et al. Is ^{18}F-fluorodeoxyglucose positron emission tomography in recurrent colorectal cancer a contribution to surgical decision making? Am J Surg 2000; 180:1-5.

132. Cohen AM, Minski BD. Aggressive surgical management of locally advanced primary and recurrent rectal cancer. Current status and future directions. Dis Colon Rectum 1990; 33:432-8.
133. Brophy PF, Hoffman JP, Eisenberg BL. The role of palliative pelvic exenteration. Am J Surg 1994; 167:386-90.
134. Gunderson LL, Sosin H. Areas of failure found at reoperation (second or symptomatic look) following "curative surgery" for adenocarcinoma of the rectum. Clinicopathologic correlation and implications for adjuvant therapy. Cancer 1974; 34:1278-92.
135. Obrand DI, Gordon PH. Incidence and patterns of recurrence following curative resection for colorectal carcinoma. Dis Colon Rectum 1997; 40:15-24.
136. Stipa S, Nicolanti V, Botti C et al. Local recurrence after curative resection of colorectal cancer: frequency, risk factors and treatment. J Surg Oncol Suppl 1991; 2:155-60.
137. Nicholls J. Large bowel cancer. In: Slevin ML, Staquet MJ eds. Randomised trials in cancer: a critical review by sites. New York, Raven Press, 1986; 241-71.
138. Levi F, Lucchini F, La Vecchia C. Worldwide patterns of cancer mortality, 1985-89. Eur J Cancer Prev 1994; 3:109-43.
139. Monnet E, Faivre J, Raymond L et al. Influence of stage at diagnosis on survival differences for rectal cancer in three European populations. Br J Cancer 1999; 81:463-8.
140. Pedersen IK, Burcharth F, Roikjaer O et al. Resection of liver metastases from colorectal cancer. Indications and results. Dis Colon Rectum 1994; 37:1078-82.
141. Cattell R. Successful removal of liver metastasis from a carcinoma of the rectum. Lahey Clinic Bull 1940; 2:7-11.
142. Ballantyne GH, Quin J. Surgical treatment of liver metastases in patients with colorectal cancer. Cancer 1993; 71:4252-66.
143. Steele G Jr, Ravikumar TS. Resection of hepatic metastases from colorectal cancer: biological perspectives. Ann Surg 1989; 210:127-38.
144. Hughes K, Simon R, Songhorabodi S et al. Resection of the liver for colorectal carcinoma metastases: a multiinstitutional study of indications for resection. Registry of hepatic metastases. Surgery 1988; 57:278-88.
145. Doci R, Gennari L, Bignami P et al. One hundred patients with hepatic metastases from colorectal cancer treated by resection: analysis of prognostic determinants. Br J Surg 1991; 78:797-801.
146. Elias D, Lasser P, Rougier P et al. Another failure in the attempt of definition of the indications to the resection of liver metastases of colorectal origin. J Chir (Paris, France) 1992; 129:59-65.
147. Van Ooijen B, Wiggers T, Meijer S et al. Hepatic resection for colorectal metastases in The Netherlands - A multiinstitutional 10-year study. Cancer 1992; 70:28-34.
148. Busch E, Kemeny MM. Colorectal cancer: hepatic-directed therapy – the role of surgery, regional chemotherapy, and novel modalities. Semin Oncol 1995; 22:494-508.
149. Young A, Rea D. ABD of colorectal cancer. Treatment of advanced disease. Br Med J 2000; 321:1278-81.
150. Nordic Gastrointestinal Tumour Adjuvant Therapy Group. Expectancy or primary chemotherapy in patients with advanced, asymptomatic colorectal cancer: a randomized trial. J Clin Oncol 1992; 10:904-11.
151. Waters J, Cunningham D. The changing face of chemotherapy in colorectal cancer. Br J Cancer 2001; 84:1-7.
152. The Meta-analysis Group in Cancer. Efficacy of intravenous continuous infusion of fluorouracil compared this bolus administration in advanced colorectal cancer. J Clin Oncol 1998; 16:301-8.
153. The Meta-analysis Group in Cancer. Toxicity of fluorouracil in patients with advanced colorectal cancer: effect of administration schedule and prognostic factors. J Clin Oncol 1998; 16:3537-41.
154. De Gramont A, Bosset JF, Milan C et al. Randomized trial comparing monthly low-dose leucovorin-5-FU bolus with bimonthly high dose leucovorin-5-Fluorouracil bolus plus

continuous infusion for advanced colorectal cancer: a French Intergroup study. J Clin Oncol 1997; 15:808-15.
155. Leichman CG, Fleming TR, Muggia FM et al. Phase II study of fluorouracil and its modulation in advanced colorectal cancer; a Southwest Oncology Group Study, J Clin Oncol 1995; 12:1303-11.
156. Buyse M, Thirion P, Carlson RW et al. Relation between tumour response to first-line chemotherapy and survival in advanced colorectal cancer: a meta-analysis. Lancet 2000; 356:373-8.
157. Mayer RJ. Moving beyond Fluorouracil for colorectal cancer. N Engl J Med 2000; 343: 963-4.
158. Hsiang YH, Hertzberg R, Hecht S et al. Camptothecin induces protein-linked DNA breaks via mammalian DNA topoisomerase 1. J Biol Chem 1987; 260:14873-8.
159. Van Cutsem E, Rougier P, Droz JP et al. Clinical benefit of irinotecan (CPT-11) in metastatic colorectal cancer (CRC) resistant to 5-FU. Proc ASCO 1997; 16:268a (abstr).
160. Rougier P, Bugat R, Douillard JY et al. Phase II study of Irinotecan in the treatment of advanced colorectal cancer in chemotherapy-naïve patients and patients pretreated with fluorouracil-based chemotherapy. J Clin Oncol 1997; 15:251-60.
161. Cunningham D, Pyrhönen S, James RD et al. Randomised trial of Irinotecan plus supportive care versus supportive care alone after fluorouracil failure for patients with metastatic colorectal cancer. Lancet;1998; 352:1413-8.
162. Douillard JY, Cunningham D, Roth AD et al. Irinotecan combined with fluorouracil compared with fluorouracil alone as first-line treatment for metastatic colorectal cancer: a multicentre randomised trial. Lancet 2000; 355:1041-7.
163. Saltz LB, Cox JV, Blanke C et al. Irinotecan plus fluorouracil and leucovorin for metastatic colorectal cancer. N Engl J Med 2000; 355:1372.
164. Biasco G, Gallerani E. Treatment of liver metastases from colorectal cancer: what is the best approach today? Digest Liver Dis 2001; 33:438-44.
165. De Gramont A, Vignoud J, Tournigand C et al. Oxaliplatin with high-dose leucovorin and 5-fluorouracil 48-hour continuous infusion in pretreated metastatic colorectal cancer. Eur J Cancer 1997; 33:214-9.
166. De Gramont A, Figer A, Seymur M et al. Leucovorin and fluorouracil with or without oxaliplatin as first-time treatment in advanced colorectal cancer. J Clin Oncol 2000; 18:2938-47.
167. Van Cutsem E, Szanto J, Roth A et al. Evaluation of the addition of oxaliplatin to the same Mayo or German 5FU regimen in advanced refractory colorectal cancer. Proc Am Soc Clin Oncol 1999; 18:234.
168. Maindrault-Goebel F, De Gramont A, Louvet C et al. High-dose oxaliplatin with the simplified 48 h bimonthly leucovorin and 5-fluorouracil, regimen in pretreated metastatic colorectal cancer. Proc Am Soc Clin Oncol 1999; 18:265a.
169. Takiuchi H, Ajani J. Uracil-tegafur in gastric carcinoma: a comprehensive review. J Clin Oncol 1998; 16:2877-2885.
170. Pazdur R, Douillard JY, Killings JR et al. Multi-center Phase III study of 5-FU or UFT in combination with Leucovorin (LV) in patients with metastatic colorectal cancer. Proc Am Soc Clin Oncol 1999; 18:1990.
171. Lamont EB, Schilsky RL. Mini-review: the oral fluoropyrimidines in cancer chemotherapy. Clin Cancer Res 1999; 5:2289-96.
172. Harper P, Van Cutsem E, Thibault A et al. A phase III trial (SO14796) of Xeloda (capecitabine) in previously untreated advanced/metastatic colorectal cancer. Proc Am Soc Clin Oncol 1999; 18:1010.
173. Baccanafi DP, Davis ST, Knick VC et al. 5-Ethynyluracil: effects on pharmacokinetics and anti-tumor activity of 5-FU. Proc Natl Acad Sci USA 1993; 90:11064-8.
174. Mani S, Beck T, Chevlen E et al. A phase II open-label study to evaluate a 28-day regimen of oral 5-FU plus 776C85 for the treatment of patients with previously untreated metastatic colorectal cancer. Proc Am Soc Clin Oncol 1998; 17:281a.

175. Zonder JA, Shields AF, Zalupski M et al. A phase II trial of Bryostatin 1 in the treatment of metastatic colorectal cancer. Clin Cancer Res 2001; 7:38-42.
176. Kennedy MJ, Prestigiacomo LJ, Tyler G et al. Differential effects of bryostatin I and phorbol ester on human breast cancer cell lines. Cancer Res 1992; 52:1278-83.
177. Kemeny MM, Goldberg D, Beatty D et al. Results of a prospective randomized trial of continuous regional chemotherapy and hepatic resection as treatment of hepatic metastases from colorectal primaries. Cancer 1986; 57:492-8.
178. Rougier P, Laplanche A, Huguier M et al. Hepatic arterial infusion of fluoxuridine in patients with liver metastases from colorectal carcinoma. Long-term results of a prospective randomized trial. J Clin Oncol 1992; 10:1112-8.
179. Allen-Mersh TG, Earlam S, Fordy C et al. Quality of life and survival with continuous hepatic-artery floxuridine infusion for colorectal liver metastases. Lancet 1994; 344: 1255-60.
180. Petrelli NJ, Barcewicz PA, Evans JT et al. Hepatic artery ligation for liver metastasis in colorectal carcinoma. Cancer 1984; 53:1347-53.
181. Gerard A, Buyse M, Pector J et al. Hepatic artery ligation with and without portal infusion of 5-FU. A randomized study in patients with unresectable liver metastases from colorectal carcinoma. Eur J Surg Onc 1991; 17:289-94.
182. Heslin MJ, Medina-Franco H, Parker M et al. Colorectal hepatic metastases. Resection, local ablation, and hepatic artery infusion pump are associated with prolonged survival. Arch Surg 2001; 136:318-23.
183. Schafer DF, Sorrell MF. Hepatocellular carcinoma. Lancet 1999; 353:1253-7.
184. Hunt TM, Flowerdew ADS, Birch SJ et al. Prospective randomized controlled trial of hepatic arterial embolization or infusion chemotherapy with 5-gluorouracil and degradable starch microspheres for colorectal liver metastases. Br J Surg 1990; 77:779-82.
185. Leibel SA, Pajak TF, Massullo V et al. A comparison of Misonidazole sensitized radiation therapy to radiation therapy alone for the palliation of hepatic metastases. Results of a Radiation Therapy Oncology Group randomized prospective trial. Int J Rad Ond Biol Phys 1987; 13:1057-64.
186. Hafström L, Naredi P, Lindnér P et al. Treatment of primary liver cancer. Eur J Surg 1998; 164:569-74.
187. Behr TM, Sharkey RM, Juweid ME et al. Phase I/II clinical radioimmunotherapy with an iodine-131-labeled anti-carcinoembryonic antigen murine monoclonal antibody IgG. J Nucl Med 1997; 38:858-70.
188. Riethmuller G, Schneider-Gadicke E, Schlimok G et al. The German Cancer Aid 17-1A Study Group. Randomised trial of monoclonal antibody for adjuvant therapy of resected Dukes' C colorectal carcinoma. Lancet 1994; 343:1177-83.
189. Behr TM, Blumenthal RD, Memtsoudis S et al. Cure of metastatic human colonic cancer in mice with radiolabeled monoclonal antibody fragments. Clin Cancer Res 2000; 6:4900-7.
190. Ward RL, Packham D, Smythe AM et al. Phase I clinical trial of the chimeric monoclonal antibody (c30.6) in patients with metastatic colorectal cancer. Clin Cancer Res 2000; 6:4674-83.
191. Chung-Faye GA, Kerr DJ, Young LS et al. Gene therapy strategies for colon cancer. Molecular Medicine Today 2000; 6:82-7.
192. Kaji M, Yonemura y, Harada S et al. Participation of c-met in the progression of human gastric cancer: anti-c-met oligonucleotides inhibit proliferation or invasiveness of gastric cancer cells. Cancer Gene Ther 1996; 3:393-404.
193. Frebourg T, Friend SH. The importance of p53 gene alterations in human cancer: is there more than circumstantial evidence? J Natl Cancer Inst 1993; 85:1554-7.
194. Chungh-Faye GA, Kerr DJ. ABC of colorectal cancer. Innovative treatment for colon cancer. Br Med J 2000; 321:1397-9.
195. Rubin J, Charboneau JW, Reading C et al. Phase I study of immunotherapy of hepatic metastases of colorectal carcinoma by direct gene transfer. Hum Gen Ther 1994; 5:1385-99.

8 Survival and Follow-up of Colorectal Cancer

Introduction

Despite the undoubted advances in early diagnosis, screening procedures and surgical treatment, the prognosis of colorectal cancer has not shown over the last 3-4 decades the remarkable improvements that could be expected [1]. Moreover, rather unexpectedly, impressive intercountry differences in survival have recently been reported [2] - even within Europe - which are difficult to explain and interpret when taking into account the well standardized therapeutic approaches [3]. These findings, however, should not obscure the fact that colorectal neoplasms remain the most treatable and probably the most preventable tumor of the digestive organs [4].

Several clinical, biological, histological and subsequently molecular variables have been investigated in survival studies, with the objective of identifying useful indicators of the clinical outcome. Although many of these have been shown to be related to prognosis, the results have often been intriguing and conflicting. Thus, nearly 60 years after its original publication [5], Dukes' staging - together with more recent staging procedures [6] - continues to represent the most reliable prognostic indicator in colonic and rectal cancer. Indeed, in terms of prognosis, no other neoplasms appear so closely related to pathological stage at diagnosis as tumors of the large bowel.

After apparently curative resection for colorectal cancer, both the patient and physician are faced with the problem of follow-up. In most instances, surgeons tend to review their patients at regular intervals. However, recent studies cast some doubts on the real value of follow-up and showed a frequent lack of consensus among surgeons about the type and intensity of follow-up [7, 8], with a consequent tendency among clinicians to devise their own surveillance protocols. The cost of follow-up and the risk of excessive "medicalization" [9] of patients render these aspects even more relevant and underscore the need of developing appropriate guidelines for the increasing number of patients who undergo bowel resection for cancer.

Factors Influencing Colorectal Cancer Survival

Gender, Age and Stage at Diagnosis

The overall 5-year cancer-specific survival for colorectal neoplasms is of the order of 50% [10]; since late mortality is unusual for this type of tumor, at present half of these patients are cured from their disease, at least in Western countries [2]. The situation is not so bright in Eastern Europe and in many Asian and African countries [2, 11], where survival rates of 30% or less have been reported, mainly as a consequence of late diagnosis.

In most investigations, no appreciable differences in survival by gender have been reported [2, 12]. In contrast, conflicting results have been found as far as site of the tumor and age of the patient at diagnosis are concerned. Various studies showed a worse prognosis for rectal malignancies [13, 14], sometimes with a markedly different survival profile [12]; in contrast, in other studies no appreciable differences in survival by site of the tumor could be detected [15, 16]. On clinical grounds, a rectal neoplasm might be diagnosed earlier, due to symptoms such as bleeding or obstruction; these tumors, however, show a more marked tendency to infiltrate surrounding tissues and organs, and their removal is undoubtedly more complex [3]. Colonic malignancies may grow without symptoms for years, but tend to be less infiltrating and can be removed more easily; in addition, there is evidence that some subsets of right-sided tumors may have a less aggressive clinical behavior [17, 18]. Thus, several clinical and biological reasons may partially explain differences in survival between colonic and rectal neoplasms.

The effect of age on the survival of patients with colonic or rectal cancer is similarly unclear and controversial [19, 20]. In some investigations, patients younger than 40 or 50 years had a more favorable prognosis in both univariate and multivariate analysis [12, 21]. The reasons for this better clinical outcome include: (A) the possibility to carry out radical surgical approaches in younger individuals; (B) the fact that these patients may tolerate better the minor side-effects of adjuvant chemotherapy or radiotherapy; (C) the inclusion of patients with hereditary non-polyposis colorectal cancer (HNPCC), who are frequently younger than 50 years old and tend to show a more prolonged survival [17]; and (D) presumably the better awareness of relatively young patients regarding symptoms of the disease, with consequently improved chances of early diagnosis.

There is no doubt, however, that stage at diagnosis is the most powerful and, according to many authors, the only relevant indicator of the clinical outcome [3, 4, 21–23]. Tumors limited to the bowel wall (stage I, Dukes' A) have an excellent prognosis, with an overall survival that approaches 100% [24]. When the neoplasm expands beyond the muscularis propria and infiltrates the perirectal (or pericolic) tissues or organs (stage II, Dukes' B), the 5-year survival after curative resection is similarly excellent, about 60%–80%. When neoplasms form deposits in the mesenteric lymph nodes (stage III, Dukes' C), nearly half of the patients can still be cured with surgery, chemotherapy or radiotherapy [3]. Finally, for patients with haematogenous metastasis in the liver, lung or other organs

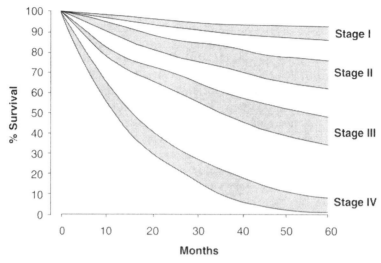

Fig. 8.1. Representative example of 5-year survival by TNM-Dukes' stage in colorectal cancer patients

(approximately 1/3–1/4 of the total) the prognosis is extremely poor despite aggressive chemotherapy, with 5-year survival not exceeding 5%–10% (stage IV, Dukes' D). Colorectal cancer survival by stage is schematically illustrated in Fig. 8.1, which reminds us that in dealing with these patients, early diagnosis remains the fundamental objective.

Morphological and Clinical Indicators

The strict dependence of survival on stage at diagnosis renders the search for prognostic markers in colorectal cancer research rather difficult. In the last 2–3 decades several biological, histological and molecular indicators of the clinical outcome have been proposed [25], but the results have been almost invariably controversial, even when supported by multivariate analysis. One might wonder why people are searching for additional prognostic markers when staging can provide us with all the information we need. A possible answer to this question is that markers may be of help in identifying patients who are best treated with surgery alone, those requiring chemotherapy and those requiring a more aggressive or even an experimental approach. Despite the many efforts, however, the choice of the most appropriate strategy is at present based almost exclusively on the stage at diagnosis [3, 26]. The search for factors affecting survival will continue therefore, especially in the direction of a molecular assessment of cancer [27], but at present none of the proposed prognostic indicators has been included in routine clinical practice.

In histological grading, pathologists try to infer tumor aggressiveness from a careful evaluation of cell and tissue characteristics. The prognostic value of histological and grade-related parameters in colorectal cancer remains highly controversial. In a series of classical studies, Jass and collaborators tried to assess the relative importance of several parameters by using multivariate analysis and creating simple scoring systems [28-30]. They and other investigators [21] suggested a prognostic value for many of these variables [31,32]. Other reports suggested the possible prognostic importance of some morphological parameters, such as degree of differentiation [33-35], venous invasion by tumor cells [35, 36], eosinophil and mast cell infiltration [37], tumor morphology [38] and lymphatic microinvasion [22]. Again, most of these observations were not confirmed by other studies; in fact, despite the rigorous definition of each variable, it is commonly accepted that histological grading is a rather subjective exercise, and that the final interpretation may vary considerably, both interindividually and intraindividually [28, 39]. These considerations may explain – at least in part – the existing controversies regarding the prognostic significance of grading and of several histological parameters.

The possible relevance of clinical variables has also been taken into account. According to some authors [40], lactic dehydrogenase levels, Karnofsky performance status and lung involvement were the best predictors of survival in patients with advanced colorectal cancer. With the same statistical approach, Hannisdal and Thorsen observed that a high erythrocyte sedimentation rate and leucocyte count were important prognostic indicators in addition to stage [41], and in more recent investigations a possible value of hemoglobin levels has been suggested [42]. Once again, the clinical relevance of these (and other) observations remains unclear, and none of the above-mentioned parameters has been accepted as a useful prognostic indicator.

The role of new surgical techniques – such as total mesorectal excision and laparoscopic surgery – and of combined chemotherapy on colorectal cancer prognosis has been discussed in chapter 7. Another factor influencing survival is the development of postoperative complications. In elective surgery, when the general condition of the patient is good and there is no relevant associated disease, postoperative mortality is negligible. The most common reasons for a fatal result are cardiac infarction and pulmonary embolism; in debilitated patients the use of subcutaneous heparin prophylaxis can prevent deep vein thrombosis, thus lowering the risk of thromboembolism [43]. Short-term complications include wound infections (common in obese and diabetic subjects), abdominal abscesses (more frequent in obese individuals and in the case of bowel perforation during surgery), anastomotic dehiscence, urinary tract infections (owing to the use of an indwelling catheter) and postoperative ileus due to adhesion, which in many cases requires a further operation [44]. Long-term postoperative complications include small-bowel obstruction, bowel dysfunction (frequent diarrhea, which may represent a problem for elderly patients) and impaired genitourinary function (such as difficulties in emptying the bladder and retrograde ejaculation). These side-effects may impair quality of life but rarely affect survival [45].

Cell Replication, Nuclear Ploidy and Colorectal Cancer Survival

Since uncontrolled cell replication is one of the main features of malignancy, it is not surprising that the proliferative activity of tumor cells has been investigated as a possible indicator of prognosis. Cell replication can be evaluated by assessing several parameters, including the number of mitoses on histological slides, the S-phase fraction (after incorporation of tritiated thymidine or bromodeoxyuridine), measurement of argyrophilic nucleolar organizer regions (AgNOR) and immunohistochemical analysis with Ki67 or PCNA (proliferating cell nuclear antigen) monoclonal antibodies [25, 46, 47].

Tanigawa et al. measured thymidine uptake by cultured tumor cells in 127 patients with colorectal carcinoma [48] and compared the influence of various parameters on survival. They found little correlation between high or low thymidine uptake and most of the patients' clinical or pathological features; however, thymidine incorporation was strongly associated with survival according to multivariate analysis. The conclusion was that thymidine uptake can predict the prognosis, independent of its relationship to other variables. However, other investigations showed that thymidine incorporation was not invariably correlated with prognosis in a large variety of neoplasms, including colorectal cancer [49, 50].

Ki-67 is an antibody directed against an antigen expressed in all phases of the cell cycle, with the exception of G-0, while PCNA is a DNA polymerase delta which interacts with cyclin D and cyclin-dependent kinases [25]. In a large study involving 293 patients with colorectal cancer, Sun et al. [51] assessed the possible prognostic role of PCNA expression. Patients were followed up for at least 5 years after surgery, and PCNA was estimated by counting immunoreactive cells in histological slides. PCNA did not correlate with survival. At variance with these results, Paradiso et al. [52] found PCNA expression independently related to survival in 71 patients with metastatic or recurrent colorectal carcinoma. Similarly inconsistent results were observed with AgNOR [47] and bromodeoxyuridine [46, 53].

An abnormal DNA content (aneuploidy) in cancer cells can be evaluated by DNA flow cytometry [46]. When compared with cell replication, ploidy determination is relatively simple and allows the rapid assessment of thousands of nuclei. For this reason, flow cytometry has been used extensively over the last two decades for assessing the possible prognostic role of aneuploidy virtually in any type of malignancy [54, 55]. In general terms, these studies suggest that patients with aneuploid tumors have a worse prognosis than individuals with diploid tumors [56, 57]. As far as colorectal carcinoma is concerned, tumor ploidy was usually correlated with other prognostic variables – including tumor stage – and consequently appeared to be of limited value as an independent prognostic indicator [58, 59].

Molecular Markers of Prognosis

Since the development of tumors is attributed to the accumulation of genetic alterations in somatic cells [60], a detailed molecular assessment of colorectal cancer in search of prognostic parameters might give valuable information which could be used in the management of these patients (Table 8.1). Most studies have focused on oncogenes, tumor suppressor genes and, more recently, microsatellite instability. Once again, the results have often been conflicting and controversial, and at present there is no single molecular test which can be proposed as a definite indicator of the clinical outcome in patients with colorectal malignancies [25]. Parameters investigated included transforming growth factors (TGF) α and β and their receptors [61], *c-myc* amplification [62], *c-erb* β2 overexpression [63], allelic losses at various chromosomes (especially 18q, where the DCC gene is located) [64], genes involved in the apoptosis pathway (such as *bcl-2*) [65] and many others [25, 46]. However, *k-ras* mutations, p53 alterations and microsatellite instability have been studied in greater detail.

The prognostic relevance of *k-ras* mutations has been assessed in several tumors, including colorectal neoplasms. The gene encodes a 21-KDa protein which is localized in the cytoplasmic membrane and exhibits GTPase activity [66]. *K-ras* is the member of a "gene family" which also includes *H-ras* and *N-ras*. Mutations of *ras* oncogenes can be detected in about 50% of colorectal cancers; the majority of these alterations are found at codon 12 (75%) and a smaller fraction at codons 13 and 62 [67]. Although there are data in the literature on *ras* mutations and survival from more than 1000 patients with colorectal neoplasms, the clinical implications of these alterations remain unclear. As recently reviewed by McLeod and Murray [25], the presence of *ras* gene mutations was associated

Table 8.1. Main biological indicators of prognosis in colorectal cancer

Marker	Type of change	Proposed effect on prognosis	Reference
Grading	Degree of differentiation	Worse prognosis for poorly differentiated tumors	[33, 34]
Venous invasion	Presence	Worse prognosis	[35, 36]
Lymphatic invasion	Presence	Worse prognosis	[22]
Cell proliferation	High replicative activity	Worse prognosis	[48]
Nuclear DNA content	Aneuploidy	Worse prognosis	[57–59]
K-ras	Point mutations	Worse prognosis	[25]
p53	Point mutations, positive immuno-histochemistry	Worse prognosis	[25, 73]
Microsatellites	Microsatellite instability	Improved prognosis	[76, 77, 81]
Micrometastases	Presence	Worse prognosis	[86, 87, 89]

with a poor clinical outcome in at least four studies, whereas in other seven investigations – carried out with a similar design and patient selection – no association between the presence of mutations and prognosis could be detected. In a more recent study limited to patients with Dukes' C tumors treated with adjuvant chemotherapy [68], *k-ras* mutations did not appear as a prognostic indicator, either alone or in association with p53 mutations.

p53 mutations have been largely investigated in colorectal cancer research, especially because some 70% of these tumors show p53 alterations, and these are considered one of the rate-limiting steps in colorectal tumorigenesis [69, 60]. Moreover, this tumor suppressor gene is mutated in several other human neoplasms, while germline mutations are associated with the phenotypic manifestations of Li-Fraumeni syndrome [70]. The encoded protein is one of the main regulators of the cell cycle; in addition, it stimulates DNA repair and modulates apoptosis [71]. These functions are lost in the presence of mutations, and the involved tissue rapidly acquires the main features of malignancy. Alterations in p53 can be evaluated through PCR-based studies or by immunohistochemistry, since the "mutated" protein has a prolonged half-life which leads to its accumulation in the nuclei [46]. Once again, studies aimed at evaluating the prognostic role of p53 have been controversial, and the body of evidence does not support the association between p53 mutations and poor clinical outcome that had been suggested in the initial investigations [25]. Indeed, in one of the largest series [72], patients with positive immunostaining (i.e. with p53 mutations in the tumors) showed a more favorable outcome. Moreover, a recent meta-analysis [73] of 28 studies involving a total of 4,416 patients with colorectal cancer showed only a borderline significant hazard associated with p53 overexpression or mutation versus wild-type. According to these authors, it is unlikely that p53 can be applied in routine clinical practice because of the presence of much more powerful indicators of prognosis, such as T stage and nodal status.

Microsatellites are repetitive genetic sequences (1–5 base pairs, repeated 15–30 times) located on non-coding regions of DNA, within genes or between genes [74]. Microsatellite instability (MSI) is defined as a frequent change of any length of these DNA sequences, due to either the insertion or deletion of repeated units. MSI is particularly frequent in HNPCC (or Lynch syndrome), where this marker can be of considerable help in identifying individuals who should be tested for constitutional mutations of DNA mismatch repair genes [17]. In addition, MSI can be detected in 10%–20% of apparently sporadic colorectal tumors, especially among patients with right-sided and mucinous lesions [74, 75]. Various studies have reported an association between MSI and improved clinical outcome [76, 77], while other investigators could not demonstrate any survival advantage for patients with unstable tumors [78, 79]. Gryfe et al. [80] studied MSI in a large series of patients ($n = 617$) with colorectal neoplasms diagnosed before the age of 50 years. Of these, 17% showed high-frequency MSI, and in multivariate analysis MSI was associated with a significant survival advantage, independently of other prognostic indicators including stage at diagnosis. Similar results were reported by Gafà et al. [81], who concluded that MSI evaluation is an essential step in the genetic characterization of colorectal malignancies, and identified a subset of neoplasms with distinct clinical and biological features. In contrast, Salahshor et al. [82] in a series of 181 unselected colorectal carcinomas (12% of which exhibited MSI) did not find any significant difference in prognosis between patients with stable or unstable tumors. Once again, the reasons for these conflicting results remain unclear.

Micrometastases and Prognosis

Until recent years, pathologists considered micrometastases as foci of neoplastic cells visible only under the microscope and, thus, measuring less than 1–2 mm. The term, however, has evolved to signify metastases detected by whatever means, provided that they were missed during routine histological examination [83]. Micrometastases can be detected with immunohistochemistry by using antibodies against cytokeratins (which recognize epithelial cells in general) or carcinoembryonic antigen (CEA, expressed by most colorectal neoplasms). More recently, genetic-based techniques have been employed to detect micrometastases in regional lymph nodes, and the available evidence suggests that these methods are more sensitive than histopathology and immunohistochemistry [84]. These techniques are mainly based on the selective PCR amplification of altered DNA sequences of genes commonly mutated in human neoplasms, such as the *ras* family and p53.

The prognostic role of micrometastases has been explored, not without controversies, in breast cancer, pancreatic carcinoma and other malignancies [83, 85]. As far as colorectal malignancies are concerned, Calaluce et al. [86] recently reviewed 11 studies, 5 of which reported that patients were upstaged by using immunohistochemical examination of regional lymph nodes, but only 2 involved prognostic significance. Adell et al., for instance, used antibodies to cytokeratin and found micrometastases in 39% of patients with stage II colorectal cancer; however, no difference in survival could be detected between patients with or without micrometastases [87]. In contrast, Liefers et al. [88] reported a worse prognosis in patients with micrometastases. Moreover, Sanchez-Cespedes and collaborators [89] used a sensitive oligonucleotide-mediated ligation assay to detect the presence of *k-ras* and p53 mutations in lymph nodes from colorectal cancer patients; 12 of the 68 evaluated lymph nodes were positive for tumor cells by molecular analysis but negative for neoplastic cells by routine histopathology and even cytokeratin immunohistochemistry. Survival analysis revealed a median survival of 1,056 days for individuals without evidence of lymph node involvement by molecular analysis as opposed to 165 days for patients with positive lymph nodes. This highly significant difference led the authors to suggest that screening for metastasis by molecular-based techniques increases the sensitivity of tumor cell detection and might represent a reliable predictor of recurrence.

In conclusion, these and other investigations clearly suggest that many patients with colorectal cancer have systematic spread of the disease even when the pathological staging indicates localized lesions. As pointed out by Keene and

Demeure [83], the observation that many patients with micrometastases do not develop recurrence and may enjoy prolonged survival clearly suggests that the immune system can suppress or prevent tumor growth and eradicate small tumor burdens. Moreover, the frequent occurrence of micrometastases is a further element in favor of adjuvant chemotherapy in colorectal malignancies.

Temporal Trends and Ethnic Differences in Colorectal Cancer Survival

One of the ways to assess whether we are making progress against tumors is the careful analysis of temporal trends in survival among different countries. As far as colorectal cancer is concerned, there is a general consensus that in most Western countries both relative and absolute survival have been gradually increasing over the last 3–4 decades, though not without differences between countries [1, 2, 4]. Data from developing countries are scanty and fragmentary, but the general impression is that the overall prognosis has changed very little over time, and that survival rates are lower than in the Western world [90–92].

In a longitudinal observational study of all patients with colon cancer observed in Sweden between 1973 and 1993 ($n = 41,700$), Blomqvist et al. [93] reported that relative survival increased substantially throughout this period, presumably owing to the net effect of health care availability, diagnostic efficacy and improved management strategies. Similarly, in an Italian population-based investigation [1, 9], there was a definite improvement in overall 5-year survival between 1984 and 1996 which was mainly attributed to a progressively more favorable clinical stage and to the recent introduction of more powerful treatments for Dukes' C and D patients [3]. Moreover, Finn-Faivre et al. [94] evaluated the management and prognosis of rectal cancer in two French regions between 1978 and 1993. Over the 16 years of observation, resection rates grew from 66.0% to 80.21% of all cases; the proportion of patients receiving adjuvant chemotherapy increased remarkably, and the fraction of patients with stage I lesions increased from 17.7% to 30.6%. All these clinical findings resulted in a significant improvement in relative survival, which was 35.4% for patients registered in 1978–1981 and was 57.0% for individuals diagnosed in 1985–1989. Finally, according to the SEER data [95], survival rates in the USA for all of the most frequent malignancies (including colorectal neoplasms) showed an improvement with calendar time between 1973 and 1990.

Thus, the available evidence indicates that most developed countries enjoyed a certain improvement of colorectal cancer prognosis over the last 30–40 years. The more favorable clinical outcome should be attributed to the concurrence of several factors, including better stage at diagnosis, the general improvement of surgical and anaesthesiological techniques (with a consequent reduction of perioperative mortality), and the more appropriate use of chemotherapy and radiotherapy.

If we are ready to accept differences in survival between well developed and less developed countries – because of the different national incomes, welfare system and medical facilities – the variations in colorectal cancer survival among

Western countries are more disturbing and require some explanation. Thus, in contrast to the above-mentioned SEER data [10, 95], Sharma et al. [96] did not report any improvement in survival among patients with colorectal cancer diagnosed in two hospitals in North Carolina (USA) between 1981 and 1995; rather surprisingly, this occurred despite the earlier stage at diagnosis over the study period. The authors tried to explain these unexpected results with the inclusion in screening programs of patients who were poor candidates for screening, or who had high risks for surgical operations. Gatta et al. [2] studied the variation in survival of colorectal cancer patients in Europe during the period 1978–1989. The study examined population-based data from 17 countries, for a total of 156,634 cases. The 5-year relative survival differed significantly between different European countries: the Nordic countries and France had the highest survival rates (52%–59%); intermediate values were seen in Italy, Spain and Germany (46%–50%), whereas Eastern European countries (especially Poland), Denmark and the United Kingdom were characterized by the lowest survival, for both colonic and rectal neoplasms (23%–43%). In a subsequent investigation [97], the authors noticed that differences among countries narrowed when corrections for stage were applied and therefore concluded that these wide differences in colorectal cancer survival across Europe should be attributed to a large extent to differences in stage at diagnosis. However, some significant variations persisted even after correcting for stage; since cancer survival reflects the global impact of the health system on a population (i.e. efficacy and effectiveness of screening programs, clinical management and follow-up), it is likely that differences in colorectal cancer survival are also related to differences in health spending [1]. Indeed, considering that in the United Kingdom survival rates for the "big killers" (lung, breast, colorectal and prostate tumors) seem to be consistently below the average for Europe, the London support group "Cancer BACUP" stressed that "If Britain could achieve the same rate of survival as the best performing European country for each of these cancers, 25,000 lives per year would be saved" [98]. Moreover, in a comparative study of survival in American and European cancer patients, Gatta et al. [99] reported that survival for most major malignancies (prostate, skin melanoma, colon, rectum, breast and endometrium) was worse in Europe than in the USA, especially for older individuals.

Clearly, variation in survival among developed countries is a complex and "slippery" topic, where scientific reasons can easily conflict with ethical and economic justifications. With the emerging importance of evidence-based medicine but with a progressive and inexorable "medicalization" of Western society, it is easy to guess that these arguments will become more and more actual for both scientists and economists.

Follow-up of Colorectal Cancer Patients

As already discussed, the clinical evolution of colorectal cancer – after apparently curative surgery – is closely dependent on the stage at diagnosis. Local recurrence is more frequent in stage III than in stages I and II individuals; moreover, recurrence is more common for rectal tumors, which may recur in up to 20%–30% of the cases [8]. The main objectives of follow-up after curative resection of colorectal cancer is two-fold: first, to detect local recurrence or distal metastasis as early as possible, so that surgery can be tried again with some probability of success; second, to find out and remove metachronous adenomas (or carcinoma), hopefully through endoscopy. Although most surgeons and oncologists are used to reviewing their patients at regular intervals after surgery, the optimal type of follow-up of patients has not yet been established. The importance of early diagnosis of recurrence is underscored by studies showing that successful resection of recurrent malignancy is directly related to early detection [100]; moreover, it has been suggested that patients with metachronous colorectal tumors enjoy increased survival when they are detected in an early, asymptomatic stage [101]. However, various studies underline the lack of consensus among surgeons about the modality and intensity of follow-up [8]. There are strong supporters of follow-up, who claim that intensive surveillance can lead to a significant reduction in death rates for colorectal cancer; on the other hand, other investigators stress the fact that the value of follow-up remains unproven.

Proposed Surveillance Programs After Colorectal Cancer Resection

All surveillance programs are based on a combination of screening procedures which include complete blood profile, CEA determination, digital rectal examination, occult blood test, colonoscopy, liver (and rectal) ultrasound, computed tomography (CT) of the liver and pelvis, chest radiographs and nuclear magnetic resonance [102]. Recently, positron emission tomography (PET) has been proposed as the technique of choice for the early detection of local recurrence [103].

In a recent investigation, Schoemaker et al. [7] defined as "standard follow-up" a program consisting of complete blood profile, CEA and occult blood testing every 3 months for 2 years, and thereafter every 6 months for 5 years until a major end-point was reached. According to this protocol, patients underwent other clinical investigations (imaging studies, colonoscopy) only if indicated by clinical or screening test abnormalities and after completing 5 years of follow-up (to exclude the possibility of undiagnosed recurrence or metastasis). The same authors defined as "intensive follow-up" the addition of chest X-ray, CT of the liver, and colonoscopy to the standard follow-up.

Other protocols were mainly based on barium enema and sigmoidoscopy during the postoperative period at 6 and 12 months, and then yearly; in addition, CEA evaluations were performed every 3 months in the 1st year and subsequently on an annual basis [104]. In a recent review, Bond [105] summarized the "current surveillance recommendations" as follows. Colonoscopy should be carried out during the perioperative period to clear the colon of all neoplasia; repeat colonoscopy should be performed at 3 years and then every 3–5 years. Digital rectal examination, proctoscopy and rectal ultrasound are reserved for patients undergoing sphincter-saving anterior resection for rectal neoplasms. In patients with stage III disease, who are at major risk of liver and lung metastasis, surveillance should also include chest radiographs (and liver ultrasound) every 6–12 months, and CEA determination at least every 3 months. The author, however, concluded that the value of this expensive and rigorous approach has not been demonstrated in terms of survival or early detection.

Controlled Studies Evaluating the Effectiveness of Follow-up

Various studies evaluated the effect of more or less intensive follow-up procedures on the clinical outcome of patients operated on for colorectal malignancies. In a Scandinavian study [106], 107 patients with colorectal carcinoma were randomized to intensive follow-up (fecal occult blood tests, serum liver profile, CEA determination, sigmoidoscopy and either barium enema or colonoscopy) or no follow-up; the recurrence rate and overall and cancer-specific survival did not show any significant difference between the two arms of the trial. Rather similar results were reported by Mákélá et al. [107] and in a larger investigation [108]: 600 patients with colorectal malignancies were randomized to intensive 6-monthly follow-up (which included repeated colonoscopy) or to clinical investigations scheduled at 5 and 10 years after surgery. The recurrence rate was similar in the two groups (20%); however, in the intensive group recurrent tumors were diagnosed earlier, often at an asymptomatic stage, and more patients underwent second-look surgery with curative intent. Surprisingly, no difference could be detected between the two groups as far as overall survival was concerned. Finally, in a recent study [7], Shoemaker et al. randomized 350 patients operated on for colorectal cancer to either intensive or standard follow-up. After 5 years, no significant difference in survival between the two groups could be detected, and the authors concluded that yearly colonoscopy, liver CT and chest X-ray did not improve survival after colorectal malignancies when added to symptoms and simple screening review.

This lack of evidence of survival benefit due to an intensive follow-up after curative surgery was also supported by meta-analysis. Bruinsvels et al. [109] assessed seven non-randomized studies (for a total of more than 3,000 patients), comparing intensive follow-up with minimal or no follow-up. Although in the intensive group more asymptomatic recurrences could be detected and more patients underwent a second, potentially curative operation, no significant difference in survival was observed.

Thus, there is no evidence – from controlled investigations – that the clinical outcome of patients with colorectal cancer can be improved through a careful or intensive follow-up after bowel resection. Yet most physicians and surgeons feel that these patients should not be abandoned and that some sort of surveillance after surgery is justified. Instinct and, presumably, moral concerns may be (on some occasions) as relevant as scientific evidence. Finally, the increasing social attention to costs of medical interventions and to evidence-based medicine requires a close evaluation of the cost-effectiveness of follow-up procedures in colorectal cancer research.

Conclusions

Colorectal cancer survival may appear unsatisfactory if we consider that thousands of individuals die each year of the disease around the world, but it is undoubtedly better than that of other neoplasms of the digestive organs. Survival remains closely related to the stage at diagnosis, and the many morphological, clinical and molecular indicators of prognosis are at present of little value in the management of these patients. Temporal trends indicate that cancer-specific survival increases over time, at least in Western countries, as a result of earlier diagnosis and of an overall improvement in surgical and anaesthesiological techniques. Rather surprisingly, significant intercountry differences in survival still exist, not only between Europe and the USA, but also within Europe. Finally, the value of follow-up after colorectal cancer surgery remains to be proven, though some sort of surveillance is usually recommended to most patients.

References

1. Ponz de Leon M, Benatti P, Di Gregorio C. et al. Staging and survival of colorectal cancer: are we making progress? Dig Liv Dis 2000; 32:312-7.
2. Gatta G, Faivre J, Capocaccia R et al. Survival of colorectal cancer patients in Europe during the period 1978-1989. Eur J Cancer 1998; 34:2176-83.
3. Galandiuk S, Mortensen N. Contributions of academic medicine to colon and rectal surgery. Dis Colon Rectum 2000; 43:1653-9.
4. Boland CR, Sinicrope FA, Brenner De et al. Colorectal cancer prevention and treatment. Gastroenterology 2000; 118:S115-S128.
5. Dukes CE. The classification of cancer of the rectum. J Path Bact 1932; 35:1489-94.
6. Hutter RVP, Sobin LH. A Universal staging system for cancer of the colon and rectum. Let there be light. Arch Pathol Lab Med 1986; 110:367-8.
7. Schoemaker D, Black R, Giles L et al. Yearly colonoscopy, liver CT, and chest radiography do not influence 5-year survival of colorectal cancer patients. Gastroenterology 1998; 114:7-14.
8. McArdle C. ABC of colorectal cancer. Effectiveness of follow up. BMJ 2000; 321:1332-5.
9. Ponz de Leon M, Benatti P, Percesepe A et al. Epidemiology of cancer of the large bowel – The 12-year experience of a specialized Registry in Northern Italy. Ital J Gastroenterol Hepatol 1999; 31:10-8.
10. Papworth DG, Lloyd RA. Cancer survival in the USA, 1973-1990: a statistical analysis. Br J Cancer 1998; 78:1514-5.
11. Shanta V, Gajalakshmi CK, Swaminathan R et al. Cancer registration in Madras Metropolitan Tumour Registry, India. Eur J Cancer 1994; 30 A:974-8.
12. Roncucci L, Fante R, Losi L et al. Survival for colon and rectal cancer in a population-based cancer registry. Eur J Cancer 1996; 32 A:295-302.
13. Wiggers T, Arends JW, Volovics A. Regression analysis of prognostic factors in colorectal cancer after curative resections. Dis Colon Rectum 1988; 31:33-41.
14. Kune GA, Kune S, Field B et al. Survival in patients with large-bowel cancer. A population-based investigation from the Melbourne Colorectal Cancer Study. Dis Colon Rectum 1990; 33:938-46.
15. Enblad P, Adami HO, Bergstrom R et al. Improved survival of patients with cancers of the colon and rectum. J Natl Cancer Inst 1988; 80:586-91.
16. Steinberg SM, Barkin JS, Kaplan RS et al. Prognostic indicators of colon tumors. The Gastrointestinal Tumor Study Group Experience. Cancer 1986; 57:1866-70.

17. Lynch HT, Smyrk T, Lynch J. An update of HNPCC (Lynch syndrome). Cancer Genet Cytogenet 1997; 93:84-99.
18. Nicholl ID, Dunlop MG. Molecular markers of prognosis in colorectal cancer. J Natl Cancer Inst 1999; 91:1267-9.
19. Chapuis PH, Dent OF, Fisher R et al. A multivariate analysis of clinical and pathological variables in the prognosis after resection of large bowel cancer. Br J Surg 1985; 72: 698-702.
20. Svendsen LB, Sorensen C, Kjersgaard P et al. The influence of age upon the survival after curative operation for colorectal cancer. Int J Colorectal Dis 1989; 4: 123-7.
21. Ponz de Leon M, Sant M, Micheli A et al. Clinical and pathologic prognostic indicators in colorectal cancer. Cancer 1992; 69:626-35.
22. Michelassi F, Block GE, Vannucci L et al. A 5- to 21-year follow-up and analysis of 250 patients with rectal adenocarcinoma. Ann Surg 1988; 208:379-89.
23. Herrera L, Luna P, Villarreal JR et al. Perspectives in colorectal cancer. J Surg Oncol 1991; 2 S:92-103.
24. Di Gregorio C, Fante R, Roncucci L et al. Clinical features, frequency and prognosis of Dukes' A colorectal carcinoma: a population-based investigation. Eur J Cancer 1996; 32 A:1957-62.
25. McLeod HL, Murray GI. Tumour markers of prognosis in colorectal cancer. Br J Cancer 1999; 79:191-203.
26. Grem JL. Current treatment approaches in colorectal cancer. Semin Oncol 1991; 18: 17-26.
27. Caldas C. Molecular assessment of cancer. BMJ 1998; 316:1360-3.
28. Jass JR, Atkin WS, Cuzick J et al. The grading of rectal cancer: historical perspectives and a multivariate analysis of 447 cases. Histopathol 1986; 10:437-59.
29. Jass JR. Lymphocitic infiltration and survival in rectal cancer. J Clin Pathol 1986; 39: 585-9.
30. Sasaki O, Atkin WS, Jass JR. Mucinous carcinoma of the rectum. Histopathol 1987; 11:259-72.
31. Stahle E, Enblad P, Pàhlman L et al. Can mortality from rectal and rectosigmoid carcinoma be predicted from histopathological variables in the diagnostic biopsy? APMIS 1989; 97:513-22.
32. Hermanek P, Guggenmoos-Holzmann I, Gall FP. Prognostic factors in rectal carcinoma. A contribution to the further development of tumor classification. Dis Colon Rectum 1989; 32(7):593-9.
33. Halvorsen TB, Seim E. Degree of differentiation in colorectal adenocarcinomas. A multivariate analysis of the influence on survival. J Clin Pathol 1988; 41:532-7.
34. Deans GT, Patterson CC, Parks TG et al. Colorectal carcinoma: importance of clinical and pathological factors in survival. Ann R Coll Surg Engl 1994; 76:59-64.
35. Bokey EL, Chapuis PH, Dent OF et al. Factors affecting survival after excision of the rectum for cancer. A multivariate analysis. Dis Colon Rectum 1997; 40:3-10.
36. Moore PA, Dilawari RA, Fidler WJ. Adenocarcinoma of the colon and rectum in patients less than 40 years of age. Am Surg 1984; 50:10-4.
37. Fisher ER, Rockette H, Jones J et al. Prognostic significance of eosinophils and mast cells in rectal cancer: findings from the national surgical adjuvant breast and bowel project (protocol R-01). Hum Pathol 1989; 20:159-63.
38. Shepherd NA, Saraga EP, Love SB et al. Prognostic factors in the colonic cancer. Histopathology 1989; 14:613-20.
39. Emedley FH, Hoile RW, Macfarlane DA. Rectal biopsies: inaccuracy of histological grading in carcinoma of the rectum. J R Soc Med 1984; 77:564-6.
40. Kemeny N, Braun DW Jr. Prognostic factors in advances colorectal carcinoma: importance of lactic dehydrogenase level, performance status, and white blood cell count. Am J Med 1983; 74:786-96.

41. Hannisdal E, Thorsen G. Regression analyses of prognostic factors in colorectal cancer. J Surg Oncol 1988; 37:109-12.
42. Graf W, Glimelius B, Påhlman et al. Determinants of prognosis in advanced colorectal cancer. Eur J Cancer 1991; 27:1119-23.
43. Lopez MJ, Monafo WW. Role of extended resection in the initial treatment of locally advanced colorectal carcinoma. Surgery 1993; 113:365-72.
44. McArdle CS, Hole D. Impact of variability among surgeons on postoperative morbidity and mortality and ultimate survival. BMJ 1991; 302:1501-5.
45. Cady B, Stone MD, McDermott WV et al. Technical and biological factors in disease-free survival after hepatic resection for colorectal cancer metastases. Arch Surg 1992; 127:561-9.
46. Bosman FT. Prognostic value of pathological characteristics of colorectal cancer. Eur J Cancer 1995; 31 A:1216-21.
47. Adachi Y, Kido A, Mori M et al. Nuclear DNA content and nucleolar organizer regions in colorectal cancer. J Surg Oncol 1995; 59:177-80.
48. Tanigawa N, Masuda Y, Muraoka R et al. Prognostic significance of in vitro thymidine uptake in patients with colorectal carcinoma. J Surg Oncol 1994; 55:209-14.
49. Hattori T, Hosokawa Y, Sugihara H et al. DNA content of diffusely infiltrative carcinomas in the stomach. Pathol Res Pract 1985; 180:615-8.
50. Meyer JS, Priolean PG. S-phase fractions of colorectal carcinomas related to pathological and clinical features. Cancer 1981; 48:1221-8.
51. Sun XF, Cartensen JM, Stal O et al. c-erb B2 oncoprotein in relation to DNA ploidy and prognosis in colorectal adenocarcinoma. APMIS 1995; 103:309-15.
52. Paradiso A, Rabinovich M, Vallejo C et al. p53 and PCNA expression in advanced colorectal cancer: response to chemotherapy and long-term prognosis. Int J Cancer 1996; 54:594-606.
53. Roncucci L, Pedroni M, Scalmati A et al. Cell kinetics evaluation of colorectal tumors after in vivo administration of Bromodeoxyuridine. Int J Cancer 1992; 52:856-61.
54. Tang R, Ho YS, You YT et al. Prognostic evaluation of DNA flow cytometric and histopathologic parameters of colorectal cancer. Cancer 1995; 76:1724-30.
55. Takanishi DM, Hart J, Covarelli P et al. Ploidy as a prognostic feature in colonic adenocarcinoma. Arch Surg 1996; 131:587-92.
56. Stewart CC. Flow cytometric analysis of oncogene expression in human neoplasias. Arch Pathol Lab Med 1989; 113:634-40.
57. Williams NN, Daly JM. Flow cytometry and prognostic implications in patients with solid tumors. Surg Gynecol Obstet 1990; 171:257-66.
58. Böttger TC, Potratz D, Stöckle M et al. Prognostic value of DNA analysis in colorectal carcinoma. Cancer 1993; 72:3579-87.
59. Yamazoe Y, Maetani S, Nishikawa T et al. The prognostic role of the DNA ploidy pattern in colorectal cancer analysis using paraffin-embedded tissue by an improved method. Surg Today 1994; 24:30-6.
60. Ponz de Leon M, Percesepe A. Pathogenesis of colorectal cancer. Digest Liver Dis 2000; 32:807-21.
61. Robson H, Anderson E, James RD et al. Transforming growth factor beta 1 expression in human colorectal tumours: an independent prognostic marker in a subgroup of poor prognosis patients. Br J Cancer 1996; 74:753-8.
62. Smith DR, Goh H-S. Overexpression of the c-myc proto-oncogene in colorectal carcinoma is associated with a reduced mortality that is abrogated by point mutation of the p53 tumor suppressor gene. Clin Cancer Res 1996; 2:1049-53.
63. Kapitanovic S, Radosevic S, Kapitanovic M et al. The expression of p185$^{HER-2/neu}$ correlates with the stage of disease and survival in colorectal cancer. Gastroenterology 1997; 112:1103-13.
64. Jen J, Kim HG, Piantadosi S et al. Allelic loss of chromosome 18q and prognosis in colorectal cancer. N Engl J Med 1994; 331:213-221.

65. Schneider HJ, Sampson SA, Cunningham D et al. Bcl-2 expression and response to chemotherapy in colorectal adenocarcinomas. Br J Cancer 1997; 75:427-31.
66. Bos JL. ras oncogene in human cancer: a review. Cancer Res 1989; 49:4682-9.
67. Duggan BD, Felix JC, Muderspach LI et al. Early mutational activation of the c-Ki-ras oncogene in endometrial carcinoma. Cancer Res 1994; 54:1604-7.
68. Bleeker WA, Hayes VM, Karrenbeld A et al. Prognostic significance of K-ras and TP53 mutations in the role of adjuvant chemotherapy on survival in patients with Dukes C colon cancer. Dis Colon Rectum 2001; 44:358-63.
69. Kinzler KW, Vogelstein B. Lessons from hereditary colorectal cancer. Cell 1996; 87: 159-70.
70. Varley JM, Evans DGR, Birch JM. Li-Fraumeni syndrome – a molecular and clinical review. Br J Cancer 1997; 76:1-14.
71. Shimamura A, Fisher DE. p53 in life and death. Clin Cancer Res 1996; 2:435-40.
72. Soong R, Grieu F, Robbins P et al. p53 alterations are associated with improved prognosis in distal colonic carcinomas. Clin Cancer Res 1997; 3:1405-11.
73. Petersen S, Thames HD, Nieder C et al. The results of colorectal cancer treatment by p53 status. Treatment-specific overview. Dis Colon Rectum 2001; 44:322-34.
74. Wheeler JMD, Bodmer WF. DNA mismatch repair genes and colorectal cancer. Gut 2000; 47:148-53.
75. Salovaara BR, Louokola A, Kristo P et al. Population-based molecular detection of hereditary nonpolyposis colorectal cancer. J Clin Oncol 2000; 18:2193-200.
76. Lothe RA, Peltomaki P, Meling GI et al. Genomic instability in colorectal cancer: relationship to clinicopathological variables and family history. Cancer Res 1993; 53: 5849-52.
77. Lukish JR, Muro K, DeNobile J et al. Prognostic significance of DNA replication errors in young patients with colorectal cancer, Ann Surg 1998; 227:51-6.
78. Ko JM, Cheung MH, Kwan MW et al. Genomic instability and alterations in Apc, Mcc and Dcc in Honk Kong patients with colorectal carcinoma. Int J Cancer 1999; 84:404-9.
79. Johannsdottir JT, Bergthorsson JT, Gretarsdottir S et al. Replication error in colorectal carcinoma: association with loss of heterozygosity at mismatch repair loci and clinicopathological variables. Anticancer Res 1999; 30:629-34.
80. Gryfe R, Kim H, Hsieh ETK et al. Tumor microsatellite instability and clinical outcome in young patients with colorectal cancer. N Engl J Med 2000; 342:69-77.
81. Gafà R, Maestri I, Matteuzzi M et al. Sporadic colorectal adenocarcinomas with high-frequency microsatellite instability. Cancer 2000; 89:2025-37.
82. Salahshor S, Kressner U,. Fischer H et al. Microsatellite instability in sporadic colorectal cancer is not an independent prognostic factor. Br J Cancer 1999; 81:190-3.
83. Keene SA, Demeure MJ. The clinical significance of micro-metastases and molecular metastases. Surgery 2001; 129:1-5.
84. Miyake Y, Yamamoto H, Fujiwara Y et al. Extensive micrometastases to lymph nodes as a marker for rapid recurrence of colorectal cancer: a study of lymphatic mapping. Clin Cancer Res 2001; 7:1350-7.
85. International (Ludwig) Breast Cancer Study Group. Prognostic importance of occult axillary lymph node micrometastases from breast cancer. Lancet 1990; 335:1565-8.
86. Calaluce R, Miedema BW, Yohannes WY. Micrometastases in colorectal carcinoma: a review. J Surg Oncol 1998; 67:194-202.
87. Adell G, Boeryd B, Frånlung B et al. Occurrence and prognostic importance in micrometastases in regional lymph nodes in Dukes' B colorectal carcinoma; an immunohistochemical study. Eur J Surg 1996; 162:637-42.
88. Liefers GJ, Cleton-Jansen AM, van de Velde CKH et al. Micrometastases and survival in stage II colorectal cancer. N Engl J Med 1998; 339:223-8.
89. Sanchez-Cespedes M, Esteller M, Hibi K et al. Molecular detection of neoplastic cells in lymph nodes of metastatic colorectal cancer patients predicts recurrence. Clin Cancer Res 1999; 5:2450-4.

90. Naeder SB, Archampong EQ. Cancer of the colon and rectum in Ghana: a 5-year prospective study. Br J Surg 1994; 81:456–9.
91. Al-Jaberi TM, Ammari F, Gharieybeh K et al. Colorectal adenocarcinoma in a defined Jordianian population from 1990 to 1995. Dis Colon Rectum 1997; 40:1089–94.
92. Tovar-Guzmán V, Flores-Aldana M, Salmeron-Castro J et al. Epidemiologic panorama of colorectal cancer in Mexico, 1980–1993. Dis Colon Rectum 1998; 41:225–31.
93. Blomqvist P, Ekbom A, Nyrén O et al. Survival after colon cancer 1973–1990 in Sweden. Ann Surg 1997; 225:208–16.
94. Finn-Faivre C, Maurel J, Benhamiche AM et al. Evidence of improving survival of patients with rectal cancer in France: a population based study. Gut 1999; 44:377–81.
95. Miller B, Ries LAG, Hankey BF et al (eds). SEER Cancer Statistics Review 1973–1990. National Cancer Institute, NIH Publication: USA 1993; 93–2789.
96. Sharma VK, Vasudeva R, Howden CW. Changes in colorectal cancer over a 15-year period in a single United States city. Am J Gastroenterol 2000; 95:3615–9.
97. Gatta G, Capocaccia R, Sant M et al. Understanding variations in survival for colorectal cancer in Europe: a EUROCARE high resolution study. Gut 2000; 47:533–8.
98. Sharp D. Trends in cancer survival in England and Wales. Lancet 1999; 353:1437–8.
99. Gatta G, Capocaccia R, Coleman MP et al. Toward a comparison of survival in American and European cancer patients. Cancer 2000; 89:893–900.
100. Martin EW Jr, Cooperman M, Carey LC et al. Sixty second-look procedures indicated primarily by rise in serum CEA antigen. J Surg Res 1980; 28:389–94.
101. Enker WE, Dragacevic S. Multiple carcinomas of the large bowel: a natural experiment in etiology and pathogenesis. Ann Surg 1978; 187:8–11.
102. Tempero M, Brand R, Holdeman K et al. New imaging techniques in colorectal cancer. Semin Oncol 1995; 22:448–71.
103. Staib L, Schirrmeister H, Reske SN et al. Is ^{18}F-fluorodeoxyglucose positron emission tomography in recurrent colorectal cancer: a contribution to surgical decision making? Am J Surg 2000; 180:1–5.
104. Barkin JS, Cohen ME, Flaxman M et al. Value of a routine follow-up endoscopy program for the detection of recurrent colorectal carcinoma. Am J Gastroenterol 1988; 88:1355–60.
105. Bond JH. Colorectal surveillance for neoplasia: an overview. Gastrointest Endosc 1999; 49:S35–40.
106. Ohlsson B, Breland U, Ekberg H et al. Follow-up after curative surgery for colorectal carcinoma: randomised comparison with no follow-up. Dis Colon Rectum 1995; 38:619–26.
107. Mákélá JT, Laitinen SO, Kairaluoma MI. Five year follow-up after radical surgery for colorectal cancer: results of a prospective randomised trial. Arch Surg 1995; 130:1062–7.
108. Kjeldsen B, Kronberg O, Fenger C et al. A prospective randomised study of follow-up after radical surgery for colorectal cancer. Br J Surg 1997; 84:666–9.
109. Bruinsvels DJ, Stiggelbout AM, Kievit J et al. Follow-up of patients with colorectal cancer: a meta-analysis. Ann Surg 1994; 219:174–82.

9 Cancer of the Anal Canal

Introduction

The anal canal is the most extreme segment of the digestive tract and extends proximally from the anal margin (which is covered by epidermis) to the rectal mucosa. Since the anal canal is almost entirely covered by squamous epithelium, neoplasms arising in this segment are usually keratinizing or non-keratinizing squamous cell carcinomas, whose biology and clinical features are rather similar.

Although cancers of the anal canal remain rare neoplasms (1%-2% of all tumors of the digestive organs), their incidence has increased markedly over the last 30-40 years, especially among women, unmarried persons and individuals living in large cities [1]. There is evidence that epidermoid anal carcinoma is somehow associated with sexually transmitted diseases and male homosexuality [2]; moreover, its incidence might also be influenced by the AIDS epidemic. Finally, many observations established a link between anal cancer and cervical carcinoma, which are both associated with human papillomavirus (HPV) infection [3].

From the above considerations, it follows that the morphological, epidemiological and - more in general - biological features of anal cancer are completely different from those of the more frequent colorectal carcinoma.

Epidemiology of Anal Cancer

Descriptive Epidemiology

Melbye et al. [1] analyzed data of the Connecticut Cancer Registry from 1940 to 1988 in order to evaluate the pattern of incidence of anal cancer in the USA. They concluded that the incidence of the disease increased remarkably during this period and that these tumors became progressively more common in women than men, in blacks than Caucasians, and in individuals resident in large cities than those in rural areas. All these data strongly suggest the importance of environmental factors and behavioral changes in anal tumor development, though it remains unclear whether the HIV epidemic affected the trends of anal cancer or whether these changes could be attributed to the simultaneous influence of other causative agents. Similar results were observed in some Scandinavian countries; thus, in Denmark (especially in the Copenhagen metropolitan area) the crude incidence of anal carcinoma increased 3 times in only 30 years among women [4]. In the USA, approximately 3,500 new cases are seen each year, for an age-adjusted incidence rate of 0.3 – 0.6/100,000/year [1, 5]. Data from specialized colorectal cancer registries [6] indicate that similar rates are observed in Western Europe.

Risk Factors

Chronic irritation of the anal region – as in the case of fistulae or hemorrhoids – has been related to cancer of the anal canal by analogy with other conditions but not on the basis of well-grounded scientific evidence [7]. Moreover, rather surprisingly, a history of inflammatory bowel diseases does not confer an increased risk for this type of tumor; among 651 patients with Crohn disease and 509 patients with ulcerative colitis, Frisch et al. [8] were not able to find one case of anal cancer.

While the role of benign lesions and of chronic inflammation remains undefined, there is evidence that sexual practices and sexually transmitted diseases are strongly associated with the development of anal cancer. It has been reported that two correlates of homosexual behavior – a past history of syphilis and never having been married – were somehow related to the risk of anal cancer [9, 10]. In a large study involving 148 patients with anal carcinoma and 166 controls with colorectal neoplasms recruited during the period 1978 – 1985, Daling et al. [11] reported that in men a history of receptive anal intercourse (usually related to homosexual behavior) was strongly associated with the risk of anal cancer, with a relative risk of 33.1. In addition, among patients with epidermoid histological type, almost half of homosexual men and one-third of heterosexual men or women reported a history of genital warts, compared with 1% – 2% among controls. The authors concluded that homosexual behavior in men has to be considered a risk factor for anal cancer, and that squamous cell carcinomas are strongly related to genital warts, thus suggesting that papillomavirus infection is a likely cause of the disease. Frisch et al. [12] were led to rather similar conclusions in their evaluation of a large cohort of 324 women and 93 men with cancer of the anal canal diagnosed between 1991 and 1994 and two control groups. A significant association was found – both in men and women – between sexual promiscuity and risk of anal cancer. Among women, receptive anal intercourse – especially before the age of 30 years – was associated with an increased risk, while 15% of the men with anal cancer reported homosexual behavior, compared with none among controls. The study suggests that anal cancer can be due to a sexually transmitted infection.

A further clue linking anal cancer to an infective agent – and in particular the oncogenic HPV – is its close association with cervical cancer. Thus, there is evidence that women with anal cancer are at increased risk for tumors of the vulva, vagina and cervix uteri [13]. Moreover, data from the SEER program [14] indicate a markedly increased risk of anal and vaginal carcinomas for women with a previous diagnosis of invasive cervical cancer.

All these epidemiological and clinical observations seem to establish a close causal association between HPV infection and cancer of the anal canal. In a recent investigation [12], high-risk types of HPV (i.e. HPV-16) could be detected in 84% of the examined anal cancer samples, while all control rectal carcinomas were negative for HPV. In another large study including 99 patients with advanced anal carcinoma, HPV-16 was detected by in situ hybridization and PCR in 84% and 52% of the tumor tissues in women and men, respectively [15]. Moreover, by studying 129 invasive or in situ anal carcinomas by PCR, Daling et al. [16] reported the presence of one or more HPV types in 70% and 67% of cancer specimens among women and men, respectively. However, we should not forget that several studies indicated that 30%–40% of adults are infected during their lives with HPV of various types [17–19], and these agents therefore appear as necessary but probably not sufficient factors for anogenital cancer development [20]. Since oncogenic HPV can be detected in intraepithelial neoplasia [16, 21], one hypothesis is that these viruses could be implicated in the initial phases of carcinogenesis, while other (unknown) factors might lead to the progression from low- to high-grade dysplasia and from in situ to infiltrating lesions.

Although it is well documented that HIV infection – and the consequent virally induced immunosuppression – increases the likelihood of HPV infections [22, 23], the association between AIDS and cancer of the anal canal remains undefined; thus, we do not know whether HIV infection by itself plays any role in the development of anal cancer. There is some evidence that the risk and the incidence of anal cancer increased concurrently with the appearance of AIDS [24, 25]. However, the sharp increase in anal cancer incidence in Denmark occurred before the appearance of the AIDS epidemic [26]. A case-control investigation of single men living in San Francisco during the 1990s showed a significant increase in the incidence of various tumors (such as Kaposi sarcoma and various lymphomas) but not of anal carcinoma throughout the observation period [27], and data from cancer registries in the USA and Puerto Rico did not show any increase of anal cancer while the cases of AIDS tended to increase sharply [28]. Moreover, a specialized Colorectal Cancer Registry of Northern Italy operating since 1984 did not record any AIDS cases among 1,849 individuals with colorectal malignancies (including 28 patients with anal carcinoma) registered between 1984 and 1995 [29]. Finally, in a recent study on the association of cancer with AIDS-related immunosuppression in adults, Frisch et al. [30] did not report any significant excess risk of anal cancer in a large series (n = 302,834) of patients aged 15–69 years with HIV/AIDS observed during the period 1978–1996.

Among other putative aetiological factors, various studies have shown that a history of cigarette smoking increases the risk of anal cancer by a factor of 2 to 3, independently of sexual behavior [31, 32].

Clinical Features and Pathology

Clinical symptoms of anal carcinoma are scanty and can be absent in up to 20% of patients. Rectal bleeding is the most frequent symptom of onset of the disease and is present in approximately half of the patients. Since bleeding from the anorectal region is rather common, patients and physicians may think of hemorrhoids, fissures or fistulas, with a consequent delay in the diagnosis of anal cancer. Other symptoms include sense of discomfort in the perineal region, pain and the clinical appreciation of a mass just above or within the anal sphincter [33]. A clinical history of genital warts is rather frequent in these patients, especially among homosexual men [5, 11].

The anal canal extends for a few centimeters from the anal margin to the rectum. Unlike the rectal mucosa, which is lined by columnar epithelium, the anal region is covered by a squamous epithelium, which is present between the anal margin and the dentate line. Above this line the epithelium consists of either transitional (urothelium-like) or columnar rectal mucosa. Neoplasms of the anal canal arising distal to the dentate line are usually keratinizing squamous carcinomas; those developing in the transitional mucosa (above the dentate line) are more often non-keratinizing squamous carcinomas [5]. The clinical and biological features of these two histological subtypes of anal cancer are rather similar.

In contrast to the more common colorectal neoplasms, whose dimensions do not seem to be related to the clinical outcome [34], the size of anal tumors has prognostic relevance. Mobile lesions of no more than 2 cm in diameter can be cured in about 80% of the cases, while the likelihood of success drops to 50% for lesions of 5 cm or more [35, 36]. Moreover, the chances of nodal involvement are directly related to the size of the primary lesion. In this respect, tumors located above the dentate line are drained by perirectal and paravertebral nodes, while below the dentate line drainage is through the inguinal and femoral nodes.

In a recent investigation, Noffsinger et al. [37] evaluated the relationship among HPV infection, cell proliferation and alterations in DNA content in 56 patients with anal squamous cell carcinoma, by using in situ hybridization, PCR, immunoperoxidase staining and flow cytometry. They found that the presence of HPV in tumor cells was strongly associated with an increased replicative activity and aneuploid status of neoplasms compared with HPV-negative lesions, thus giving further support to the hypothesis that viral proteins could lead to deregulation of the cell cycle and genomic instability [38].

Finally, Goldman and co-workers [39] analyzed the possible prognostic significance of many clinical and biological parameters in a large series of patients with epidermoid carcinoma of the anal canal; either stage at diagnosis or degree of differentiation was significantly related to the clinical outcome. Moreover, it was noted that patients primarily treated with radiotherapy (with or without chemotherapy) had a more favorable prognosis than patients treated with surgery alone.

Treatment of Cancer of the Anus

As for most tumors of the digestive organs, radical surgery has been the treatment of choice for many years [5]. Local excision was usually sufficient for small and well-demarcated masses; in contrast, abdominoperineal excision became the standard treatment for large and infiltrating lesions. This radical approach required the removal of the anorectal region with a permanent colostomy; the overall probability of surviving 5 years after this type of operation was about 40%–70% [40, 41].

Radiotherapy Alone

During the past few decades there have been suggestions that radiotherapy could possess at least the same potential for curing as surgery, while avoiding colostomy in many cases [42, 43]. Thus, Green et al. [44] showed that external beam irradiation therapy alone was associated with survival rates of up to 75% at 3 years, while James and co-workers [45] favored interstitial irradiation and obtained local control of tumors in 40%–50% of the cases. It is noteworthy that with these procedures not only more than half of the patients survived for 5 years, but most of them maintained an adequate sphincter function. Further investigations revealed that radiation therapy (either as external beam or as interstitial irradiation) was associated with complete eradication of anal carcinomas in 70%–80% of selected patients [46, 47], though the probability of cure was markedly reduced in the case of nodal involvement or neoplasms larger that 5 cm [48]. The optimal dose of radiation therapy is a matter of debate; high doses (50–55 Gy) are probably more effective in inducing a permanent eradication of the tumor [49] but are more often associated with side-effects such as anal ulcers, stenosis and necrosis which may lead to subsequent colostomy [50]. John et al. [51] developed a dose-escalation treatment by giving 36 Gy initially and 23 Gy 2 weeks later, in an attempt to reduce the risk of adverse reactions; unfortunately, this approach resulted in reduced tumor control and had no favorable effect on toxicity.

Combination Therapy

This novel approach was proposed by Norman Nigro and other investigators from Wayne State University (Detroit, USA) in 1974 [52] in an attempt to improve the clinical outcome and to convert inoperable cases into candidates for surgery. The authors treated three patients with anal carcinoma with multimodality therapy consisting of irradiation, chemotherapy with 5-fluorouracil and mitomycin C, followed by abdominoperineal resection. Rather surprisingly, no residual tumor could be detected in the surgical specimens of two patients, and the third subject – who refused surgery – was free of disease at the time of the report, 14 months later. As the authors increased their experience, they no longer recommended that their patients undergo radical surgery, but limited the intervention to excision of the primary carcinoma after chemotherapy and irradiation. Subsequently, they eliminated even this minor surgical procedure [53, 54].

The same approach was subsequently adopted by other investigators and has resulted in a colostomy-free survival rate of 60%–70%. Patients who were not free of tumor after combination treatment with chemotherapy and irradiation – or in whom the disease recurred – could undergo abdominoperineal resection, with a subsequent probability of success of about 60%–90% [55–57].

Finally, the results of three randomized clinical trials [58–60] provided definite evidence of the value of combined chemotherapy and radiation therapy over irradiation alone. In the largest of these investigations [60], 585 patients with squamous cell anal carcinoma were randomized to receive either 45 Gy radiotherapy over 4.4 weeks or the same dose of radiotherapy plus 5-fluorouracil by continuous infusion during the first and the last weeks of radiotherapy, and mitomycin on day 1 of the first course. After a median follow-up of 42 months, 164 of the 279 (59%) patients receiving radiotherapy alone had a local failure, as opposed to 101 of 283 (36%) who were given combination therapy. These findings correspond to a 46% reduction in the risk of local failure ($p < 0.0001$) and to a lower probability of a subsequent colostomy owing to persistent disease. The authors concluded that the standard treatment for most patients with anal carcinoma should consist of a combination of radiotherapy and infused 5-fluorouracil and mitomycin, with surgery reserved for those patients in whom control of the disease was not achieved by this regimen.

Local recurrence and distant metastases are closely related to the size and spread of the tumor at diagnosis [35, 36]. For patients with locally recurrent disease, abdominoperineal resection appears to be the treatment of choice, with a probability of success of about 50% [61]. Distant metastasis developed in 10%–20% of patients treated with combination therapy [59, 60]; the liver is the most frequent site, and there is no curative treatment in such cases [62].

Conclusions

Through cancer of the anal canal is a rare disease, its biology and response to treatment render this neoplasm rather peculiar compared with other tumors of the digestive organs. In fact, it is now widely accepted that the majority of cases are closely related to (if not caused by) HPV infection, as a consequence of sexual promiscuity in both women and men. It follows that in most cases the disease is potentially preventable and in the future could be treated with vaccine or antiviral therapy. Moreover, at sharp variance with all other neoplasms of the digestive tract – which still require surgery as the initial and fundamental treatment – in anal carcinoma a combination therapy with external-beam irradiation and chemotherapy represents the standard approach, with surgery limited to those patients who fail to achieve local control.

References

1. Melbye M, Rabkin C, Frisch M et al. Changing patterns of anal cancer incidence in the United States, 1940-1989. Am J Epidemiol 1994; 139:772-80.
2. Holly EA, Whittemore AS, Aston DA et al. Anal cancer incidence: genital warts, anal fissure or fistula, hemorrhoids, and smoking. J Natl Cancer Inst 1989; 81:1726-31.
3. Melbye M, Sprøgel P. Aetiological parallel between anal cancer and cervical cancer. Lancet 1991; 338:657-9.
4. Frisch M, Melbye M, Moller H. Trends in incidence of anal cancer in Denmark. BMJ 1993; 306:419-22.
5. Ryan DP, Compton CC, Mayer RJ. Carcinoma of the anal canal. N Engl J Med 2000; 342: 792-800.
6. Ponz de Leon M, Di Gregorio C, Roncucci L et al. Epidemiologia dei tumori del colon-retto. Incidenza, mortalità, sopravvivenza e familiarità nella ex U.S.L. di Modena, 1984-1995. Pagine 1-58. Università di Modena, 1998.
7. Holmes F, Borek D, Owen-Kummer M et al. Anal cancer in women. Gastroenterology 1988; 95:107-11.
8. Frisch M, Olsen JH, Bautz A et al. Benign anal lesions and the risk of anal cancer. N Engl J Med 1994; 331:300-2.
9. Daling JR, Weiss NS, Klopfenstein LL et al. Correlates of homosexual behaviour and the incidence of anal cancer. JAMA 1982; 247:1988-90.
10. Austin DF. Etiologic clues from descriptive epidemiology: squamous carcinoma of the rectum or anus. Bethesda, MD: National Cancer Institute, 1982:89-90.
11. Daling J, Weiss NS, Hislop G et al. Sexual practices, sexually transmitted diseases, and the incidence of anal cancer. N Engl J Med 1987; 317:973-7.
12. Frisch M, Glimelius B, van den Brule AJC et al. Sexually transmitted infection as a cause of anal cancer. N Engl J Med 1997; 337:1350-8.
13. Frisch M, Olsen JH, Melbye M. Malignancies that occur before and after anal cancer: clues to their etiology. Am J Epidemiol 1994; 140:12-9.
14. Rabkin CS, Biggar RJ, Melbye M et al. Second primary cancers following anal and cervical carcinoma: evidence of shared etiologic factors. Am J Epidemiol 1992; 136: 54-8.
15. Holm R, Tanum G, Karlsen F et al. Prevalence and physical state of human papillomavirus DNA in anal carcinoma. Mod Pathol 1994; 7:449-53.
16. Daling JR, Sherman KJ, Hislop TG et al. Cigarette smoking and the risk of anogenital cancer. Am J Epidemiol 1992; 135:180-9.
17. Schneider A, Hotz M, Gissmann L. Increased prevalence of human papillomavirus in pregnant women. Int J Cancer 1987; 40:198-201.
18. De Villiers EM, Wagner D, Schneider A et al. Human papillomavirus infections in women with and without abnormal cervical cytology. Lancet 1987; 2:703-6.
19. Zur Hausen H. Papillomavirus in anogenital cancer: the dilemma of epidemiologic approaches. J Natl Cancer Inst 1989; 81:1680-2.
20. Zur Hausen H. Papillomavirus in anogenital cancer as a model to understand the role of viruses in human cancers. Cancer Res 1989; 49:4677-81.
21. Fenger C. Anal neoplasia and its precursors: facts and controversies. Semin Diagn Pathol 1991; 8:190-201.
22. Caussy D, Goedert JJ, Palefsky J et al. Interaction of human immunodeficiency and papilloma viruses: association with anal epithelial abnormality in homosexual men. Int J Cancer 1990; 46:214-9.
23. Williams AB, Darragh TM, Vranizan K et al. Anal and cervical human papillomavirus infection and risk of anal and cervical epithelial abnormalities in human immunodeficiency virus-infected women. Obstet Gynecol 1994; 83:205-11.
24. Melbye M, Cote TR, Kessler L et al. High incidence of anal cancer among AIDS patients. Lancet 1994; 343:636-9.

25. Biggar RJ, Burnett W, Mikl J et al. Cancer among New York men at risk of acquired immunodeficiency syndrome. Int J Cancer 1989; 43:979-85.
26. Goldman S, Glimelius B, Nilsson B et al. Incidence of anal epidermoid carcinoma in Sweden 1970-1984. Acta Chir Scand 1989; 155:191-7.
27. Biggar RJ, Horm J, Goederet JJ et al. Cancer in a group at risk of acquired immunodeficiency syndrome (AIDS) through 1984. Am J Epidemiol 1987; 126:578-86.
28. Goedert JJ, Cote TR, Virgo P et al. Spectrum of AIDS-associated malignant disorders. Lancet 1998; 351:1833-9.
29. Ponz de Leon M, Benatti P, Percesepe A et al. Epidemiology of cancer of the large bowel – The 12-year experience of a specialized Registry in Northern Italy. Ital J Gastroenterol Hepatol 1999; 31:10-8.
30. Frisch M, Biggar RJ, Engels EA et al. Association of cancer with AIDS-related immunosuppression in adults. JAMA 2001; 285:1736-45.
31. Daniell HW. Re: causes of anal carcinoma. JAMA 1985; 21:254-358.
32. Trevathan E, Layde P, Webster LA et al. Cigarette smoking and dysplasia and carcinoma in situ of the uterine cervix. JAMA 1983; 250:499-502.
33. Singh R, Nime F, Mittelman A. Malignant epithelial tumors of the anal canal. Cancer 1981; 48:411-5.
34. Ponz de Leon M, Sant M, Micheli A et al. Clinical and pathologic prognostic indicators in colorectal cancer. Cancer 1992; 69:626-35.
35. Schlienger M, Krzisch C, Pene F et al. Epidermoid carcinoma of the anal canal treatment results and prognostic variables in a series of 242 cases. Int J Radiat Oncol Biol Phys 1989; 17:1141-51.
36. Touboul E, Schlienger M, Buffat L et al. Epidermoid carcinoma of the anal canal: results of curative-intent radiation therapy in a series of 270 patients. Cancer 1994; 73:1569-79.
37. Noffsinger AE, Hui YZ, Suzuk L et al. The relationship of human papillomavirus to proliferation and ploidy in carcinoma of the anus. Cancer 1995; 75:958-67.
38. Woodworth CD, Cheng S, Simpson S et al. Recombinant retrovirus encoding human papillomavirus type 18 E6 and E7 genes stimulate proliferation and delay differentiation in human keratinocytes early after infection. Oncogene 1992; 7:619-26.
39. Goldman S, Glimelius B, Påhlman L et al. Anal epidermoid carcinoma: a population-based clinico-pathological study of 164 patients. Int J Colorect Dis 1988; 3:109-18.
40. Greenall MJ, Quan SH, Urmacher C et al. Treatment of epidermoid carcinoma of the anal canal. Surg Gynecol Obstet 1985; 161:509-17.
41. Dougherty BG, Evans HL. Carcinoma of the anal canal: a study of 79 cases. Am J Clin Pathol 1985; 83:159-64.
42. Papillon J, Mayer M, Montbarbon J. A new approach to the management of epidermoid carcinoma of the anal canal. Cancer 1983; 51:1830-7.
43. Cummings B. The place of radiation therapy in the treatment of carcinoma of the anal canal. Cancer Treat Rev 1982; 9:125-47.
44. Green J, Schaupp W, Cantril S. Anal carcinoma: therapeutic concepts. Am J Surg 1980; 140:151-5.
45. James R, Pointon R, Martin S. Local radiotherapy in the management of squamous carcinoma of the anus. Br J Surg 1985; 72:282-5.
46. Doggett SW, Green JP, Cantril ST. Efficacy of radiation therapy alone for limited squamous cell carcinoma of the anal canal. Int J Radiat Oncol Biol Phys 1988; 15:1069-72.
47. Martenson JA Jr, Gunderson LL. External radiation therapy without chemotherapy in the management of anal cancer. Cancer 1993; 71:1736-40.
48. Eschwege F, Lasser P, Chavy A et al. Squamous cell carcinoma of the anal canal: treatment by external beam irradiation. Radiother Oncol 1985; 3:145-50.
49. Constantinou EC, Daly W, Fung CY et al. Time-dose consideration in the treatment of anal cancer. Int J Radiat Oncol Biol Phys 1997; 39:651-7.

50. Allal AS, Mermillod B, Roth AD et al. Impact of clinical and therapeutic factors on major late complications after radiotherapy with or without concomitant chemotherapy for anal carcinoma. Int J Radiat Oncol Biol Phys 1997; 39:1099–105.
51. John M, Pajak T, Flam M et al. Dose escalation in chemoradiation for anal cancer: preliminary results of RTOG 92–08. Cancer J Sci Am 1996; 2:205–11.
52. Nigro ND, Vaitkevicius VK, Considine B Jr. Combined therapy for cancer of the anal canal: a preliminary report. Dis Colon Rectum 1974; 17:354–6.
53. Nigro N, Seydel H, Considine B et al. Combined preoperative radiation and chemotherapy for squamous cell carcinoma of the anal canal. Cancer 1983; 51:1826–9.
54. Nigro N. An evaluation of combined therapy for squamous cell cancer of the anal canal. Dis Colon Rectum 1984; 27:763–6.
55. Sischy B, Remington JH, Hinson EJ et al. Definitive treatment of anal-canal carcinoma by means of radiation therapy and chemotherapy. Dis Colon Rectum 1982; 25:685–8.
56. Johnson D, Lipsett J, Leong L et al. Carcinoma of the anus treated with primary radiation therapy and chemotherapy. Surg Gynecol Obstet 1993; 177:329–34.
57. Martenson JA, Lipsitz SR, Lefkopoulou M et al. Results of combined modality therapy for patients with anal cancer (E7283): an Eastern Cooperative Oncology Group study. Cancer 1995; 76:1731–6.
58. Flam M, John M, Pajak TF et al. Role of mitomycin in combination with fluorouracil and radiotherapy, and of salvage chemoradiation in the definitive nonsurgical treatment of epidermoid carcinoma of the anal canal: results of a phase III randomized intergroup study. J Clin Oncol 1996; 14:2527–39.
59. Bartelink H, Roelofsen F, Eschwege F et al. Concomitant radiotherapy and chemotherapy is superior to radiotherapy alone in the treatment of locally advanced anal cancer: results of a phase III randomized trial of the European Organization for Research and Treatment of Cancer Radiotherapy and Gastrointestinal Cooperative Group. J Clin Oncol 1997; 15:2040–9.
60. UKCCCR Anal Cancer Trial Working Party. Epidermoid anal cancer: results from the UKCCCR randomised trial of radiotherapy alone versus radiotherapy, 5-fluorouracil, and mitomycin. Lancet 1996; 348:1049–54.
61. Longo WE, Vernava III AM, Wade TP et al. Recurrent squamous cell carcinoma of the anal canal. Predictors of initial treatment failure and results of salvage therapy. Ann Surg 1994; 220:40–9.
62. Tanum G, Tveit K, Karlsen KO et al. Chemotherapy and radiation therapy for anal carcinoma: survival and late morbidity. Cancer 1991; 67:2462–6.

10 Hereditary Non-polyposis Colorectal Cancer (Lynch Syndrome)

Introduction

A definite fraction of colorectal malignancies are inherited through a Mendelian pattern of genetic transmission; this includes not only familial adenomatous polyposis (FAP) and related polyposis syndromes [1], but also hereditary non-polyposis colorectal cancer (HNPCC or Lynch syndrome). HNPCC is characterized by the early manifestation of colorectal cancer – which is more often localized in the proximal colon (from caecum to the splenic flexure) – by the frequent occurrence of multiple tumors of the large bowel (both synchronous and metachronous) and by the association with neoplasms of other organs, especially endometrium, small bowel, stomach, urothelium and ovary [2]. In typical cases, aggregation of neoplasms in various branches of a given family and striking "verticality" (the apparent transmission of cancer from parent to offspring) can be observed.

At least some of the individuals with clinical features of HNPCC inherit a constitutional mutation in one of the several genes controlling DNA mismatch repair [3]. When a somatic mutation inactivates the corresponding wild-type allele, the affected cell accumulates new mutations at a very high rate, and this results in a generalized genomic instability, particularly evident at microsatellite loci [4]. Microsatellite instability (MSI) is therefore a marker of the disease and can be detected in the large majority of tumors from affected individuals.

Lynch syndrome has been extensively investigated in the last two decades, especially because the disease provides an almost unique model for the study of the interaction between environmental factors and genetic background in the development of malignancy of various organs. Despite these efforts, in many cases the identification of HNPCC is complex, and many families may be overlooked. Moreover, several clinical and biological aspects of the disease remain unclear or controversial, and are at present the object of intensive investigation.

Brief History of HNPCC

Aldred Warthin, an American pathologist, reported the first case of HNPCC in 1913 [5]. The family was that of a seamstress working in his house; the author noticed that the woman was depressed because she felt – from her family history – that she would die of cancer. In fact, malignancies of various organs – and especially female organs, stomach and bowel – had already developed in several members of the family. Her suspicions were, unfortunately, correct, and she died of endometrial carcinoma at a young age. Warthin gathered further information from the family and described his "Family G", which was characterized by the occurrence of gastric, colorectal and endometrial carcinomas spanning three generations. Various other tumors were also present in the family; moreover, Warthin noticed the tendency of these neoplasms to develop at an earlier age when compared with sporadic carcinomas. Further reports on the same family appeared in 1931 [6] and 1936 [7]. The significance of this aggregation of neoplasms was appreciated only 30 years later, when Lynch and associates [8] described two large kindreds – with a tumor spectrum similar to that of Family G – defined as "Cancer Family Syndrome". Because of the continuing efforts of Henry T. Lynch – over the last 30 years – in extending and revising the genealogical trees of many HNPCC families and in promoting basic and clinical research virtually in all possible directions, the disease is also referred to as Lynch syndrome.

A further advance in our knowledge of HNPCC was reached in the early 1990s, when an international research group cloned and sequenced a class of genes responsible – when mutated – for the complete clinical spectrum of the disease [9, 10]. The same studies led to the definition of MSI, a type of alteration closely related to the DNA mismatch repair system, which further contributed to the characterization of the complex HNPCC phenotype.

Epidemiology and Frequency of Lynch Syndrome

Lynch syndrome has been described in many races and populations, including North Americans, Europeans, Australians, Japanese, Filipinos [11], Native Americans [12] and Latin Americans [13], but the real prevalence of the disease remains difficult to determine. One of the main problems is that until recently the diagnosis of HNPCC rested on descriptive clinical criteria, some of which may be absent in part of these families. In 1991, the International Collaborative Group on HNPCC proposed the so-called "Amsterdam Criteria" (Table 10.1) as the minimum requisites that should be satisfied for the diagnosis of Lynch syndrome [14]. After a few years, it was recognized that the Amsterdam criteria were rather restrictive, inadequate for small families and, more generally, did not take into account extracolonic tumors, which in most families represent an important component of the syndrome. It is not surprising, therefore, that estimates of the frequency of HNPCC based on these criteria tended to be low. In 1999, the same group proposed new clinical criteria for HNPCC [15] (Table 10.1) which seem more appropriate for defining the syndrome but which should not be considered a guide to exclude suspected families from further investigations.

With the discovery of the mismatch repair genes and of their role in the pathogenesis of Lynch syndrome [3, 4], new problems arose in establishing the frequency of HNPCC. In fact, the list of genes responsible for the HNPCC phenotype includes at least 5 genes but is presumably incomplete, since mutations

Table 10.1. Clinical criteria used for the definition of HNPCC

Amsterdam I criteria [14], 1991:
Three or more relatives in a family should have histologically verified colorectal cancer
One of these should be first-degree relative to the other two
Colorectal cancer should affect at least two generations
One or more colorectal cancer cases should be diagnosed before the age of 50 years
FAP should be excluded

Amsterdam II criteria [15], 1999:
There should be at least three relatives with an HNPCC-associated cancer (colorectum, endometrium, small bowel, ureter or renal pelvis)
One should be a first-degree relative of the other two
At least two successive generations should be affected
At least one cancer should be diagnosed before age 50 years
FAP should be excluded
Tumors should be verified by pathological examination

are found in 30%–80% of families with features of classic HNPCC [2, 4, 16]. Clearly, these are conditions under which estimates based on clinical features will provide frequency values that do not correspond to the estimates obtained through molecular investigations [17]. This discrepancy could be due to a lack of efficacy of the available techniques in detecting all existing mutations of known mismatch repair genes; alternatively, other genes (either related or unrelated to the DNA repair system) could be responsible for the disease phenotype in a given proportion of HNPCC.

Mecklin et al. [18, 19] evaluated the frequency of HNPCC through the data of the Finnish Cancer Registry during the period 1970–1979; according to their estimates, a well-grounded suspicion of Lynch syndrome could be established in 3.8%–5.5% of all patients with colorectal cancer. Rather similar results were obtained by Westlake et al. [20] in southern Alberta (Canada), who reported a frequency of 3.4%, and by Ponz de Leon and collaborators [17, 21, 22], who estimated the frequency of HNPCC in northern Italy to be about 2.6%–4.5% of all registered patients with colorectal malignancies. Rather interestingly, in southern Italy the frequency of HNPCC was less than 1% [23]; since the diet and lifestyle are different in these regions, the findings could be explained by possible differences in the interaction between environmental factors and genetic background. A similar gradient exists in the UK, where a frequency of HNPCC as low as 1% of all colorectal cancers has been reported in some regions (Northern Ireland), while in England the estimate was about 4.0% [24, 25].

More recent studies on the frequency of HNPCC tended, as a whole, to give lower estimates. Aaltonen et al. [26] screened tumor specimens from 509 consecutive patients with colorectal tumors for MSI. Sixty-three patients showed MSI, and in 10 of them constitutional mutations of either MLH1 or MSH2 genes were detected. All individuals with germline alterations had some clinical features of Lynch syndrome. The authors concluded that with their approach the frequency of HNPCC in Finland was at least 2% of all colorectal neoplasms. In a further investigation [27], the same research group evaluated a larger population with a similar approach; the reported frequency of HNPCC was 2.8%. Through the data of a colorectal cancer registry [28], Percesepe et al. screened 389 individuals with neoplasms of the large bowel for MSI and subsequent search of constitutional mutations of MLH1 and MSH2 genes. The observed frequency of HNPCC was much lower than that reported by the Finnish group, about 0.5% of all patients [29]. With a mixed clinical and molecular approach, Peel et al. [30] assessed the frequency of HNPCC in 1,134 American patients with colorectal cancer; on the basis of their data, the authors concluded that the prevalence of the disease in the general population was closer to 1% than to 5%. Finally, Hemminki and Li [31] evaluated the frequency of HNPCC through the nationwide Swedish Family-Cancer Database of 9.6 million subjects. Depending on the assumptions that were made, the prevalence of Lynch syndrome corresponded to 1% or 2.5% of all colorectal malignancies developing among individuals from 0 to 61 years of age.

In summary, clinical studies presumably overestimate the real prevalence of HNPCC among patients with colorectal cancer; this can be due to the frequency of phenocopies and to the chance occurrence of cancer aggregation. On the other hand, it is likely that molecular studies underestimate the frequency of HNPCC, since germline mutations are detectable in only a fraction of typical HNPCC families [32, 33]. As shown in Table 10.2, the real prevalence of HNPCC remains undefined, but almost 15 years of investigations clearly suggest that it should range between 1% and 5% of all colorectal malignancies. If we consider the lower estimate, this means some 300 new cases per year in countries such as Italy or Britain, and some 1,800 cases in countries such as the USA.

Table 10.2. Frequency of HNPCC expressed as percentage of all colorectal malignancies

Study	Evaluation		Reference
	Clinical	Molecular	
Mecklin (1987)	3.8%–5.5%	–	[19]
Westlake (1991)	3.4%	–	[20]
Ponz de Leon (1993)	2.6%–4.5%	–	[17, 21]
Kee (1991)	1.0%	–	[24]
Stephenson (1991)	4.0%	–	[25]
Aaltonen (1998)	–	2.0%	[26]
Salovaara (2000)	–	2.8%	[27]
Percesepe (2001)	–	0.5%	[29]
Peel (2000)	–	~1.0%	[30]

Formal Genetics and the Role of Family History

From the initial reports on HNPCC, its genetic nature became apparent by the simple inspection of the most representative pedigrees. In typical cases, vertical transmission and aggregation of early onset cancer can be observed in all affected branches of these families. However, familial aggregation of colorectal cancer can be the result of hereditary as well as non-hereditary factors, such as environmental determinants (i.e. diet, lifestyle, exposure to carcinogens) shared by family members. The first scientific evidence that a genetic factor underlies at least a fraction of HNPCC came from segregation analysis. Bailey-Wilson and collaborators [34] analyzed 11 HNPCC families comprising 2,762 individuals; the observed findings indicated segregation of a major autosomal dominant gene. Between 71% and 79% of the putative gene carriers were affected by cancer, at an age that was normally distributed with a mean of about 47 years. The results, therefore, favored autosomal dominant transmission with an elevated penetrance, whereas both recessive and polygenic models were rejected. Ponz de Leon et al. [35] came to similar conclusions by studying 28 families with a clinical diagnosis of HNPCC. A few years later, the same authors – using sophisticated analytical procedures – suggested a two-loci model for explaining genetic transmission in HNPCC [36], in which the segregation of a major locus is compatible with co-dominant transmission, and both alleles of a pair are fully expressed on the heterozygote. The estimated gene frequency was 0.0044, which is not far from the figure of 0.006 given by Houlston et al. in 1992 [37], and the lifetime penetrance 0.728 for the heterozygotes. Burt et al. [38, 39] performed segregation analysis in 34 Utah kindreds with clustering of colorectal cancer and adenomatous polyps among close relatives; the results showed that an autosomal dominant type of inheritance could explain the susceptibility to both cancers and polyps.

Thus, the available evidence clearly suggests an autosomal dominant transmission of a highly penetrant gene in classic HNPCC families. This contention is further confirmed by anecdotal reports. In one of these [40], an asymptomatic "obligate carrier" was identified in a large Lynch kindred; the father of this subject had multiple tumors (colon and bladder), while the son developed colon cancer at age 28. When this obligate carrier underwent colonoscopy, a partially obstructing carcinoma of the transverse colon was detected. The situation of an obligate carrier is further illustrated in Fig. 10.1, showing a family that at a first visit had only a suspicion of HNPCC, but that developed full-blown disease after the occurrence of colorectal cancer in an obligate carrier [41]. These case reports underscore the crucial importance of taking an accurate family history for the diagnosis of HNPCC. Indeed, this remains one of the most powerful and cost-effective diagnostic tools, which is frequently overlooked by physicians and surgeons. The family history, however, may not be impressive in many HNPCC families, especially in these times of smaller and more mobile families. These considerations should stimulate the interest of physicians – and especially of family doctors – in gathering all possible information concerning an apparently vague history of cancer running in a family [2]. In a recent study, Johnson et al.

196   Hereditary Non-polyposis Colorectal Cancer (Lynch Syndrome)

PANEL A

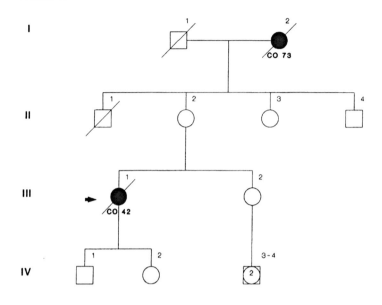

PANEL B

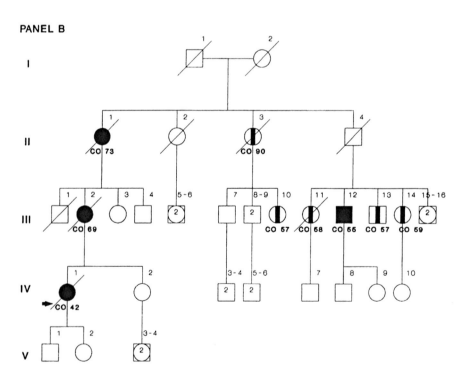

Fig. 10.1 A, B. Legend see page 197

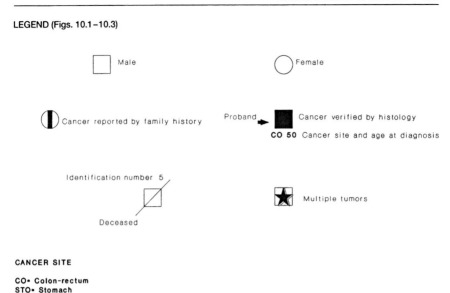

Fig. 10.1 A, B. Obligate carrier in HNPCC family. A Cancer develops in the proband at age 42 years; at this time there are no features of HNPCC. Three years later, colorectal cancer develops in the obligate carrier II-2. Extension of the pedigree (**B**) shows distinctive features of Lynch syndrome

[42] showed that among a general practitioner's practice of 2,000 patients, 40 to 50 of them should have at least one first-degree relative with either breast, ovarian, colorectal or endometrial carcinoma. Moreover, in some European countries, one or two patients every month per family doctor discuss their family history of cancer or other common disease [43]. Thus, there is evidence of an increased public awareness of genetic and familial diseases, and this should lead physicians to a closer evaluation of family history.

Clinical Features of HNPCC

Lynch syndrome is characterized by early age of cancer onset (younger than 45-50 years), proximal predominance of colorectal lesions (70% in most reports), frequency of multiple tumors (both synchronous and metachronous) and excess of extracolonic malignancies, including endometrial, gastric, small bowel, ovarian and transitional cell carcinoma of the ureter and renal pelvis (Table 10.3) [2, 3].

Table 10.3. Extracolonic tumor spectrum in Lynch syndrome

Cancer type	
Integral HNPCC phenotype	*Associated with HNPCC in some families*
Endometrial carcinoma	Haematologic malignancy
Gastric cancer	Soft-tissue tumors
Urothelial cancer (ureter and pelvis)	Laryngeal carcinoma
Small-bowel cancer	Brain tumors
Hepatobiliary tumors	Breast carcinoma
Ovarian tumors	

Age at Diagnosis and Preferential Location in the Right Colon

Although early age of cancer onset in HNPCC is extremely frequent, this cannot be considered an absolute requirement. In most families, patients with tumors (of the colon or other target organs) detected at an early age coexist with individuals in whom tumors develop in their sixties or seventies. In the Lynch series, the average age at diagnosis of the first colorectal cancer was 44 years [2]. In other series, however, the mean age of onset of colorectal neoplasms was slightly different (between 45 and 55 years), with only 30%–40% of tumors being diagnosed before the age of 50 [44–46]. So far, the youngest affected patient reported in the literature was 13 years old [47]. In general, in all patients who developed colorectal cancer before the age of 45 years, the diagnosis of HNPCC should be suspected. Aside from an accurate family history, further investigations include MSI and immunohistochemical expression of MLH1 and MSH2 gene proteins (see below). Even in the absence of a strong familiality, the occurrence of a MSI+ colorectal tumor before the age of 45 should suggest a search for possible germline mutations of the DNA mismatch repair genes. However, we should not forget that the majority of patients with colorectal cancer diagnosed prior to 45 years will not have HNPCC [20, 48].

In the Lynch experience, about 70% of colorectal carcinomas in HNPCC, versus 30% of sporadic tumors, are located proximal to the splenic flexure [2]. In other series this proportion tended to be lower: 42% in an Italian study [44, 49], 60% and 50%, respectively, in Dutch and Finnish series [45, 46]. These differences could be due to the method of selection of families, to diversities in the populations investigated, and to the effect of phenocopies [44]. The reasons for the preferential location of HNPCC tumors in the proximal colon remain unexplained. The fact that most MSI+ lesions occur in the right colon extends the observation but does not provide an explanation. In effect, proximal carcinomas, HNPCC-associated tumors, and MSI+ lesions share some characteristics, such as a higher frequency of poorly differentiated carcinomas and of mucinous carcinomas [2, 3].

Multiple Tumors

Multiple tumors are relatively frequent in some types of cancer that may be associated with a good prognosis, such as colorectal and breast carcinomas. The reasons why a subgroup of patients develops more than one neoplasm remain unclear and represent a challenge for cancer researchers. By definition, two or more tumors occurring simultaneously are designated as synchronous, whereas tumors occurring at various intervals of time are known as metachronous. Multiple tumors (both synchronous and metachronous) are rather frequent in the large bowel, in which they may represent up to 10% of all malignancies [50, 51]. In HNPCC, multiple malignancies of the large bowel are particularly frequent, an observation which led various investigators to propose subtotal colectomy and ileorectal anastomosis as the most appropriate surgical approach, because of the risk of a second or third tumor [52, 53]. In the Lynch series, 21 of 116 patients (in 10 HNPCC kindreds) presented with multiple cancers in the colorectum; even more significant was the fact that the 10-year cumulative incidence of metachronous neoplasms was 40%, when the first cancer was not treated with subtotal colectomy [54]. Similarly, Mecklin and Jarvinen [52] reported multiple malignancies in 29 of 81 HNPCC patients who survived at least 1 year after the index colorectal carcinoma, corresponding to a cumulative annual risk of 3.2%. Although lower frequencies of multiple lesions were reported in other HNPCC series [55, 56], as a general tendency the incidence of multiple lesions in HNPCC

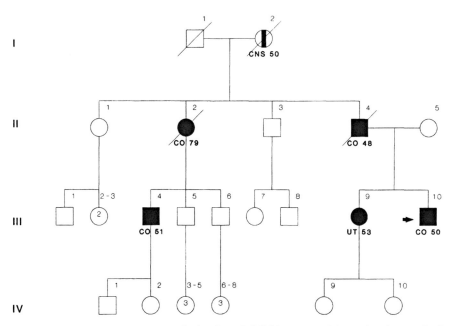

Fig. 10.2. Representative pedigree of a family with full-blown HNPCC meeting the standard criteria of Table 10.1. A MSH2 gene truncating mutation co-segregates with the neoplastic phenotype. (For explanation of labels see Fig. 10.1, p. 197)

was appreciably higher than that observed among patients with common colorectal tumors. In one of these studies, the interval between the first and the second malignancy ranged between 1 and 18 years, with an average of 9 years [56]. The reasons for the proclivity to multiple lesions in HNPCC patients is presumably related to the underlying constitutional mutation in one of the DNA mismatch genes and to the consequent generalized genomic instability [3, 4]. Figure 10.2 shows a representative family with full-blown HNPCC.

Tumor Spectrum

In addition to colorectal tumors, several extracolonic malignancies can be observed in the majority of HNPCC families [3]. At present, the HNPCC tumor spectrum includes endometrial carcinoma, gastric cancer, tumors of the small bowel (not concentrated in the periampullar region, as in FAP), tumors of the hepatobiliary tract, transitional cell carcinoma (of the ureter and renal pelvis), pancreatic and ovarian tumors [2, 3]. There is also evidence that soft-tissue tumors (fibrous histocytoma, neurofibroma), laryngeal carcinoma and breast cancer should also be included in the spectrum, though their occurrence is limited to a small number of families [57, 58]. Finally, various skin tumors (sebaceous adenomas and carcinomas, keratoacanthomas) characterize the Muir-Torre syndrome [59], a clinical variant of HNPCC.

The tumor spectrum of Lynch syndrome has been largely investigated, especially in American and European series. Fitzgibbons et al. [53] examined the distribution of 334 cancers diagnosed in 10 extended HNPCC kindreds. They found that colorectal tumors represented 55% of all cancers, and endometrial carcinomas 14%; both tumor types were markedly more frequent than the rates observed in the general population. Vasen and collaborators [55] described the tumor spectrum of 324 Dutch HNPCC families; as expected, colorectal carcinoma was the most frequent malignancy and was the only cancer type observed in four families. Among extracolonic lesions, endometrial, gastric and urinary tract carcinomas were detected more frequently than expected, leading the authors to conclude that these cancer types were integral to the hereditary tumor spectrum of HNPCC. Rather similar tumor spectra were reported by Mecklin and Jarvinen [52] in a study of 22 Finnish HNPCC kindred and by Benatti et al. [22] in an Italian series of 28 families. In another large Italian kindred, Cristofaro et al. [60] reported a marked excess of gastric carcinomas (almost as frequent as colorectal cancer, and with an early age of onset in all cases) and of chronic gastritis of the antrum. In a more recent report by the Lynch group [61], the frequency of specific cancer types was evaluated in 23 large kindreds with HNPCC. By comparing the observed number of cancers to the expected rates from tumor registries, the authors showed that tumors of the stomach, small intestine, hepatobiliary system, urinary tract, endometrium and ovary all occurred significantly more often in HNPCC family members than in the general population.

Other tumor types have been described in Lynch families, but it is not yet clear whether this is a coincidental association or should be considered part of the HNPCC phenotype. These neoplasms include haematologic malignancies [62], brain tumors [63], laryngeal carcinoma [64], soft-tissue tumors [58,65] and breast carcinoma [57]. Cancer of the stomach is usually included in the Lynch spectrum, though it is much more common in older generations of American and European HNPCC families [2, 52, 55, 44], and in HNPCC kindreds from Eastern Asia (Japan and Korea), where the risk is high enough to justify close surveillance [66].

There is some evidence that differences in the frequency of extracolonic involvement might exhibit a genetic basis. Mecklin et al. [67] evaluated the tumor occurrence in 28 HNPCC families with MLH1 gene mutations and in 19 families with MSH2 mutations; in the former group, 27% of all tumors were extracolonic compared with 42% in the latter group. Similar observations were reported by Liu et al. [68], who found extracolonic cancers in 33% of HNPCC patients carrying a MSH2 constitutional mutation, but in only 12% of patients with MLH1 mutations. From these preliminary observations it seems probable that the phenotypic expression of MSH2 alterations includes a broader spectrum of lesions, an observation which might be of relevance in the screening, surveillance and follow-up of affected individuals.

Pathology of HNPCC

Lynch syndrome is referred as "non-polyposis" colorectal cancer; this definition underscores the concept that HNPCC and FAP are different diseases but does not mean that adenomas do not play any role in the pathogenesis of malignancy. As a matter of fact, there are various observations indicating that common adenomatous polyps are more frequent in HNPCC than in a control population of the same age [69, 70]. Moreover, Jass and co-workers [71, 72] showed that these lesions – in HNPCC families – tend to be large and with a villous configuration. The observation led to the concept of "aggressive adenomas" in HNPCC; in effect, there is evidence that adenomas in HNPCC progress to carcinoma at a more rapid rate than in the general population and that this accelerated progression can be attributed to loss of DNA repair proficiency [4, 73]. Further confirmation of this hypothesis was provided by Ponz de Leon et al. in a recent study [70]. The authors evaluated colonoscopic reports in 86 high-risk individuals from 31 HNPCC families; one or more colorectal lesions were found in 40.7% of HNPCC asymptomatic family members compared with 17.4% in matched controls. Adenomatous lesions in high-risk subjects were significantly larger (9.1 vs 5.8 mm, $p < 0.02$) and more frequently showed a tubulovillous pattern and a high degree of dysplasia. The authors concluded that the high incidence of neoplastic lesions in asymptomatic HNPCC family members, their distribution in the large bowel and the possible aggressive behavior suggest screening by colonoscopy only and at intervals of 1–2 years.

Colorectal carcinomas arising in HNPCC have been extensively investigated with the purpose of identifying distinctive features from common malignancies of the large bowel. As a matter of fact, there is no single morphological parameter which can differentiate tumors occurring in Lynch syndrome from their sporadic counterpart; however, certain histopathologic findings show a higher prevalence in individuals with HNPCC. These include poorly differentiated carcinoma, mucinous tumors, signet ring cell carcinoma, and medullary or undifferentiated lesions [2, 3, 74, 75]. According to some observations [74], the mucinous histological type is present in 30%-40% of HNPCC tumors as opposed to 10%-15% of sporadic colorectal cancers: in addition, mucinous lesions appear to aggregate in certain families [75]. "Poorly differentiated", "undifferentiated" or "medullary" carcinomas can be observed more frequently in HNPCC than in sporadic colorectal tumors; these histological types seem to be closely associated with lesions of the right colon and exhibit MSI [76]. A recent study [77] suggested that poor differentiation in general was a particularly prominent features of colorectal cancer from HNPCC families with MSH2 mutations, whereas MLH1-associated tumors are more likely to elicit a Crohn's-like lymphoid response.

Two flow cytometric studies showed a definite prevalence of diploid tumors in HNPCC patients (70% versus 30% in sporadic tumors), thus suggesting that this could be one of the distinctive features of colorectal carcinoma in Lynch syndrome [78, 79]. Since diploid lesions are usually associated with a better prognosis than aneuploid tumors, predominance of the diploid pattern might explain the more favorable outcome of colorectal malignancies in HNPCC (see below). Low cell replication activity (assessed with the AgNOR technique) and poor vascularization of tumors have also been reported in HNPCC [80].

Taken together, can these morphological parameters be of help in the identification of HNPCC? Unfortunately, none of these markers showed a clear-cut result in defining HNPCC. However, when evaluating a suspected HNPCC, the presence of a diploid pattern in tumor fragments, associated with low cell kinetics, poor differentiation or medullary histological type, and abundant mucin secretion, may reinforce the suspicion, thus suggesting further investigations, such as MSI and MSH2/MLH1 proteins immunohistochemical expression.

Molecular Biology of HNPCC

The greatest discoveries to date in the molecular genetics of common inherited neoplasms relate primarily to breast, ovarian and colorectal carcinomas [81]. Lynch syndrome, therefore, exemplifies the main problems inherent in identifying the genetic components of diseases of common occurrence in the population. The confounding factors include chance aggregation of cancers in families, the possible influence of exogenous factors (such as diet and lifestyle), genetic heterogeneity and frequency of phenocopies [4]. Despite these problems, in the last 10 years a new class of genes has been discovered, and new molecular mechanisms of tumorigenesis have been proposed [2,3]. The importance of these new findings are not limited to HNPCC but, more generally, concern the process of colorectal tumor development in humans. Since most patients with HNPCC inherit a constitutional mutation in one of the genes responsible for repairing DNA mismatch errors, we should begin with a schematic description of the mismatch repair mechanisms.

DNA Mismatch Repair in Bacteria

The DNA mismatch repair is a cellular activity capable of recognizing abnormal base pairs and correcting the sequence on one strand to obtain a normal A-T or G-C pairing. This activity also corrects stretches of unpaired bases that result from the insertion or deletion of nucleotides on one of the two DNA strands [2, 3, 82]. Studies in *Escherichia coli* showed the existence of multiple mismatch repair pathways and, among these, two pathways termed "Long Patch" and "Very Short Patch" repair, for the different lengths of DNA sequence excised during repair [83]. Three main proteins are involved in mismatch repair: mut S, mut L and mut H; these proteins are encoded by the corresponding "mutator" genes *Mut S, Mut L* and *Mut H* [84, 85]. The mut S protein binds to mismatched DNA sequences; mut H identifies the newly created DNA strand by differences in methylation between the template and the new strand; mut L and mut H then cooperate with mut S to remove the mismatched nucleotides. It has been subsequently determined that the bacterial methyl-directed mismatch repair system requires several proteins acting in the following three steps [3, 85]:

1. *Recognition of the mismatched DNA.* mut S protein binds to the mismatch, and mut H to hemimethylated GATC sequences; a homodimer of mut L forms a complex with mut S and mut H; this binding potentiates the endonuclease activity of mut H, which cleaves the DNA at the GATC site on the unmethylated strand [86].
2. *Excision of the newly synthesized strand.* An enzyme removes a segment of the incised strand extending from the nick of the GATC site to just beyond the mismatch [86].
3. *Replacement of the excised DNA and ligation.* The unpaired DNA is stabilized with single-strand binding protein, as DNA polymerase III resynthesizes the complementary strand, thus correcting the mismatch [87].

   Eukaryotic cells follow a very similar bacterial pathway, characterized by strand-specificity, bidirectional excision capability and employment of the replicative DNA polymerase alpha [88].

Human Mismatch Repair Genes in Lynch Syndrome

Although DNA mismatch repair genes have been well characterized in yeast and bacteria, until the 1990s there was little evidence that similar mechanisms were operating in humans. The first human mismatch gene to be cloned was *hMSH2* (MSH2), the homologue of yeast *MSH2* and *Escherichia coli Mut S*. Peltomaki et al. [9, 10], through linkage studies, mapped hMSH2 to chromosome 2p15–16 in two large HNPCC families, and constitutional mutations co-segregating with the disease phenotype were subsequently identified [89]. Most of these mutations result in truncated polypeptides and, consequently, could be detected by a coupled in vitro transcription-translation assay (protein truncation test) [90].

The second human mismatch gene (*hMLH1*) was mapped to chromosome 3p21.3 and showed striking homologies to yeast *MLH1* and *E. coli Mut L* [91]. Constitutional mutations in MLH1 were identified in affected members of HNPCC families and linked to chromosome 3p; most of these germline mutations appeared to alter the size of the MLH1 protein [92]. It was also found that most Finnish HNPCC families showed an ancestral MLH1 mutation indicative of a founder effect [93]. Two additional mut L-related genes were subsequently identified and designated as *hPMS1* and *hPMS2*, owing to homology to the yeast mut L homologue *PMS* [94]. Although HNPCC patients with constitutional alterations in *PMS1* or *PMS2* have been identified, mutations at these genetic loci are much less prevalent than mutations in either *MLH1* or *MSH2* [93, 95]. Another MUT S homologue, termed *GTBP* (for G-T binding protein) or *MSH6*, has been identified [96] and constitutional mutations detected in some HNPCC families [97, 98]. Finally, germline variants (mostly missense mutations) in the recently cloned human MLH3 gene have been reported in 12 patients suspected of HNPCC [98a] (Table 10.4).

From the above-mentioned investigations, it became clear that tumor development in many HNPCC families was strongly associated with constitutional mutations of human homologues of *Mut S* or *Mut L* bacterial genes designated as hMSH2, hMLH1, hPMS1, hPMS2, GTBP/hMSH6 [3, 4] and probably hMLH3. Additional *Mut S* and *Mut L* homologues have been identified, but their role in human diseases remains unsettled [3, 99]. Although this new class of genes ("mismatch repair" or "mutator" genes) is different from the well-known oncogenes and tumor suppressor genes, the mechanism of action in inducing tumor development shows similarities with that of tumor suppressor genes. In fact, both alleles need to be inactivated for the cell to display a mutator phenotype

Table 10.4. Genes involved in HNPCC

Main DNA mismatch repair genes	Homologue (*E. coli*)	CDNA (bp)	Amino acids	Chromosome
hMSH2	Mut S	3,111	934	2p16
hMLH1	Mut L	2,484	–	3p21–23
hPMS1	Mut L	3,063	756	2q31–33
hPMS2	Mut L	2,771	932	7q22
GTBP/hMSH6	Mut S	4,200	832	2p16
hMLH3	Mut L	–	–	–
Other genes				
MED 1 [141]	Glycosylase/lyase	–	–	3q21–22
CRAC 1 [140]	–	–	–	15q14–22
EXO 1 [142]	Yeast exonuclease 1	–	–	1q42–43

with consequent MSI, a situation that is clearly reminiscent of Knudson's "two-hit" hypothesis for tumor suppressor genes [100]. As suggested for other rare or common inherited tumors, cells carrying a constitutional alteration in a tumor suppressor gene acquire the second "hit" through inactivating mutations, loss of heterozygosity or methylation of the other allele [100]. In accordance with this reasoning, Hemminki et al. [101] provided evidence that loss of the wild-type allele accompanies tumor development in HNPCC.

Microsatellite Instability: the MSI+ Phenotype

The identification and characterization of mutator genes favored some critical work on DNA microsatellites. Microsatellites are repeating sequences of DNA that are distributed throughout the human genome, most commonly (A)n/(T)n and (CA)n/(GT)n. Their function remains poorly understood, but they are useful in linkage analysis owing to their degree of polymorphism [3, 4].

During linkage studies which led to the identification of the main DNA mismatch genes, a new genetic alteration was identified in HNPCC tumors. Shifts in the electrophoretic mobility of microsatellite markers were usually present in tumor DNA compared with normal DNA from the same patient [10, 102]. These mobility shifts were due to the deletion or expansion of one or more repeat units at several loci and occurred mostly within dinucleotide or trinucleotide repeats (especially CAn). Microsatellites display a mutation rate higher than other genomic loci, but they are stably inherited across generations and mutate appreciably only on an evolutionary scale. Thus, the results were interpreted as genomic instability leading to replication errors. Since almost all tumors from HNPCC patients showed MSI in at least two loci, the main conclusion was that mutations in the DNA mismatch repair genes are responsible for genomic instability through a generalized defect in the replication/repair processes [103].

MSI can also be detected in 8%-15% of sporadic colorectal malignancies [104]. In these cases, somatic inactivation (usually by hypermethylation of the promoter region) of both alleles in one of the mutator genes (more often MLH1) has been demonstrated [105, 106]. Sporadic colorectal cancers with MSI show several similarities with HNPCC tumors, such as prevalent localization in the proximal colon, normal nuclear ploidy, frequent mucinous histological type and a tendency to an overall better prognosis [107, 108]. After the description of MSI in hereditary and sporadic colorectal tumors, various reports have been published describing this type of genetic alteration in several other human cancers, such as breast and lung carcinomas [109, 110], and tumors included in the HNPCC spectrum, in particular gastric, pancreatic and endometrial malignancies [111-113]. The observation of the MSI phenotype in such a broad range of neoplasms pointed out the need for establishing standardized procedures to assess MSI, both in terms of the number and type of loci investigated and of the minimal number of altered loci necessary to define a tumor as unstable [114, 115].

Microsatellite Instability and Cancer Development

The discovery that a defective DNA repair system – with the consequent development of the MSI phenotype – is involved in the pathogenesis of HNPCC (and, presumably, of a fraction of sporadic colorectal tumors) clarified the role that an increased mutation rate plays in tumor induction and progression.

As already mentioned, upon inheritance of a mutant allele, the normal allele may supply normal mismatch function to the cell; however, a second mutation (somatic) of the corresponding allele may later arise, thus disabling the mismatch repair function of the cell [100, 101]. DNA mismatch repair deficiency leads to a high level of MSI, and cells tend to accumulate mutations at an accelerated rate [116]. This elevated mutation rate may affect tumor development in at least two ways. First, the generalized genomic instability may enhance the likelihood of inducing mutations in known oncogenes or tumor suppressor genes, thus facilitating tumor growth. Second, it has been shown that certain "crucial genes" are particularly prone to replication defects upon impairment of the repair machinery [3, 85]. One of these presumably crucial mutations was reported by Parsons et al. [117] and by Markowitz et al. [118] who found that some 90% of colorectal carcinomas with MSI contain mutations of the transforming growth factor-β (TGF-β) type II receptor gene. This particular receptor gene can be preferentially mutated in patients with defective mismatch repair since the gene contains a sequence of 10 consecutive A bases, and long-repeat sequences are susceptible to mismatch errors. Since TGF-β inhibits the growth of colonic epithelial cells, the authors suggested that these mutations could represent a critical step in tumor progression. Subsequent studies showed that several other genes have repetitive tracts in their coding sequences and are frequently mutated in colorectal cancers in HNPCC or sporadic cancer with MSI. These include IGF2R, BAX, CDX-2, E2F-4 and caspase 5 [119–123], which participate in the control of cell replication, differentiation and apoptosis. Moreover, two mismatch repair genes – hMSH3 and hMSH6 – have repeat sequences in their coding regions, and various mutations have been detected in HNPCC carcinomas and sporadic cancers with MSI [124]. Somatic mutations of additional mismatch repair genes may serve as secondary mutators, thus accelerating the accumulation of further MSI and coding region mutations [125]. Perucho et al. [126] described this phenomenon as "the mutator which mutates other mutators".

Thus, colorectal tumorigenesis in HNPCC, and in sporadic colorectal carcinomas showing MSI, follows a molecular pathway that differs in many steps from the sequence of events which have been proposed for common colorectal cancers [4, 127]. This "DNA mismatch repair pathway", though defined in the late 1990s, was predicted by Loeb in 1991 [128]. The author hypothesized that the multistage model of carcinogenesis required more mutations than could be expected for cells subject to the observed spontaneous mutation rate and suggested that an early mutation in a multistep process could be one that confers a mutator phenotype on affected cells.

Frequency of Mutations in HNPCC Families

Although at least six genes (Table 10.4) have been associated with DNA mismatch repair, most of the mutations found in humans were detected in either hMSH2 or hMLH1 genes. The contribution of hPMS1, hPMS2 and hMSH6 remains undefined; however, the available evidence suggests that they account for less than 5% of all constitutional alterations detected in HNPCC families [129]. The majority of mutations in hMSH2 and hMLH1 genes are evenly distributed, with some clustering in MSH2 exon 12 and MLH1 exon 16. Most MSH2 alterations consist of frameshift (60%) or missense mutations (31%). Although most of these molecular changes were unique, a few common recurring mutations were found [129]. On the transcriptional/translational level, mutations in MLH1 and MSH2 genes were predicted to result in changes of the reading frame, translation termination (owing to the introduction of a stop codon), substitution of an amino acid, or deletion of one or more amino acids with the basic reading frame unchanged (in-frame deletions) [129, 130].

The search for constitutional mutations depends closely on the criteria adopted for the selection of families. When the Amsterdam criteria (I or II) are applied (Table 10.1) [14, 15], the available literature suggests that MLH1 or MSH2 mutations can be found in 30%-70% of the investigated families [131-134]. When other selection criteria were used - "suspected" HNPCC on a clinical basis, Bethesda criteria [115] - germline mutations are detected in no more than 5%-20% of the families [135, 136]. In a recent study, Wjinen et al. [137] evaluated the prevalence of MSH2 and MLH1 mutations in 184 kindreds with familial clustering of colorectal cancer or other tumors of the HNPCC spectrum [53]. Mutations could be detected in 47 of 184 families (26%). Multivariate analysis showed that a younger age at diagnosis of colorectal cancer, fulfillment of the Amsterdam criteria, and presence of endometrial cancer in the kindred were independent predictors of germline mutations. These investigations confirm that the identification of HNPCC families remains problematic - despite our knowledge about the genetic basis of the disease - and that the Amsterdam criteria represent the most accurate method for selecting families to be tested for the presence of constitutional mutations. Benatti et al. [138] evaluated whether the presence of germline mutations in MSH2 or MLH1 genes and MSI could identify distinct clinical subgroups among HNPCC families. Twenty-nine families selected on the basis of the Amsterdam criteria were divided into three groups: those with constitutional mutations in one of the genes (group 1, $n = 10$), those with MSI but without mutations (group 2, $n = 10$), and those with neither MSI nor constitutional mutations (group 3, $n = 9$). When compared with group 3, group 1 and 2 families showed a similar tumor spectrum, an earlier age of onset of colorectal cancer, a higher risk of cancer during follow-up, and an overall better prognosis. The authors concluded that molecular analysis could distinguish - within HNPCC families clinically defined - different subgroups which could be followed with specific surveillance programs. The close similarities between group 1 and group 2 families suggest the probable involvement of DNA mismatch repair genes, even when mutations are not detectable.

In summary, a fraction of patients with HNPCC defined by the Amsterdam criteria do not harbor mutations in the mismatch repair genes. This might depend on the presence of "cryptic" alterations which are not easily detectable with the available techniques; as an alternative, these families could have mutations in other, not yet identified genes. Chance aggregation of cancer and phenocopies cannot be excluded, though this event seems unlikely, especially in large families with several affected generations.

New Genes Predisposing to HNPCC

Since germline mutations in the known mismatch repair genes have been detected in only a fraction of HNPCC families, various investigators attempted to evaluate the possible existence of other colorectal cancer susceptibility genes (Table 10.4). The indirect evidence for additional genes is further supported by the presence of families with clinical features of HNPCC that show evidence against linkage to the known loci [139].

Tomlinson et al. [140] evaluated, by linkage analysis, a large Ashkenazi family in which several members developed multiple colorectal adenomas, while some were affected by colorectal or pancreatic carcinomas. The authors provided evidence for a new colorectal cancer susceptibility gene (denominated CRAC1, for colorectal adenoma and carcinoma) mapping to chromosome 15q14–22. This chromosomal region contains several genes (such as the human homologue of RecA gene, BCL8, FGF7 and others) that might be considered candidates. Additional studies are needed, however, to confirm the localization of this putative gene and to evaluate its contribution to hereditary colorectal cancer. Riccio et al. [141] identified a new mismatch repair gene (MBD4 or MED1, for methyl-binding endonuclease 1) that encodes a MLH1 interactor. Somatic mutations of MED1 have been detected in 11 of 42 colorectal carcinomas with MSI; these alterations consisted of 1- or 2-bp deletions or 1-bp insertions causing frameshifts and premature stop codons. Constitutional mutations of MED1 have not been detected so far in HNPCC families; with regard to the possible role of this new gene in regulating genomic instability, the authors proposed that MED1 alterations may represent mutator's mutations that contribute to the progressive unfolding of MSI in colorectal carcinoma.

A human exonuclease 1 (EXO1) homologue to yeast exonuclease 2 has recently been cloned [142]. The gene comprises 14 exons and 13 introns that span approximately 42 kilobases of genomic DNA at chromosome 1q42–43. The protein product of the human EXO1 interacts with the human MSH2 protein, thus suggesting a possible involvement in the process of mismatch repair [143]. Wu et al. [144] analyzed all exons of EXO1 for mutations in index patients from 33 families with HNPCC fulfilling the Amsterdam II criteria [15] and in 225 index patients suspected of HNPCC. Constitutional variants of EXO1 could be detected in 14 patients, but not in more than 200 control individuals; all EXO1 variants were identified in families in which no germline MSH2, MLH1 or MSH6 mutation had been found. About half of the tumors with EXO1 alterations showed

MSI. The authors concluded that these preliminary results indicate a possible association of EXO1 germline variants with classical and suspected HNPCC.

Further studies are needed to evaluate the possible contribution of CRAC1, MED1, EXO1 and presumably other genes in the pathogenesis of HNPCC.

Diagnosis of HNPCC

Until the discovery of mismatch repair genes and MSI, the only approach to the identification of HNPCC was based on a close analysis of pedigrees with the selective extension of those showing a clinical suspicion of the disease. At present, the situation is much more favorable, since molecular tests are now available which can indicate in many cases whether or not probands and their close relatives are predisposed to tumor development. Being costly and time consuming, however, these molecular techniques can hardly be applied to the entire population of colorectal cancer patients, but only to highly selected groups. Thus, one of the main tasks for researchers and physicians dealing with hereditary cancer syndromes is the recognition and classification of patients with colorectal cancer according to different levels of genetic risk.

Identification of HNPCC

At present, there are three major strategies for selecting individuals at risk of genetically determined colorectal tumors. The first approach is mainly based on pedigree analysis. Several research groups [22, 25, 53, 55] developed clinical criteria which were used for stratifying and classifying patients with colorectal tumors into different subgroups, according to a more or less likely genetic component. Ponz de Leon et al. [17, 145] subdivided all tumors developed in the general population into five major classes based on the data of a colorectal cancer registry: HNPCC (on a clinical basis), suspected HNPCC, juvenile cases (individuals with cancer diagnosis before the age of 50 years), familial tumors (i.e. aspecific cancer aggregation) and sporadic cases. In the two groups who were at higher risk of genetically determined disease (HNPCC and suspected HNPCC), MSI was assessed, and MSI-positive patients were studied for constitutional alterations of the major DNA mismatch repair genes (MSH2 and MLH1). Mutations were found only in families meeting the Amsterdam criteria [14], and their frequency (16.6% of all families with clinical features of HNPCC) was lower than that reported in previous investigations [131, 132].

Since the large majority of neoplasms developing in HNPCC show MSI, de la Chapelle and collaborators [26] proposed an alternative approach for the identification of the disease. All colorectal malignancies arising in a given population could be analyzed for MSI; from the available literature, there should be 10%–15% positive tests. All patients showing instability should then be screened for constitutional mutations of MSH2, MLH1 and, possibly, other DNA mismatch repair genes. Although rather straightforward, this approach demands considerable laboratory work and is best implemented in areas covered by cancer registries. Recent observations with these procedures [27, 29] indicate an overall incidence of the HNPCC phenotype of the order of 0.5%–3.0% of all registered colorectal malignancies.

A third approach can take advantage of the fact that most MSH2 and MLH1 mutations cause truncation of the proteins or absence of the transcripts [146], and that monoclonal antibodies have been developed which react with the proteins encoded by the two genes. Immunohistochemistry, therefore, can be used to identify homozygous inactivation of either MSH2 or MLH1 by the absence of immunoreactive cells in tumor tissue. This can allow the screening of a large number of colorectal tumors and the search for possible constitutional mutations of the major mismatch repair genes in patients whose neoplasms are negative to immunostaining. Since this approach cannot differentiate somatic from constitutional mutations, it is likely that – as with the MSI testing – only a small proportion of the tumors lacking immunoreactive staining will represent HNPCC. In a recent study, Terdiman et al. [147] analyzed MSI and MSH2 and MLH1 immunostaining in 114 families at high-risk for hereditary colorectal cancer. In patients showing MSI or absence of immunoreactivity in tumor cells, constitutional mutations of MSH2 and MLH1 were looked for. The authors found that detection of MSI and loss of MSH2 or MLH1 immunostaining in colorectal cancer are both useful criteria for selecting high-risk patients who should be tested for germline mutations of the major mismatch repair genes.

Despite the availability of several approaches, the identification of HNPCC families remains difficult owing to the existence of several problems, such as presence of phenocopies, small size of most families, variability in the clinical expressivity, and possible reduced penetrance [2,3]. Nonetheless, the use of molecular techniques represents a considerable advance in the diagnosis of Lynch syndrome.

Suspected HNPCC

In current clinical practice, it is frequent to observe families not fulfilling the Amsterdam criteria (Table 10.1) who nevertheless maintain a strong clinical suspicion of HNPCC because of cancer aggregation, "verticality" or development of colorectal cancer at a very young age [49]. Moreover, the availability of genetic tests for the genes responsible for HNPCC allowed the identification of many cases of Lynch syndrome solely based on the genetic diagnosis. Thus, various reports described constitutional mutations in MLH1 or MSH2 genes in colorectal cancer patients and families who do not fulfil the Amsterdam criteria, but in whom a genetic basis was strongly suspected [148, 149]. These findings clearly indicate that there are families not fulfilling the standard clinical criteria but in whom constitutional mutations of the mismatch repair genes can be detected. These families, therefore, represent true HNPCC, in which the full-blown clinical spectrum has not yet developed. The situation is not surprising, since cancers develop over the course of many years, and it is likely that certain kindreds require

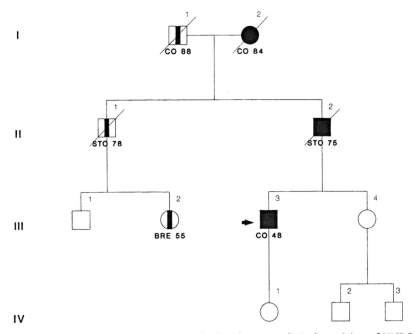

Fig. 10.3. Representative pedigree of a kindred with strong clinical suspicion of HNPCC, though not fulfilling the Amsterdam criteria (Table 10.1). (For explanation of labels see Fig. 10.1, p. 197)

Table 10.5. Clinical criteria suggested by the International Collaborative Group on HNPCC for the definition of suspected HNPCC [151]

Criteria I: At least one item from both Category 1 and Category 2 should be fulfilled:

Category 1: Vertical transmission of colorectal cancer. At least two siblings affected by colorectal cancer in a family

Category 2: Multiple colorectal tumors (including adenomas). At least one colorectal carcinoma diagnosed before the age of 50. Development of extracolonic cancers of the Lynch spectrum in family members

Criteria II: One colorectal cancer patient with at least one of the following:

Early age of onset (< 40 years)

Endometrial, urinary tract or small intestine cancer in the index patient or a sibling (one aged 50 years)

Two siblings with other integral HNPCC extracolonic cancers (one aged < 50 years)

---

an observation period of many years before being diagnosed as HNPCC. In the meantime, these families should be labeled as suspicious and followed up with a surveillance strategy similar to that adopted for true HNPCC [44].

Several authors used clinical criteria for defining suspected HNPCC [17, 150]. In 1996, the International Collaborative Study Group on HNPCC proposed some criteria which summarize the experience of various investigators, which are listed in Table 10.5. Figure 10.3 shows the representative pedigree of a family with a strong clinical suspicion of hereditary colorectal cancer, though not fulfilling the Amsterdam criteria. Park et al. [151] evaluated the frequency of mutations in the mismatch repair genes in suspected HNPCC kindreds subdivided into families meeting criteria I or II (Table 10.5). The results of this study showed that families meeting criteria I often had germline mutations (19 of 67, 28%), whereas these were much rarer (5 of 56) among families meeting criteria II. The former, therefore, should be offered genetic testing, while the low mutation rate of the latter renders the test impractical.

Genetic Counseling in HNPCC

In the process of genetic counseling, the counselor (the family doctor, a clinical geneticist, a physician expert in hereditary cancer syndromes) acquires from the proband all information regarding the family, with particular attention – in case of HNPCC – to the age of tumor occurrence, tumor location in the large bowel, histological type and biological characterization, and the tumor spectrum. During counseling, the patient should be informed about the natural history of the cancer syndrome, the availability of surveillance and management opportunities, and the potential risk of any choice made. Moreover, the physician should assist the patient in making informed decisions on the crucial questions that arise in the genetic testing process. The patient should realize the potential psychological burden of knowing that DNA studies indicate mutations of MSH2, MLH1 or other genes and the equally likely psychologic burden for those found negative for mutations, the so-called survivor's guilt [2, 152].

Since HNPCC is curable and preventable, genetic counseling should be offered to all patients and family members at risk, including individuals from suspected families. The situation is clearly different from that of other hereditary cancer syndromes (such as Li-Fraumeni syndrome) or genetic diseases (such as Huntington chorea) for which prevention and early treatment can hardly be implemented.

Before the identification of the mismatch repair genes and of their role in HNPCC, the best estimate that physicians could make of the cancer risk in hereditary colorectal cancer was that a family member in such a kindred would have a lifetime risk for cancer of approximately 50% [36].

The introduction of DNA testing for constitutional mutations of the responsible genes has changed this situation. In fact, individuals at risk in families meeting the Amsterdam criteria, or with a strong suspicion of HNPCC, will be candidates for mutation testing. If the test shows that a subject carries the deleterious mutation, then the lifetime risk of cancer will change to that of the penetrance of the gene, which may be as high as 80%–100% [37, 38]. Alternatively, if the test shows that mutations are absent, then the risk of cancer for that individual reverts to that of the general population, which is about 4%–6% [153].

Moreover, in HNPCC kindreds, the detection of a constitutional mutation in an index patient is a prerequisite for the identification of other heterozygote family members at risk for colorectal cancer. These individuals should be offered counseling and, in case of positive testing, should be maintained under close surveillance. On the other hand, individuals ascertained as not being carriers of predisposing mutations should be excluded from monitoring programs. Thus, surveillance and prevention efforts will be focused on mutation carriers, allowing a more rational application and a more accurate interpretation of the results, especially in terms of psychological consequences, and a reduction of cancer morbidity and mortality [2, 3].

At present, genetic testing for germline mutations of mismatch repair genes should be proposed – after appropriate counseling – only to family members of kindreds with clinical features of HNPCC (Table 10.1) or with a strong suspicion of it (Table 10.5). In both cases, the search for mutations should be preceded by MSI evaluation in tumor samples. When DNA testing is carried out randomly in the general population – or in the presence of a vague and aspecific familiality – there is a possibility of identifying genetic polymorphisms, i.e. DNA changes that do not contribute to cancer susceptibility, but that may mimic cancer-associated mutations. Indeed, the best evidence that a constitutional DNA alteration represents a true deleterious mutation is provided by its close cosegregation with the neoplastic phenotype through various generations and in all affected branches of the family.

On some occasions, genetic counseling may be a difficult task, and particular attention must be given to the patient's culture, beliefs and traditions. Lynch et al. [154] provided genetic counseling to a large Navajo Indian kindred in which a germline mutation in the MLH1 gene had been identified. Reaction to counseling ranged from complete acceptance of the genetic implications to traditional Navajo reasoning, such as attributing colon cancer risk to the fact that the family had been cursed in previous generations. But the experience reported by Lerman et al. [155] was even more surprising. The authors evaluated the utilization of genetic testing in members of families in which constitutional mutations in any of the mismatch repair genes had been detected. In the total sample of 208 eligible participants (from 4 extended HNPCC families), 90 individuals (43%) received test results and 118 (57%) declined. The existence of depression and low education were significantly related to reduced rates of genetic test use. It was concluded that despite the elevated risk of colorectal cancer, a relatively small proportion of HNPCC family members are likely to take advantage of genetic testing.

Management and Survival

In dealing with HNPCC patients, physicians should take into account the genetic nature of the disease (in particular, the risk for other family members) and some of the biologic characteristics of the syndrome (such as the tendency to multiple and recurrent tumors).

Treatment and Follow-up

To date, there is no known preventive or chemopreventive approach that can reduce the risk of tumor development in HNPCC. Oral calcium supplementation has been evaluated in HNPCC, but with little or no effect on the clinical outcome [156]. Since in vitro studies suggested that aspirin may inhibit the growth of cells with MSI, the CAPP 2 study (for Concerted Action on Polyposis Prevention) is evaluating aspirin and other chemopreventive compounds as a possible strategy for tumor prevention in HNPCC [157], but the results are not yet available.

Surgery remains the most important approach for HNPCC. The optimal treatment for a newly detected colorectal cancer includes two main options. The first is subtotal colectomy with ileorectal anastomosis: in this case, the risk of metachronous tumors is limited to the rectum, but cannot be considered negligible [158]. The second approach is right or left hemicolectomy, an intervention that should be followed by close endoscopic surveillance of the remaining large bowel, owing to the risk of recurrent lesions [52, 53]. Prophylactic subtotal colectomy, especially in carriers of deleterious germline mutations, should be mentioned as a further options for patients who are reluctant to undergo regular endoscopic controls [2, 73]. Owing to the high risk of endometrial carcinoma in affected women, prophylactic hysterectomy, at the time of surgery for colorectal cancer, has been proposed [2].

With the knowledge currently available, there is no consistent reason for adopting different strategies in adjuvant chemotherapy. Thus, HNPCC patients with Dukes' C lesions should follow the protocols which are usually recommended to patients with sporadic tumors (5-fluorouracil + levamisole or folinic acid) [159]. However, preliminary studies suggest that mismatch repair-deficient cells might be susceptible to killing by alkylating agents [160], though there is evidence that adjuvant chemotherapy in MSI+ patients is at least as effective as in common colorectal neoplasms [161]. Clearly, further studies are needed to evaluate the possible role of new chemotherapy regimens in HNPCC.

Although there is a general consensus that individuals at risk of cancer in HNPCC families should be followed at regular intervals, no standard guidelines have been developed. Thus, the strategies adopted by various centers may differ in relation to: availability of resources, medical and cultural traditions, observed tumor spectrum, and pattern of cancer occurrence in the follow-up [53, 60, 62, 63]. However, the main recommendations for the follow-up of affected or high-risk individuals in HNPCC families can be summarized as follows [44, 49, 17]: (1) pancolonoscopy should be proposed to all first-degree relatives of affected patients, usually starting at age 20–25, and the examination repeated every 2–3 years. If the results of genetic testing are available, follow-up can be limited to gene carriers; (2) upper gastrointestinal endoscopy is suggested only for those families in which several cases of gastric carcinoma have occurred, especially with an early age of onset; (3) gynecological investigations (including lower abdominal ultrasound or, according to some authors, transvaginal ultrasound) are usually suggested to all women at risk; it should be noted, however, that the real benefit of screening for endometrial and ovarian carcinoma remains undefined; (4) other, more specific clinical investigations (such as urography, endoscopic retrograde cholangiography or computed tomography) are usually recommended in selected cases and families; (5) since the genetic nature of HNPCC does not exclude the possible contribution of environmental factors in tumor development, some authors [44] recommend modification of dietary habits (i. e. increasing the amount of fiber, fruit and vegetables, and reducing the intake of animal fat and meat), avoiding obesity, and spending more time in physical activity.

In a recent investigation [162], Jarvinen et al. evaluated the efficacy of a 15-year endoscopic screening in 22 Finnish families with HNPCC. Eight colorectal carcinomas developed in screened individuals as opposed to 19 in control subjects ($p = 0.014$). All cancers in the study group were localized, causing no deaths, compared with 9 deaths caused by colorectal tumors among controls. The authors concluded that endoscopic screening at 3-year intervals in HNPCC family members reduces the risk of colorectal carcinoma, prevents cancer-related deaths, and decreases the overall mortality by approximately 65%.

Survival

Lynch and collaborators [163] - mostly on the basis of anecdotal reports - proposed that patients with HNPCC could have a more favorable clinical outcome than patients with sporadic colorectal carcinoma. The issue may appear rather paradoxical, since some morphological features usually associated with a more aggressive clinical course - such as mucinous histological type and poor degree of differentiation - are more frequent in HNPCC than in the sporadic counterpart [3, 74, 75]. Since then, other investigations confirmed this tendency towards a better prognosis. Thus, Sankila et al. [164] compared the colorectal cancer survival of 175 HNPCC patients with that of 14,086 patients with colorectal malignancies from the Finnish population-based registry. The 5-year survival rate was 65% in HNPCC and 44% in controls; curiously, this survival advantage was observed only in women. A significant overall better prognosis was also reported by Watson et al. [165] in 274 patients with HNPCC (from 98 kindreds) compared with an unselected colorectal cancer series. The more favorable outcome might be attributed to the frequency of Crohn's-like peritumoral lymphoid reaction in HNPCC [166], which may be indicative of a host defense mechanism. A more likely explanation could be related to the profound genomic instability that is present in almost all HNPCC cases; indeed, several studies reported a better survival associated with MSI [167, 168], although the biological basis of these findings remains unclear.

Finally, other studies could not find any clear-cut survival advantage in HNPCC patients. Percesepe et al. [169] evaluated a large series of patients with HNPCC selected on the basis of the Amsterdam I criteria (Table 10.1). When compared with controls, patients with Lynch syndrome showed a slightly increased 5-year survival, which was of borderline significance; moreover, multivariate analysis revealed that this more favorable outcome was strongly related to the preferential location of tumors in the right colon. Similarly, no survival advantage was reported by Bertario et al. [170] in a large Italian series of HNPCC patients.

Conclusions

HNPCC is an example of how advances in cancer genetics could affect clinical medicine. According to the model of hereditary cancer syndromes, progress in understanding gene-environment interactions will lead the traditional pattern of care based on diagnosis and therapy slowly towards prediction and prevention. Indeed, the prodigious advances in molecular genetics are changing how hereditary colorectal cancer and its integral extracolonic spectrum of tumors are diagnosed and managed. However, there are several observations about HNPCC that have yet to be explained by clinicians and biologists, such as the preferential involvement of the proximal colon, the reasons for tumor occurrence in certain organs, and the possible more favorable outcome. The explanations for these phenomena might tell us much about tumorigenesis and, in particular, the interaction between environmental carcinogens and highly susceptible cells.

References

1. Haggitt RC, Reid BJ. Hereditary Gastrointestinal Polyposis Syndromes. Am J Surg Pathol 1986; 10:871–87.
2. Lynch HT, Smyrk T. Hereditary Nonpolyposis Colorectal Cancer (Lynch syndrome). Cancer 1996; 78:1149–67.
3. Bellacosa A, Genuardi M, Anti M et al. Hereditary Nonpolyposis Colorectal Cancer: review of clinical, molecular genetics, and counseling aspects. Am J Med Genet 1996; 62:353–64.
4. Kinzler KW, Vogelstein B. Lessons from Hereditary Colorectal Cancer. Cell 1996; 87: 159–70.
5. Warthin AS. Heredity with reference to carcinoma. Arch Int Med 1913; 12:546–55.
6. Warthin AS. Heredity of carcinoma in man. Ann Intern Med 1931; 4:681–96.
7. Hauser IJ, Weller CV. A further report on the cancer family of Warthin. Am J Cancer 1936; 26:434–49.
8. Lynch HT, Shaw MW, Magnuson CW et al. Hereditary factors in cancer. Study of two large midwestern kindreds. Arch Intern Med 1966; 117:206–12.
9. Peltomaki P, Lothe RA, Aaltonen LA et al. Microsatellite instability is associated with tumors that characterize the hereditary nonpolyposis colorectal carcinoma syndrome. Cancer Res 1993; 53:5853–5.
10. Aaltonen LA, Peltomaki P, Leach FS et al. Clues to the pathogenesis of familial colorectal cancer. Science 1993; 260:812–6.
11. San Jose BA, Navarro NS, Doble F. Hereditary nonpolyposis colorectal cancer: an awareness. JMMS 1989; 25:37–8.
12. Lynch HT, Drouhard TJ, Schuelke Gs et al. Hereditary nonpolyposis colorectal cancer in a Navajo Indian family. Cancer Genet Cytogenet 1985; 15:209–13.
13. Sarroca C, Alfano N, Tedesco Bendin G et al. Hereditary Nonpolyposis Colorectal Cancer (Lynch syndrome II) in Uruguay. Dis Colon Rectum 2000; 43:353–62.
14. Vasen HFA, Mecklin JP, Meerakhan P et al. The international collaborative group on hereditary nonpolyposis colorectal cancer. Dis Colon Rectum 1991; 34:424–5.

15. Vasen HFA, Watson P, Mecklin JP et al. New clinical criteria for Hereditary Nonpolyposis Colorectal Cancer (HNPCC, Lynch syndrome) proposed by the International Collaborative Group on HNPCC. Gastroenterology 1999; 116:1453-6.
16. Lynch HT, Smyrk TC. Identifying hereditary nonpolyposis colorectal cancer. N Engl J Med 1998; 338:1537-8.
17. Ponz de Leon M, Pedroni M, Benatti P et al. Hereditary colorectal cancer in the general population: from cancer registration to molecular diagnosis. Gut 1999; 45:32-8.
18. Mecklin JP, Jarvinen HJ, Peltokallio P. Cancer family syndrome: genetic analysis of 22 Finnish kindreds. Gastroenterology 1986; 90:328-33.
19. Mecklin JP. Frequency of hereditary colorectal carcinoma. Gastroenterology 1987; 93: 1021-5.
20. Westlake PJ, Bryant HE, Huchcroft SA et al. Frequency of hereditary nonpolyposis colorectal cancer in Southern Alberta. Dig Dis Sci 1991; 36:1441-7.
21. Ponz de Leon M, Sassatelli R, Benatti P et al. Identification of HNPCC in the general population. Cancer 1993; 71:3493-501.
22. Benatti P, Sassatelli R, Roncucci L et al. Tumour spectrum in HNPCC and in suspected HNPCC: a population based study in Northern Italy. Int J Cancer 1993; 54:371-7.
23. Modica S, Roncucci L, Benatti P et al. Familial aggregation of tumors and detection of hereditary non-polyposis colorectal cancer in 3-year experience of 2 population-based colorectal-cancer registries. Int J Cancer 1995; 62:685-90.
24. Kee F, Collins BJ. How prevalent is cancer family syndrome? Gut 1991; 32:509-12.
25. Stephenson BM, Finan JP, Gascoyne J et al. Frequency of familial colorectal cancer. Br J Surg 1991; 78:1162-6.
26. Aaltonen LA, Salovaara R, Kristo P et al. Incidence of hereditary nonpolyposis colorectal cancer and the feasibility of molecular screening for the disease. N Engl J Med 1998; 338:1481-7.
27. Salovaara R, Loukola A, Kristo P et al. Population-based molecular detection of hereditary nonpolyposis colorectal cancer. J Clin Oncol 2000; 18:1-8.
28. Ponz de Leon M, Sassatelli R, Scalmati A et al. Descriptive epidemiology of colorectal cancer in Italy: the 6-year experience of a specialised registry. Eur J Cancer 1993; 29 A: 367-71.
29. Percesepe A, Borghi F, Menigatti M et al. Molecular screening for Hereditary Non Polyposis Colorectal Cancer (HNPCC): a prospective, population-based study. J Clin Oncol 2001; 19:3944-50.
30. Peel DJ, Ziogas A, Fox EA et al. Characterization of Hereditary Nonpolyposis Colorectal Cancer families from a population-based series of cases. J Natl Cancer Inst 2000; 92:1517-22.
31. Hemminki K, Li X. Familial colorectal adenocarcinoma and hereditary nonpolyposis colorectal cancer: a nationwide epidemiological study from Sweden. Br J Cancer 2001; 84:969-74.
32. Tannergård P, Lipford JR, Kolodner et al. Mutation screening in the hMLH1 gene in Swedish hereditary nonpolyposis colon cancer families. Cancer Res 1995; 55: 6092-6.
33. Han HJ, Yuan Y, Ku JL et al. Germline mutations of hMLH1 and hMSH2 genes in Korean hereditary nonpolyposis colorectal cancer. J Natl Cancer Inst 1996; 88:1317-9.
34. Bailey-Wilson JE, Elston RC, Schuelke GS et al. Segregation analysis of hereditary nonpolyposis colorectal cancer. Genet Epidemiol 1986; 3:27-38.
35. Ponz de Leon M, Scapoli C, Zanghieri G et al. Genetic transmission of colorectal cancer: exploratory data analysis from a population based registry. J Med Genet 1992; 29:531-8.
36. Scapoli C, Ponz de Leon M, Sassatelli R et al. Genetic epidemiology of hereditary nonpolyposis colorectal cancer syndromes in Modena, Italy: results of a complex segregation analysis. Ann Hum Genet 1994; 58:275-95.
37. Houlston RS, Collins A, Slack J et al. Dominant genes for colorectal cancer are not rare. Ann Hum Genet 1992; 56:99-103.

38. Burt RW, Bishop TD, Cannon LA et al. Dominant inheritance of adenomatous colonic polyps and colorectal cancer. N Engl J Med 1985; 312:1540-4.
39. Cannon-Albright L, Skolnick MH, Bishop TD et al. Common inheritance of susceptibility to colonic adenomatous polyps and associated colorectal cancers. N Engl J Med 1988; 319:533-7.
40. Lynch HT, Albano WA, Ruma TA et al. Surveillance/management of an obligate gene carrier:the cancer family syndrome. Gastroenterology 1983; 84:404-8.
41. Ponz de Leon M, Benatti P, Pedroni M et al. Problems in the identification of hereditary nonopolyposis colorectal cancer in two families with late development of full-blown clinical spectrum. Am J Gastroenterol 2000; 95:2110-5.
42. Johnson N, Lancaster T, Fuller A et al. The prevalence of a family history of cancer in general practice. Fam Pract 1995; 12:287-9.
43. Emery J, Watson E, Rose P et al. A systematic review of the literature exploring the role of primary care in genetic services. Fam Pract 1999; 16:426-45.
44. Evans DG, Wu CL, Walsh S et al. Characterization of Hereditary Nonpolyposis Colorectal Cancer families from a population-based series of cases. J Natl Cancer Inst 2001; 93:716-7.
45. Mecklin JP, Jarvinen HJ. Tumor spectrum in cancer-family syndrome (hereditary nonpolyposis colorectal cancer). Cancer 1991; 68:1109-12.
46. Vasen HFA, Offerhaus GJA, den Hartog J et al. The tumour spectrum in hereditary nonpolyposis colorectal cancer: a study of 24 kindreds in the Netherlands. Int J Cancer 1990; 46:31-4.
47. Faragher IG, Cox CJ, Stevenson A. Hereditary nonpolyposis colorectal cancer (Lynch syndrome I) in a 13-year-old male. Aust N Z J Surg 1993; 63:494-6.
48. Isbister WH, Fraser J. Large-bowel cancer in the young: a national survival study. Dis Colon Rectum 1990; 33:363-6.
49. Ponz de Leon M, Benatti P, Pedroni M et al. Risk of cancer revealed by follow-up of families with hereditary non-polyposis colorectal cancer: a population-based study. Int J Cancer 1993; 55:202-7.
50. Enker WE, Dragacevic S. Multiple carcinomas of the large bowel: a natural experiment in etiology and pathogenesis. Ann Surg 1978; 187:8-11.
51. Robinson E, Nasrallah S, Adler Z et al. Clinical, demographic, and follow-up characteristics of patients with two primary metachronous tumors, one of them being in the colon. Dis Colon Rectum 1992; 35:457-61.
52. Mecklin JP, Jarvinen HJ. Clinical features of colorectal carcinoma in cancer family syndrome. Dis Colon Rectum 1986; 29:160-4.
53. Fitzgibbons RJ, Lynch HT, Stanislav GV et al. Recognition and treatment of patients with hereditary non polyposis colorectal cancer (Lynch syndrome I and II). Ann Surg 1987; 206:289-94.
54. Lynch HT, Watson P, Kriegler M et al. Differential diagnosis of hereditary nonpolyposis colorectal cancer (Lynch syndrome I and Lynch syndrome II). Dis Colon Rectum 1988; 31:372-7.
55. Vasen HFA, Offerhaus GJA, Jager H et al. The tumour spectrum in hereditary nonpolyposis colorectal cancer: a study of 24 kindreds in the Netherlands. Int J Cancer 1990; 46:31-4.
56. Fante R, Roncucci L, Di Gregorio C et al. Frequency and clinical features of multiple tumors of the large bowel in the general population and in patients with hereditary colorectal carcinoma. Cancer 1996; 77:2013-21.
57. Risinger JI, Barrett JC, Watson P et al. Molecular genetic evidence of the occurrence of breast cancer as an integral tumor in patients with the Hereditary Nonpolyposis Colorectal Carcinoma syndrome. Cancer 1996; 77:1836-43.
58. Sijmons R, Hofstra R, Hollema H et al. Inclusion of malignant fibrous histiocytoma in the tumour spectrum associated with Hereditary Non-Polyposis Colorectal Cancer. Genes Chromosom Cancer 2000; 29:353-5.

59. Lynch HT, Fusaro RM. Muir-Torre syndrome: heterogeneity, natural history, diagnosis, and management. Probl Gen Surg 1993; 113:295-301.
60. Cristofaro G, Lynch HT, Caruso L et al. New phenotypic aspects in a family with Lynch syndrome II. Cancer 1987; 60:51-8.
61. Watson P, Lynch HT. Extracolonic cancer in hereditary nonpolyposis colorectal cancer. Cancer 1993; 71:677-85.
62. Love RR. Small bowel cancers, B-cell leukemia, and six primary cancers with metastases and prolonged survival in the Cancer Family Syndrome of Lynch. Cancer 1985; 55:499-502.
63. Hamilton SR, Liu B, Parsons RE et al. The molecular basis of Turcot's syndrome. N Engl J Med 1995; 332:839-47.
64. Lynch HT, Kriegler M, Christiansen TA et al. Laryngeal carcinoma in a Lynch syndrome II kindred. Cancer 1988; 62:1007-13.
65. Wang Q, Lasset C, Desseigne F et al. Neurofibromatosis and early onset of cancers in hNLH1-deficient children. Cancer Res 1999; 59:294-7.
66. Park JY, Shin KH, Park JG. Risk of gastric cancer in Hereditary Nonpolyposis Colorectal Cancer in Korea. Clin Cancer Res 2000; 6:2994-8.
67. Mecklin JP. Molecular genotype/clinical phenotype relationship in HNPCC. (abstract) Genetics of FAP and HNPCC. Proceedings of the fifth workshop, Budapest, Hungary. Khan PM & Mohr J (eds). 1994; 38-9.
68. Liu KM, Shashidharan M, Ternent CA et al. Colorectal and extracolonic cancer variations in MLH1/MSH2 Hereditary Nonpolyposis Colorectal Cancer kindreds and the general population. Dis Colon Rectum 1998; 41:428-33.
69. Lanspa SJ, Lynch HT, Smyrk TC et al. Colorectal adenomas in the Lynch syndromes: results of a colonoscopy screening program. Gastroenterology 1990; 98:1117-22.
70. Ponz de Leon M, Della Casa G, Benatti P et al. Frequency and type of colorectal tumors in asymptomatic high-risk individuals in families with Hereditary Nonpolyposis Colorectal Cancer. Cancer Epidemiol Biomarkers Prev 1998; 7:639-41.
71. Jass JR. Colorectal adenomas in surgical specimens from subjects with hereditary nonpolyposis colorectal cancer. Histopathol 1995; 108:1590-2.
72. Jass JR, Stewart SM, Stewart J et al. Hereditary non-polyposis colorectal cancer: morphologies, genes and mutations. Mutation Res 1994; 290:125-33.
73. Lynch HT, Smyrk T, Lynch J. An update of HNPCC (Lynch syndrome). Cancer Genet Cytogenet 1997; 93:84-99.
74. Mecklin JP, Svensen LB, Peltomaki P et al. Hereditary Nonpolyposis Colorectal Cancer. Scand J Gastroenterol 1994; 29:673-7.
75. Jass JR, Smyrk TC, Stawart SM et al. Pathology of hereditary nonpolyposis colorectal cancer. Anticancer Res 1994; 14:1631-4.
76. Lanza G, Gafà R, Matteuzzi M et al. Medullary-type poorly differentiated adenocarcinoma of the large bowel: a distinct clinicopathologic entity characterized by microsatellite instability and improved survival. J Clin Oncol 1999; 17:2429-38.
77. Shashidharan M, Smyrk T, Lin K et al. Histologic comparison of Hereditary Nonpolyposis Colorectal Cancer associated with MSH2 and MLH1 and colorectal cancer from the general population. Dis Colon Rectum 1999; 42:722-6.
78. Kouri M, Laasonen A, Mecklin JP et al. Diploid predominance in HNPCC evaluated by flow cytometry. Cancer 1990; 65:1825-9.
79. Frei JV. Hereditary nonpolyposis colorectal cancer: diploid malignancies with prolonged survival. Cancer 1992; 69:1109-1111.
80. Losi L, Fante R, Di Gregorio C et al. Biologic characterization of Hereditary Non-Polyposis Colorectal Cancer. Nuclear ploidy, AgNOR count, microvessel distribution, oncogene expression and grade-related parameters. Am J Clin Pathol 1995; 103:265-70.
81. Emery J, Lucassen A, Murphy M. Common hereditary cancers and implications for primary care. Lancet 2001; 358:56-63.

82. Marra G, Boland CR. Hereditary Nonpolyposis Colorectal Cancer: the syndrome, the genes, and historical perspectives. J Natl Cancer Inst 1995; 87:1114-25.
83. Modrich P. Mechanisms and biological effects of mismatch repair. Ann Rev Genet 1991; 25:229-53.
84. Glickman BW, Radman M. Escherichia coli mutator mutants deficient in methylation-instructed DNA mismatch correction. Proc Natl Acad Sci USA 1980; 77:1063-7.
85. Rhyu MS. Molecular mechanisms underlying Hereditary Nonpolyposis Colorectal Cancer. J Natl Cancer Inst 1996; 88:240-51.
86. Grilley M, Griffith J, Modrich P. Bidirectional excision in methyl-directed mismatch repair. J Biol Chem 1993; 268:11830-7.
87. Lahue RS, Au KG, Modrich P. DNA mismatch correction in a defined system. Science 1989; 245:160-4.
88. Holmes J Jr, Clark S, Modrich P. Strand-specific mismatch correction in nuclear extracts of human and Drosophila melanogaster cell lines. Proc Natl Acad Sci USA 1990; 87:5837-41.
89. Leach FS, Nicolaides NC, Papadopoulos N et al. Mutations of a mutS homolog in hereditary nonpolyposis colorectal cancer, Cell 1993; 75:1216-25.
90. Xia L, Shen W, Ritacca F et al. A truncated hMSH2 transcript occurs as a common variant in the population: implications for genetic diagnosis. Cancer Res 1996; 56:2289-92.
91. Bronner CE, Baker SM, Morrison PT et al. Mutation in the DNA mismatch repair gene homologue hMLH1 is associated with hereditary non-polyposis colon cancer. Nature 1994; 368:258-61.
92. Papadopoulos N, Nicolaides NC, Wei YF et al. Mutation of mutL homolog in hereditary colon cancer. Science 1994; 263:1625-9.
93. Nystrom-Lahti M, Sistonen P, Mecklin JP et al. Close linkage to chromosome 3p and conservation of ancestral founding haplotype in hereditary nonpolyposis colorectal cancer families. Proc Natl Acad Sci USA 1994; 91:6054-8.
94. Nicolaides NC, Papadopoulos N, Liu B et al. Mutations of two PMS homologues in hereditary nonpolyposis colon cancer. Nature 1994; 371:75-80.
95. Viel A, Novella E, Genuardi M et al. Lack of PMS2 gene-truncating mutations in patients with hereditary colorectal cancer. Int J Oncol 1998; 13:565-9.
96. Palombo F, Gallinari P, Iaccarino I et al. GTBP, a 160-kilodalton protein essential for mismatch-binding activity in human cells. Science 1995; 268:1912-4.
97. Akiyama Y, Sato H, Yamada T et al. Germ-line mutation of the hMSH6/GTBP gene in an atypical hereditary nonpolyposis colorectal cancer kindred. Cancer Res 1997; 57:3920-3.
98. Miyaki M, Konishi M, Tanaka K et al. Germline mutation of MSH6 as the cause of hereditary nonpolyposis colorectal cancer. Nature Genet 1997; 17:271-2.
98a. Wu Y, Berends MJW, Sijmons RH et al. A role for MLH3 in hereditary nonpolyposis colorectal cancer. Nature Genet 2001; 29:137-8.
99. Fujii H, Shimada T. Isolation and characterization of cDNA clones derived from the divergently transcribed gene in the region upstream from the human dihydrofolate reductase gene. J Biol Chem 1989; 264:10057-64.
100. Knudson AG. Hereditary cancer: theme and variations. J Clin Oncol 1997; 15:3280-7.
101. Hemminki A, Peltomaki P, Mecklin JP et al. Loss of the wild type MLH1 gene is a feature of hereditary nonopolyposis colorectal cancer. Nature Genet 1994; 8:405-10.
102. Ionov Y, Peinado MA, Malkhosyan S et al. Ubiquitous somatic mutations in simple repeated sequences reveal a new mechanism for colonic carcinogenesis. Nature 1993; 363:558-61.
103. Aaltonen LA, Peltomaki P, Mecklin JP et al. Replication errors in benign and malignant tumors from hereditary non-polyposis colorectal cancer patients. Cancer Res 1994; 54:1645-8.
104. Thibodeau SN, Bren G, Schaid D. Microsatellite instability in cancer of the proximal colon. Science 1993; 260:816-9.

105. Fleisher AS, Esteller M, Harpaz N et al. Microsatellite instability in inflammatory bowel disease-associated neoplastic lesions is associated with hypermethylation and diminished expression of the DNA mismatch repair gene, hMLH1. Cancer Res 2000; 60:4864-8.
106. Malik K, Brown KW. Epigenetic gene deregulation in cancer. Br J Cancer 2000; 83: 1583-8.
107. Gafà R, Maestri I, Matteuzzi M et al. Sporadic colorectal adenocarcinoma with high-frequency microsatellite instability. Pathobiologic features, hMLH1 and hMSH2 expression, and clinical outcome. Cancer 2000; 89:2025-37.
108. Menigatti M, Di Gregorio C, Borghi F et al. Methylation pattern of different regions of the MLH1 promoter and silencing of gene expression in hereditary and sporadic colorectal cancer. Genes Chromosom Cancer 2001; 31:357-61.
109. Yee CJ, Roodi N, Verrier CS et al. Microsatellite instability and loss of heterozygosity in breast cancer. Cancer Res 1994; 54:1641-4.
110. Shridhar V, Siegfried J, Hunt J et al. Genetic instability of microsatellite sequences in many non-small cell lung carcinomas. Cancer Res 1994; 54:2084-7.
111. Mironov NM, Aguelon MA-M, Potapova GI et al. Alterations of (CA)n DNA repeats and tumor suppressor genes in human gastric cancer. Cancer Res 1994; 54:41-4.
112. Han HJ, Yanigasawa A, Kato Y et al. Genetic instability in pancreatic cancer and poorly differentiated type of gastric cancer. Cancer Res 1993; 53:5087-9.
113. Risinger JI, Berchuck A, Kohler MF et al. Genetic instability of microsatellites in endometrial carcinoma. Cancer Res 1993; 53:5100-3.
114. Dietmaier W, Wallinger S, Bocker T et al. Diagnostic microsatellite instability: definition and correlation with mismatch repair protein expression. Cancer Res 1997; 57: 4749-56.
115. Rodriguez-Bigas MA, Boland CR, Hamilton SR et al. A national cancer institute workshop on Hereditary Nonpolyposis Colorectal Cancer syndrome: meeting highlights and Bethesda guidelines. J Natl Cancer Inst 1997; 89:1758-62.
116. Shibata D, Peinado MA, Ionov Y et al. Genomic instability in repeated sequences is an early somatic event in colorectal carcinoma cell lines. Nature Genetics 1994; 6:273-81.
117. Parsons R, Myeroff L, Liu B et al. Microsatellite instability and mutations of the transforming growth factor β type II receptor gene in colorectal cancer. Cancer Res 1995; 55:5548-50.
118. Markowitz S, Wang J, Myeroff L et al. Inactivation of the type II TGF-β receptor in colon cancer cells with microsatellite instability. Science 1995; 268:1336-8.
119. Souza RF, Appel R, Yin J et al. Microsatellite instability in the insulin-like growth factor II receptor gene in gastrointestinal tumors. Nature Genet 1996; 14:255-7.
120. Rampino N, Yamamoto H, Ionov Y et al. Somatic frameshift mutations in the BAX gene in colon cancers in the microsatellite mutator phenotype. Science 1997; 275:967-9.
121. Wicking C, Simms LA, Evans T et al. CDX2, a human homologue of Drosophila caudal, is mutated in both alleles in a replication error positive colorectal cancer, Oncogene 1998; 17:657-9.
122. Fujiwara T, Stolker JM, Watanabe T et al. Accumulated clonal genetic alterations in familial and sporadic colorectal carcinomas with widespread instability in microsatellite sequences. Am J Pathol 1998; 153:1063-78.
123. Schwartz S, Yamamoto H, Navarro M et al. Frameshift mutations at mononucleotide repeats in caspase-5 and other target genes in endometrial and gastrointestinal cancer of the microsatellite mutator phenotype. Cancer Res 1999; 59:2995-3002.
124. Yamamoto H, Sawai H, Perucho M. Frameshift somatic mutations in gastrointestinal cancer of the microsatellite instability mutator phenotype. Cancer Res 1997; 57: 4420-6.
125. Iino H, Simms L, Young J et al. DNA microsatellite instability and mismatch repair protein loss in adenomas presenting in hereditary non-polyposis colorectal cancer. Gut 2000; 47:37-42.

126. Perucho M. Microsatellite instability: the mutator that mutates the other mutator. Nature Med 1996; 2:630-1.
127. Ponz de Leon M, Percesepe A. Pathogenesis of colorectal cancer. Digest Liver Dis 2000; 32:807-21.
128. Loeb LA. Mutator phenotype may be required for multistage carcinogenesis. Cancer Res 1991; 51:3075-9.
129. Peltomaki P, Vasen HFA, the International Collaborative Group on Hereditary Nonpolyposis Colorectal Cancer. Mutations predisposing to Hereditary Nonpolyposis Colorectal Cancer: database and results of a collaborative study. Gastroenterology 1997; 113:1146-58.
130. Viel A, Genuardi M, Capozzi E et al. Characterization of MSH2 and MLH1 mutations in Italian families with hereditary nonpolyposis colorectal cancer. Genes Chromosom Cancer 1997; 18:8-18.
131. Vasen HFA, Wjinen JT, Menko FH et al. Cancer risk in families with hereditary nonpolyposis colorectal cancer diagnosed by mutation analysis. Gastroenterology 1996; 110:1020-7.
132. Luce MC, Marra G, Chauhan DP et al. In vitro transcription/translation assay for the screening of hMLH1 and hMSH2 mutations in familial colon cancer. Gastroenterology 1995; 109:1368-74.
133. Liu B, Parsons TR, Papadopoulos N et al. Analysis of mismatch repair genes in hereditary non-polyposis colorectal cancer patients. Nature Med 1996; 2:169-74.
134. Scott RJ, McPhillips M, Meldrum CJ et al. Hereditary Nonpolyposis Colorectal Cancer in 95 families: differences and similarities between mutation-positive and mutation-negative kindreds. Am J Hum Genet 2001; 68:118-27.
135. Beck NE, Tomlinson JPM, Homfray TFR et al. Frequency of germline hereditary nonpolyposis colorectal cancer gene mutations in patients with multiple or early onset colorectal adenomas. Gut 1997; 41:235-8.
136. Park JG, Park YJ, Wujnen JT et al. Gene-environment interaction in Hereditary Nonpolyposis Colorectal Cancer with implications for diagnosis and genetic testing. Int J Cancer 1999; 82:516-9.
137. Wijnen JT, Vasen HFA, Meera Khan P et al. Clinical findings with implications for genetic testing in families with clustering of colorectal cancer. N Engl J Med 1998; 339: 511-8.
138. Benatti P, Roncucci L, Ganazzi D et al. Clinical and biological heterogeneity of HNPCC. Int J Cancer 2001; 95:323-28.
139. Lewis CM, Neuhausen SL, Daley D et al. Genetic heterogeneity and unmapped genes for colorectal cancer. Cancer Res 1996; 56:1382-88.
140. Tomlinson I, Rahman N, Frayling I et al. Inherited susceptibility to colorectal adenomas and carcinomas: evidence for a new predisposition gene on 15q14-q22. Gastroenterology 1999; 116:789-95.
141. Riccio A, Aaltonen LA, Godwin AK et al. The DNA repair gene MBD4 (MED1) is mutated in human carcinomas with microsatellite instability. Nature Genet 1999; 23: 266-8.
142. Wilson DM III, Carney JP, Coleman MA et al. Hex1: a new human Rad2 nuclease family member with homology to yeast exonuclease 1. Nucleic Acids Res 1998; 26: 3762-8.
143. Schmutte C, Marinescu RC, Sadoff MM et al. Human exonuclease I interacts with the mismatch repair protein hMSH2. Cancer Res 1998; 58:4537-42.
144. Wu Y, Berends MJW, Post JG et al. Germline mutations of EXO1 gene in patients with hereditary nonpolyposis colorectal cancer (HNPCC) and atypical HNPCC forms. Gastroenterology 2001; 120:1580-7.
145. Ponz de Leon M, Benatti P, Roncucci L. Inheritance and susceptibility to tumours of the large bowel: a new classification of colorectal malignancies. Eur J Cancer 1996; 32 A:2206-11.

146. Peltomaki P. Genetic basis of hereditary nonpolyposis colorectal carcinoma (HNPCC). Ann Med 1994; 26:215-9.
147. Terdiman JP, Gum JR, Conrad PG et al. Efficient detection of Hereditary Nonpolyposis Colorectal Cancer gene carriers by screening for tumor microsatellite instability before germline genetic testing. Gastroenterology 2001; 120:21-30.
148. Liu B, Farrington SM, Petersen GM et al. Genetic instability occurs in the majority of young patients with colorectal cancer. Nature Med 1995; 1:348-52.
149. Han HJ, Yuan Y, Ku JL et al. Germline mutations of hMLH1 and hMSH2 genes in Korean hereditary nonpolyposis colorectal cancer. J Natl Cancer Inst 1996; 88:1317-9.
150. Yuan Y, Han HJ, Zheng S et al. Germline mutations of hMLH1 and hMSH2 genes in patients with suspected hereditary nonpolyposis colorectal cancer and sporadic early onset colorectal cancer. Dis Colon Rectum 1998; 41:434-40.
151. Park JG, Vasen HFA, Park KJ et al. Suspected hereditary nonpolyposis colorectal cancer. International Collaborative Group on Hereditary Non-Polyposis Colorectal Cancer (ICG-HNPCC) criteria and results of genetic diagnosis. Dis Colon Rectum 1999; 42: 710-6.
152. Petersen GM, Brensinger JD, Johnson KA et al. Genetic testing and counseling for hereditary forms of colorectal cancer. Cancer 1999; 86:1720-30.
153. Ponz de Leon M, Benatti P, Rossi G et al. Epidemiologia dei tumori del colon-retto. Incidenza, mortalità, familiarità e sopravvivenza, nella ex U.S.L. di Modena, 1984-1998. 2001, University of Modena.
154. Lynch HT, Drouhard T, Vasen HFA et al. Genetic counseling in a Navajo hereditary nonpolyposis colorectal cancer kindred. Cancer 1996; 77:30-5.
155. Lerman C, Hughes C, Trock BJ et al. Genetic testing in families with hereditary nonpolyposis colon cancer. JAMA 1999; 17:1618-22.
156. Cats A, Kleibeuker JH, van der Meer R et al. Randomized, double-blinded, placebo-controlled intervention study with supplemental calcium in families with hereditary nonpolyposis colorectal cancer. J Natl Cancer Inst 1995; 87:598-603.
157. Hawk E, Lubet R, Limburg P. Chemoprevention in Hereditary Colorectal Cancer. Cancer 1999; 86:1731-43.
158. Rodriguez-Bigas MA, Vasen HFA, Mecklin JP et al. Rectal cancer risk in Hereditary Nonpolyposis Colorectal Cancer after abdominal colectomy. Ann Surg 1997; 225: 202-7.
159. Fuchs CS, Mayer RJ. Adjuvant chemotherapy for colon and rectal cancer. Semin Oncol 1995; 22:472-87.
160. Branch P, Hampson R, Karran P. DNA mismatch binding defects, DNA damage tolerance, and mutator phenotypes in human colorectal carcinoma cell lines. Cancer Res 1995; 55:2304-9.
161. Hemminki A, Mecklin JP, Jarvinen H et al. Microsatellite instability is a favorable prognostic indicator in patients with colorectal cancer receiving chemotherapy. Gastroenterology 2000; 119:921-8.
162. Jarvinen HJ, Aarnio M, Mustonen H et al. Controlled 15-year trial on screening for colorectal cancer in families with Hereditary Nonpolyposis Colorectal Cancer. Gastroenterology 2000; 118:829-34.
163. Lynch HT, Bardawil WA, Harris RE et al. Multiple primary cancers and prolonged survival: familial colonic and endometrial cancers. Dis Colon Rectum 1978; 21: 165-8.
164. Sankila R, Aaltonen LA, Jarvinen HJ et al. Better survival rates in patients with MLH1-associated hereditary colorectal cancer. Gastroenterology 1997; 110:682-7.
165. Watson P, Lin KM, Rodriguez-Bigas MA et al. Colorectal carcinoma survival among hereditary nonpolyposis colorectal carcinoma family members. Cancer 1998; 83: 259-66.
166. Graham DM, Appelman HD. Crohn's-like lymphoid reaction and colorectal carcinoma: a potential histological prognosticator. Mod Pathol 1990; 3:332-5.

167. Gryfe R, Kim H, Hsied ETK et al. Tumor microsatellite instability and clinical outcome in young patients with colorectal cancer. N Engl J Med 2000; 342:69–77.
168. Wheeler JMD, Bodmer WF, Mortensen NJ McC. DNA mismatch repair genes and colorectal cancer. Gut 2000; 47:148–53.
169. Percesepe A, Benatti P, Roncucci L et al. Survival analysis in families affected by hereditary non-polyposis colorectal cancer. Int J Cancer 1997; 71:373–6.
170. Bertario L, Russo A, Sala P et al. Survival of patients with Hereditary Colorectal Cancer: comparison of HNPCC and colorectal cancer in FAP patients with sporadic colorectal cancer. Int J Cancer 1999; 80:183–7.

11 Familial Adenomatous Polyposis

Introduction

Although the description of the first patient occurred more than 100 years ago, familial adenomatous polyposis (FAP or adenomatosis coli) continues to be the object of several convergent lines of scientific and medical interest. Familial gastrointestinal polyposis includes various rare syndromes with the common features of numerous polyps (often adenomatous) scattered in the various tracts of the large bowel and an autosomal dominant pattern of genetic transmission [1, 2]. The occurrence of other clinical manifestations will determine the development of specific phenotypes; thus, for instance, in Gardner's syndrome (which is considered a variant of FAP) colorectal adenomas are associated with osteomas of the skull and mandible, epidermoid cysts and soft-tissue tumors [3].

FAP is the most common among the polyposis syndromes and the one most extensively investigated. The disease represents an ideal model for the study of colorectal tumorigenesis, and its scientific interest derives from various considerations. FAP shows a clear Mendelian basis, usually with a high penetrance; it follows that accurate pedigree analysis (coupled with genetic testing) may allow the identification of individuals at risk and the implementation of close endoscopic surveillance. In fact, FAP represents an "absolute" precancerous condition, in the sense that affected patients who are not treated in due time develop malignancies of the large bowel with almost absolute certainty. However, when the disease is diagnosed before the appearance of cancer – and this occurs much more frequently than in the past [4] – surgery can be curative in almost all cases, though the frequency of extracolonic changes points out that clinical investigations should not be limited to the large bowel. Finally, the gene responsible for FAP was localized in 1986, after cytogenetic and linkage studies, and mapped to chromosome 5q 21–22 [5, 6], a region suspected of harboring genes implicated in colorectal cancer because of the frequent losses of heterozygosity [7]. The gene – called APC, for adenomatous polyposis coli – plays a fundamental role not only in FAP but also in sporadic colorectal tumor development [8].

Definition and Historical Overview

In its classical presentation, FAP is characterized by the development of hundreds to thousands of adenomatous polyps scattered throughout the various segments of the colorectum that usually appear in the second decade of life [1]. The disease is associated with several extracolonic manifestations, including polyps in the stomach, duodenum and jejunal-ileal tract, typical retinal spots, dental abnormalities, desmoid tumors, epidermoid cysts, cranial and mandibular osteomas, and thyroid tumors. In the presence of many of these changes (in particular, skull and mandible osteomas, epidermoid cysts and soft-tissue tumors), many authors use the eponym "Gardner's syndrome". However, on clinical grounds a sharp distinction between FAP and Gardner's syndrome is often impossible, since a careful investigation of families with an initial diagnosis of FAP can lead to the detection of individuals with features of Gardner's syndrome. Moreover, some patients with FAP may not show clinical signs of Gardner's syndrome initially, but these can be revealed by more appropriate techniques (for example, dental abnormalities and small osteomas can often be detected only by radiographs). Finally, the identification and characterization of the APC gene clearly showed that FAP and Gardner's syndrome are both associated with molecular alterations consisting in small deletions, insertions or point mutations which introduce premature protein termination signals [9, 10]. Thus, the available evidence clearly indicates that they are not distinct nosologic entities, but that the latter represents the full-blown manifestation of a spectrum of clinical features due to the effect of a pleiotropic gene.

On the other extreme, in the attenuated form of adenomatosis coli (AFAP) there is only a small number of colorectal adenomatous lesions (less than 100, and often less than 50) and usually a later onset of malignant changes, compared with typical, full-blown FAP [11, 12].

Adenomatosis coli was described for the first time independently by various authors at the end of nineteenth century [13–15]. In 1925, a Polyposis Coli Registry was established at St. Mark's Hospital [16], and since then this institution has contributed largely to the progress of our understanding of the disease. The genetic features of FAP and the main surgical strategies were defined in successive years [17,18]. In the 1950s, Gardner and collaborators [19–21] described the association of multiple colorectal adenomas with cutaneous cysts and multiple osteomas of the skull and mandible in a large American family. In the 1980s, a new surgical procedure was developed (i.e. restorative proctocolectomy with an ileal reservoir and anal anastomosis) which offered several advantages over the existing techniques, in particular, the prevention of tumor recurrence in the rectal stump [22, 23]. In the same decade, several extracolonic lesions were described or further characterized, such as polyps in the stomach and small bowel, desmoid tumors, and congenital hypertrophy of the retinal pigmented epithelium [24–26]. Waddell et al., in 1983, showed that sulindac (an anti-inflammatory compound) could induce a marked regression of colorectal polyps [27]; many years later, similar results were obtained with celecoxib, a selective cyclo-oxygenase-2 inhibitor [28]. Finally, between 1986 and 1991, through cytogenetic studies, linkage analysis and sophisticated molecular techniques, the FAP locus was mapped to chromosome 5q 21-22, and the deleterious gene was identified and characterized [5, 6, 29, 30]. In the last decade, the main efforts of the investigators have been aimed at evaluating genotype-phenotype correlations [31] and elucidating the biological role and properties of the APC protein [8].

Epidemiology and Formal Genetics

The large majority of FAP families and index cases have been described in Western countries and Japan [32, 33]. However, the disease is presumably ubiquitous, and the lack of reports from many countries can be attributed to the limited interest of the local physicians in this rare clinical condition. The incidence of adenomatosis coli is usually expressed as frequency at birth of individuals with the FAP phenotype; estimates are of the order of 1 in 8,000-20,000 [33, 34]. Data from the Finnish Cancer Registry indicate that the prevalence of FAP in this country is between 1.6 and 2.4 cases per million inhabitants and that 5-10 new cases could be expected every year [35]; these figures are rather similar to those reported by Bulow et al. [36] in Denmark. Although it is commonly believed that about 1% of all colorectal malignancies develop in patients with FAP [3, 31], data from specialized Colorectal Cancer Registries indicate that this fraction in much lower, about 0.1%-0.2% [37, 38].

The examination of hundreds of genealogical trees clearly indicates that the inheritance pattern in adenomatosis coli is consistent with an autosomal dominant type of genetic transmission [25, 26]. The FAP gene is considered to have a high degree of penetrance. A careful estimation of penetrance has been published based on a large Utah kindred plus 160 additional sibships from the literature [39]. The results indicated that penetrance was virtually 100%, though there was a considerable variation in expressivity of the gene. However, in the majority of cases polyps are disseminated throughout the large bowel, and this phenotypic hallmark facilitated the clinical diagnosis. Figure 11.1 shows a representative pedigree in which the deleterious gene is segregated through three successive generations with a degree of penetrance close to 100%. The risk of "skipped generations" is negligible in the large majority of these families, providing that patients are fully evaluated.

As expected for autosomal dominant transmission, the ratio between affected male and female individuals should be close to 1.0, and this has actually been reported in most studies [33, 36]. However, in a large Japanese series of 534 FAP patients, the male:female ratio was 1.70 [23], and a similar ratio was subsequently reported in an Italian series [40, 41]. A tentative explanation is the possible existence of an X-linked modifier gene which might accelerate the development of adenomas in the large bowel [42]. The FAP gene does not seem to impair the biological fitness of affected individuals, so that fertility is not reduced in these patients [3, 43].

There is a large variation in the age of appearance of colorectal adenomas both within and between families. Through a close endoscopic evaluation of

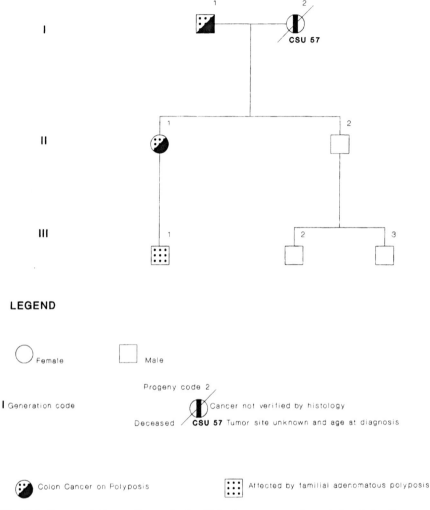

Fig. 11.1. Representative pedigree of a familial adenomatous polyposis (FAP) family spanning three generations

asymptomatic children at risk of adenomatosis coli, Alm concluded that the most frequent time of appearance of the complete phenotype is in the late teens or early twenties [33]. However, the study included a 2-year-old girl with a diagnosis of FAP who was operated on at the age of 4 owing to severe symptoms; moreover, the development of adenomas in infants has also been reported by other authors [24]. Similarly, although malignant lesions are considered rare below the age of 20, colorectal carcinoma has been reported in patients as young as 9 years [26].

In the majority of cases, adenomatosis coli is diagnosed in families segregating the phenotypic trait through various generations. However, some 20%–40% of all patients with FAP present as solitary cases, i.e. with only one affected member in a given family [40, 41, 43]. The most likely explanation for these "single cases" is that they represent new mutations, though it cannot be excluded that in some cases the deleterious gene has been transmitted through a parent who died at a very young age or in whom symptoms did not develop because of variable expressivity. Since FAP may remain asymptomatic (or "paucisymptomatic") for many years, the recognition of single patients before the appearance of clinical signs or symptoms of the disease is difficult, since there is no reason to suspect a given family. It follows that quite often solitary cases are diagnosed when the cancer has already developed [33, 41]. As fertility is not reduced in FAP, solitary cases can transmit the disease to their descendants, thus changing into segregating families.

Diagnosis, Clinical Features and Morphology

In an ideal situation, all new patients with FAP should be diagnosed by endoscopic screening of family members at risk by their position in the family tree or who tested positive for APC mutations. In fact, there is evidence that prophylactic screening and subsequent surgery reduce the morbidity and improve survival [44]. This, however, does not occur in all cases, either because individuals at risk may be reluctant to undergo endoscopic examination or in the case of solitary cases. It follows that in many cases the diagnosis is based on the occurrence of symptoms, such as rectal bleeding, diarrhea and abdominal discomfort; these usually manifest around the age of 30 years. When the diagnosis of FAP is based on symptom appearance, the probability of having developed a colorectal carcinoma is of the order of 60%–70% [33, 35]. More rarely, the disease is diagnosed by symptoms of metastatic spread to the liver or other organs.

Colorectal Lesions

Classical adenomatosis coli is characterized by the presence of at least 100 polyps throughout the entire large bowel (Fig. 11.2). The number 100 derives from the fact that in the St. Mark's series, all patients with FAP had more than 100 adenomas, and genetic transmission of the disease was not observed in patients with less than 100 polyps [45]. The large majority of these lesions are tubular or tubulovillous adenomas with mild to severe dysplasia; their density varies from 0.15 to 3.0 adenomas/cm^2, with an increasing density from the proximal colon to the rectosigmoid region [32, 33]. Utsunomiya and Iwama [32] described two types of polyp distribution among the Japanese – the "dense" and the "coarse" types – depending on the absolute number and density of adenomas. In the St. Mark's series, the mean polyp count was about 1,000 (range 104–5,000), thus confirming that in most typical cases the entire colorectal tract is virtually carpeted with polyps of various dimensions [45].

Attenuated adenomatous polyposis is a less severe variant of FAP in which fewer than 100 polyps are found in the large bowel [11, 12], that might be asso-

230 Familial Adenomatous Polyposis

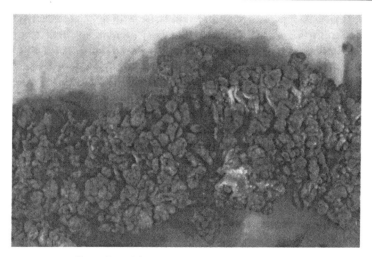

Fig. 11.2. A segment of large bowel from a FAP patient: the mucosa is carpeted with adenomatous polyps of various dimensions

ciated with specific APC mutations (see below). Individuals with attenuated FAP should undergo the same close endoscopic surveillance as "classical" FAP patients. Moreover, an accurate genealogical tree should be drawn up, and close relatives of affected patients should be advised to undergo clinical and endoscopic examinations. It should be noted, however, that there are difficulties in the phenotypic subclassification of adenomatosis coli, and some authors [46] proposed the existence of a broad spectrum of lesions, from very attenuated to attenuated, sparse, classical and profuse polyposis.

In a large series of individuals who developed features of polyposis while under endoscopic surveillance, the mean age of polyp detection was 22 years (range 11–53 years), and it is likely that the large majority of subjects carrying a mutated allele of the APC gene will develop polyps by the age of 25 years [24, 33], while the risk of developing full-blown polyposis after the age of 35 years is small. However, there is an extreme variability in the age of onset of adenomas: a high-risk individual who had a negative endoscopy result at the age of 70 years developed diffuse polyposis and rectal cancer at age 74 years [24].

When prophylactic surgery is not carried out, colorectal carcinoma usually develops in the fourth decade of life [33, 40]. The distribution of malignant lesions is similar to that of sporadic cancer, with 70%–80% of neoplasms localized in the descending colon and the rectosigmoid region. Grading, staging and other morphologic features of carcinomas developing in adenomatosis coli do not differ from those of the commonly observed sporadic malignancies of the large bowel.

Normal-appearing colorectal mucosa in FAP patients has been extensively investigated in the attempt to identify early changes indicative of an increased susceptibility to tumor formation. Various types of subtle alterations have been described, including (a) abnormalities of sialomucin content and properties

[47]; (b) expansion of the proliferative zone of colonic crypts from the base towards the luminal surface [48]; (c) an increased density of aberrant crypt foci [49]; and (d) various numerical chromosomal aberrations or changes of the banding pattern [50, 51]. These borderline alterations, however, are of limited help in the recognition of individuals at risk.

Extracolonic Manifestations

The effects of a malfunctioning APC gene are not limited to the colorectum, but involve several other organs and tissues (Table 11.1); thus, while initially adenomatosis coli was considered a organ-specific disease, subsequent studies led us to reconsider FAP as a generalized disorder of tissue growth regulation, and the list of additional lesions continues to increase [52]. The importance of extracolonic manifestations is threefold: first, they may antedate the appearance or the discovery of colorectal adenoma, thus being of help in the diagnosis of the underlying intestinal lesions. Second, though many of these lesions are essentially benign, some of them may become malignant (duodenal adenomas) or may assume a locally aggressive behavior (desmoid tumors), thus rendering more complex the follow-up of affected patients. Third, there is evidence that some extracolonic lesions can be correlated to specific APC mutations (see below), an observation which might shed light on the molecular mechanisms of the disease.

In most European series, gastric polyps have been found in 50%–70% of patients undergoing endoscopic investigations [53, 54]. Most of these lesions, however, show features of fundic gland hyperplasia (which is believed to have no malignant potential), while adenomatous changes are observed in no more than 10% of these patients [55]. In accordance with this contention, gastric cancer is rare in FAP. At variance with these observations, in Japanese series gastric adenomas are diagnosed in approximately half of the patients with adenomatosis coli, and gastric malignancies are not a rare event [56, 57]. These differences are

Table 11.1. Main extracolonic manifestations observed in FAP patients

Benign conditions	Severe or malignant conditions
Gastric hyperplastic polyps	Periampullary carcinoma
Duodenal adenomas	Desmoid tumors
Jejunal and ileal polyps	Thyroid carcinoma
Epidermoid cysts	Hepatoblastoma
Osteomas	Adrenal carcinoma
Dental abnormalities	
Congenital hypertrophy of the retinal pigment epithelium	
Adrenal adenomas	

difficult to explain if one considers the similar underlying molecular defect; however, they can tentatively be attributed to different diet and lifestyle and to the high background gastric cancer rate in Japan. The issue is further complicated by the recent observations of gastric carcinoma and dysplasia in fundic gland hyperplastic polyps in American patients with attenuated polyposis [58, 59]. Thus, gastric lesions in FAP individuals may possess or acquire – in some circumstances – an aggressive behavior, and these patients should be followed up with regular endoscopic controls.

Duodenal lesions are present in 90% or more of the patients with familial polyposis [53, 60] and their frequency increases with age; histological examination almost invariably shows adenomatous features, which are similar to those of the colorectum [25]. Moreover, biopsy specimens from apparently normal duodenal mucosa may show early adenomatous changes at histology, thus suggesting that the incidence of these lesions is even higher than that usually reported [53, 61]. Adenomas are relatively few in the first portion of the duodenum, but their density increases in the second and third portions, particularly in the periampullary region. The fact that their distribution mirrors the pattern of mucosal exposure to bile led to the suggestion that some biliary components might be implicated in the pathogenesis of upper gastrointestinal polyps [53, 55]. Spigelman et al. developed a "staging" system of duodenal polyps based on clinical and histological assessment [53]; stages I and II indicate mild duodenal polyposis, whereas stages III and IV signify severe disease. In keeping with these observations, the duodenum and periampullary region are the most common sites of extracolonic malignancy, which occurs in approximately 4% of FAP patients [62]; indeed, the risk of periampullary carcinoma in these patients is 100-fold greater than that of the general population, with a relative risk of 331 [63]. It is likely, therefore, that duodenal tumorigenesis – at least in FAP patients – follows the same adenoma-carcinoma sequence well characterized in the large bowel [64]. The high prevalence of duodenal adenomas and the elevated risk of periampullary carcinoma have resulted in widespread recommendations for routine endoscopic surveillance in FAP patients [65]. However, the fact that almost all individuals with adenomatosis coli show duodenal adenomatous polyps but that only a few of them develop into infiltrating carcinoma clearly suggests that the majority of these lesions tend to remain stable or to progress slowly. Prospective endoscopic studies on the natural history of untreated duodenal adenomas [55, 66, 67] showed that progression in the number and size of polyps occurred in 10%–50% of patients, but that histological progression was usually mild and less apparent. An endoscopic surveillance interval of 3–5 years seems therefore appropriate for the majority of these patients, whereas individuals with more advanced disease (stages III–IV) probably require a closer follow-up (6- to 12-month intervals).

When the entire small bowel could be explored through intraoperative endoscopy, jejunal or ileal adenomatous polyps were found in 20%–50% of FAP patients [41, 60]; however, malignant lesions at these anatomical sites are relatively infrequent in untreated patients [68]. Multiple adenomas have been detected in the ileal pouch of patients previously treated with total proctocolectomy and ileoanal anastomosis [69, 70]. Indeed, in recent investigations prevalence rates as high as 40%-60% have been reported, with a median follow-up of 5-7 years after surgery [71, 72]. Moreover, there are several reports of cancer arising from ileal mucosa in the pouches of patients with FAP [73, 74]; thus, restorative proctocolectomy does not exclude the risk of tumor development in the terminal ileum.

Epidermoid cysts are frequent in FAP patients. Since these lesions are usually not found until after puberty, their presence in a prepuberal individual should suggest an examination for the possible presence of adenomatosis coli [1]. Osteomas are another stigmata of Gardner's syndrome and are more frequent in the skull and mandible. Panoramic dental radiographs may detect several occult radiopaque lesions in FAP patients [75, 76], such as odontomas, supernumerary teeth, dentigerous cysts and abnormal mandibular bone sculpture. All these alterations are usually benign and do not cause symptoms or discomfort to patients; again, especially when occurring at an early age, they can be a good predictor of polyp development in FAP families.

In 1980, Blair and Trempe [77] were the first to report hypertrophy of the retinal epithelium associated with adenomatosis coli. In subsequent years, other investigators described these lesions [78, 79], which were defined as "congenital hypertrophy of the retinal pigment epithelium" (CHRPE) and which can be detected in the majority of individuals with adenomatosis coli. At ophthalmoscopy, these lesions are darkly pigmented, usually round or oval shaped, and extremely variable in number (from 1 to 20 or more), dimensions (from 0.1 to more than 1 optic disk), and distribution (unilateral or bilateral). Figure 11.3 shows a large area of CHRPE which developed in a 25-year-old patient with FAP. Histologically, CHRPE consists of a single layer of hypertrophic cells filled with

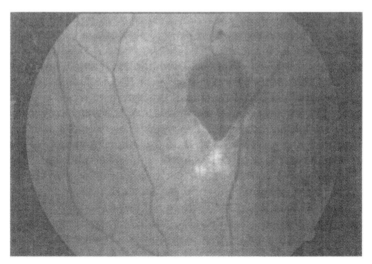

Fig. 11.3. A pigmented spot (congenital hypertrophy of the retinal pigment epithelium, CHRPE) diagnosed in a FAP patient

granules of pigment. According to most series, CHRPE are found in 70%–80% of individuals with adenomatosis coli, while they are extremely rare in the general population [80]. Thus, these lesions – especially when multiple and bilateral – seem to represent a sensitive and specific phenotypic biomarker for the identification of FAP; their absence, however, does not exclude the diagnosis of adenomatosis coli. Finally, genotype-phenotype correlation studies [31] suggest that the tendency to develop CHRPE in FAP families may depend on the site of APC germline mutations (see below).

Desmoid tumors are locally invasive, non-metastasizing, fibrous neoplasms which are part of the spectrum of lesions frequently observed in adenomatosis coli [1, 33]. Among extracolonic changes, desmoid tumors are of particular relevance, since these invasive proliferations of fibroblasts cause increased morbidity in FAP patients and may represent one of the main causes of death [81]. These lesions arise in the muscular-aponeurotic structures, especially in the anterior abdominal wall after surgical trauma (i.e. on the site of the laparotomy wound), mesentery and retroperitoneum. Extremely rare in the general population, these tumors are at least 100 times more common in FAP patients [82, 83], in whom lesions as large as 20 cm have been reported. Although desmoids are essentially benign – with minimal metastatic potential – they infiltrate contiguous organs and tissues and tend to recur after surgical removal [84]; it follows that complications of desmoids – such as intestinal obstruction, fistulas and bleeding – represent the second most common cause of death (after colorectal cancer) in adenomatosis coli [81, 85]. Desmoids are more frequently observed in the female sex, and their overall incidence is of the order of 5%–15% of all patients with FAP, with a marked tendency to aggregate in some families [86, 87]. Treatment of desmoid tumors is basically surgical, with the objective of complete excision of the lesion; surgery, however, is often unsatisfactory and is accompanied by a high rate of complications and recurrences [84–86]. Moreover, resection of desmoid tumors in the mesentery usually requires extensive excision of the intestine and the maintenance of patients on total parenteral nutrition. For these reasons, intestinal transplantation has recently been proposed for the management of otherwise untreatable FAP patients with complicated desmoid lesions [88, 89]. Several medical treatments have also been evaluated, including tamoxifen, ascorbic acid, doxorubicin-based chemotherapy and, more recently, anti-inflammatory drugs [84, 86, 90–92]. All these approaches, however, have been of limited value, and the optimal treatment for desmoid tumors remains poorly defined.

There are studies suggesting that thyroid carcinoma (especially of the papillary histological type) should be included among the additional neoplastic lesions observed more frequently in FAP patients than in the general population [93–95]. The risk of developing thyroid carcinoma in a female FAP patient is 100–160 times higher than in the background population [96]. Although the prognosis of these lesions is usually good, various authors recommended regular screening controls (including palpation, ultrasound and, when necessary, fine needle biopsy) for thyroid tumors in FAP patients [97, 98]. More recent studies, however, did not recommend regular screening for these lesions, since it is unlikely to result in a reduction of mortality [99].

Other neoplasms that occur with an increased frequency in patients with familial polyposis include hepatoblastoma [100], carcinoma of the pancreas and biliary tract [101, 102], adrenal adenomas and carcinomas [103, 104]. All these lesions confirm the generalized disorder of cell growth and differentiation which is associated with constitutional mutations of the APC gene. Finally, Matsuo et al. [105] recently reported the development of a bladder adenocarcinoma in a 50-year-old FAP patient who was operated on for rectal cancer at the age of 24 years. Clinical investigations led to the conclusion that the bladder tumor was actually due to colonic mucosa that had migrated to the bladder lumen through a rectovesical fistula, and subsequently had become cancerous.

Molecular Biology of FAP

The identification of the APC gene represents one of the major advances not only in the study of adenomatosis coli but also for our understanding of colorectal tumor development. Although the genetic nature of FAP has been recognized for many years by the simple observation of polyp and cancer occurrence in families, the underlying molecular defect associated with the FAP phenotype has been fully characterized only in the last 15 years.

The APC Gene and Its Functions

In 1986, Herrera et al. [5] described the clinical case of a 42-year-old man with adenomatosis coli, mental retardation and an interstitial deletion removing part of the long arm of chromosome 5. The attention of many investigators, therefore, focused on this chromosome, and 1 year later two independent research groups localized the FAP locus gene at 5q 21–22 by linkage analysis [6, 106]. Further investigations led to the detection of constitutional mutations in the coding sequence in FAP patients but not in unaffected controls [29, 30]. The genetics of FAP and its similarity to other syndromes of site-specific tumor predisposition – such as retinoblastoma and Wilms' tumor – led to the designation of this gene (called APC, for adenomatous polyposis coli) as a tumor suppressor gene. Sequencing of the APC gene revealed an open reading frame of 8,535 nucleotides for a predicted sequence of 2,843 amino acids encoded by 15 exons. With a length of 6,578 nucleotides, exon 15 of APC is one of the largest of all known exons [29, 30, 107]. More than 1,400 mutations in APC – both germline and somatic – have been described [108]; these alterations include single base substitutions leading to amino acid change or stop codon, and small base-pair deletions (5–15 bases) leading to frameshift. A small number of missense mutations have also been detected, whose pathogenic role can only be inferred by evaluating their co-segregation with the FAP phenotype in a given kindred. Two of the most common mutations are 5-base-pair deletions at codons 1309 and 1061 (exon 15) that account for 18% and 12%, respectively, of all constitutional APC mutations. The majority of these alterations (approximately 80%) are localized within exon 15 [107, 109].

The APC gene encodes a 311.8-KDa protein that has limited homologies to intermediate filament structural proteins, such as myosin and keratin; the protein has multiple functional domains that mediate both oligomerization and binding to many intracellular proteins, such as β-catenin, tubulin, γ-catenin [110]. The main function of the APC product is to modulate the Wingless/Wnt signal pathway through its effects on cellular levels of β-catenin. Moreover, APC affects several other physiological processes (from cell cycle control to differentiation and apoptosis) in a number of cell types and organisms [108]. Normal APC forms complexes with β-catenin and axin; through these phosphorylated complexes, β-catenin is normally degraded following an ubiquitin-mediated proteasomal pathway [111]. APC mutations result in truncation of the encoded protein and in the disruption of complex formation, with consequently increased cytoplasmic levels of β-catenin. Undegraded β-catenin is translocated into the nucleus, where it interacts with T-cell factor 4; the activation of this transcriptional factor in colonic epithelial cells leads to the up-regulation of several cancer-related genes, including *c-myc, c-jun, fra*-1 and cyclin D1 [112,113]. Thus, as recently suggested by Chung [8], it is likely that β-catenin (whose increased nuclear expression is a consequence of APC mutations) is a "driver" that up-regulates genes critical for the replication and differentiation of colonic epithelial cells.

In addition to their role in the Wingless/Wnt signaling pathway [8, 108, 110], there is evidence that APC/β-catenin play a role in controlling cell cycle progression [114], in the process of epithelial cell adhesion and migration [115] and, presumably, in regulating intestinal cell differentiation and apoptosis [116, 117]. The APC gene, therefore, participates in several cellular processes in the colonic epithelium, and some of these functions can be due to its ability to regulate β-catenin levels [108]. Immunohistochemical studies of the APC gene product in normal colonic epithelium indicate that the protein is concentrated at the basolateral portion of crypt cells. As colonocytes progress from the base of the gland to the luminal surface, APC immunostaining gradually increases, thus suggesting an association between APC expression and cell differentiation [118].

Genotype-Phenotype Correlations

Constitutional mutations of the APC gene are currently detected in the large majority (80%–90%) of individuals with clinical features of FAP; this fraction, however, does not reach 100%. It is of interest that in a recent study [119] FAP families without detected APC gene mutations showed a milder disease phenotype than APC-positive families, thus suggesting that different genetic factors could be implicated.

Several studies analyzed the possible correlation between clinical expression of FAP and type of constitutional mutation. As a general impression, some of the correlations have been confirmed by numerous investigators and can be considered as well established; however, several uncertainties still persist, and caution should be used in attributing a given phenotype too easily to a specific mutation, especially when this may influence therapeutic decisions [120, 121].

Constitutional mutations occurring within the first 4 coding exons of the APC gene have been correlated with the so-called attenuated APC [10–12]; in these patients the number of colorectal adenomas is smaller than in florid polyposis, and the disease shows a late onset and a slow progression to cancer. Spirio et al. proposed that a specific "phenotypic boundary" exists between attenuated polyposis and FAP, residing in codons 157–168 of exon 4 [122, 123]. It has been suggested that mutations at this site result in the expression of unstable mRNA, with a consequently unstable encoded peptide that does not dimerize efficiently with wild-type products. However, it should be noted that not all mutations occurring within the first 4 exons of the gene result in an attenuated disease, and that this phenotype may also develop in association with alterations occurring in other portions of the gene. Thus, Nasioulas et al. [124] recently reported a three-generation family with a 5 bp deletion at codon 116–118 – causing premature termination of protein synthesis – which was associated with profuse adenomatosis coli in two affected individuals. Moreover, Rozen et al. [120] described a family with an 11-bp insertion in exon 9 (nucleotide 1060) of the APC gene – causing frameshift and a stop codon – in which the phenotypic manifestations of FAP varied from profuse polyposis to a complete absence of clinical or endoscopic signs of disease in four individuals with confirmed germline mutation. A similar variation of clinical expressivity was reported by Presciuttini et al. [125] in two Italian FAP families.

There are several reports indicating that mutations occurring in the central part of the APC gene – between codons 1250 and 1464 – are associated with a uniformly severe polyposis phenotype [126–128], with profuse adenomatosis of the colon, early age of onset of adenomas, and rapid progression to malignancy. These features are particularly evident with the 5-bp deletion at codon 1309, which represents the most common APC mutation (18% of all cases). Because of the frequent occurrence of cancer of the rectal stump in FAP patients with mutations in the central portions of the gene, various authors [127, 129] suggested that restorative proctocolectomy with ileoanal anastomosis should be the treatment of choice in these individuals. It has been suggested that the 1309 mutation might generate a protein product acting more efficiently as dominant-negative through its ability to interact with products of the wild-type allele [10]. However, in a recent large study of 680 German, unrelated FAP families [121], a large phenotypic variation was observed even among patients with identical constitutional alterations and including individuals with the 1309 mutation. The authors concluded that molecular analysis is of limited value for predicting the clinical course of the disease and for therapeutic choices in individual patients; it follows that decisions on treatment of these patients should be mainly based on clinical symptoms and signs and, in particular, on the degree of colonic adenomatosis and the nature of extraintestinal manifestations.

The presence of pigmented ocular fundus lesions (CHRPE) also seems to depend on the location of constitutional mutations in the APC gene. There is

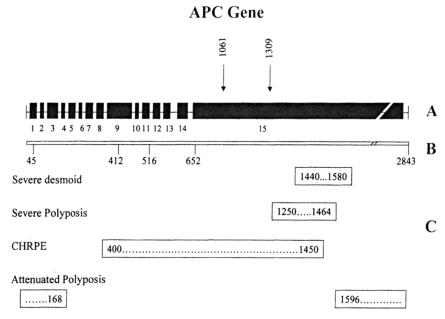

Fig. 11.4A–C. Adenomatous polyposis coli (APC) gene mutations and clinical features of FAP. A The *black boxes* represent the APC coding region split into 15 exons; B the APC protein, constituted of 2,844 amino acids; C *white boxes* assign mutated regions of APC to the main clinical manifestations of the disease

evidence that CHRPE are strongly associated with mutations between codons 400 and 1445 [10, 108, 130]. Mutations around codon 400 (exon 9) tend to show variable expression of CHRPE, presumably in relation to the type and location of the molecular changes in the exon, which is subjected to alternative splicing.

APC mutations downstream of codon 1440 up to codon 1580 (exon 15) are frequently associated with features of Gardner's syndrome [131], such as osteomas, epidermoid cysts and desmoid tumors. Severe manifestations of desmoids seem restricted to mutations between codons 1444 through 1580 [132, 133], though this does not exclude the occurrence of desmoids in association with mutations located in other portions of the gene [134]. Rather interestingly, patients with high numbers of desmoids but without features of adenomatosis coli have been identified and carry constitutional mutations at the 3' end of the APC gene [135].

Finally, no consistent associations have been reported between type or site of mutations and the development of upper gastrointestinal polyps [10, 55, 108]. Figure 11.4 shows a schematic representation of the main genotype-phenotype correlations described in FAP patients.

Methods for Study of the APC Gene

Although direct mutation analysis of the APC gene is at present the technique of choice for the identification of gene carriers in FAP families, presymptomatic diagnosis of adenomatosis coli can also be achieved by demonstrating co-inheritance of the responsible allele with one or more genetic markers flanking the gene. Several informative markers are available for the diagnosis of FAP through linkage studies [136, 137]; however, as these markers are located 1-10 centimorgans from the APC gene, they seem of limited usefulness for family studies. The identification of a highly polymorphic marker located only 30-70 kb from the gene increased remarkably the accuracy of linkage analysis in FAP families [138]. Using this biomarker, Spirio et al. were able to determine the carrier status for 20 of 31 individuals at risk in 14 investigated families [138, 139].

The standard methods used for detecting APC mutations include single strand conformation polymorphism analysis [140], denaturing gradient gel electrophoresis [141], RNAse protection assay [142] and heteroduplex analysis [143]. In addition, since most identified mutations introduce premature termination of protein translation, various laboratories developed efficient methods ("protein truncation tests") that can analyze large portions of the coding sequence for the presence of premature stop codons [144, 145]. These techniques, however, do not provide information on the sequence of mutations and therefore require further analysis to determine the nucleotide sequence of the mutant allele.

With these techniques, the frequency of APC mutations detected among FAP families varies with the method used, but in no case has it been more than 80%. The reasons for the inability to identify genetic alteration in a substantial proportion of these kindreds is unclear, but it is likely that there are APC mutations which are difficult to detect by standard mutation analysis. Laken et al. [146] recently described a new method (monoallelic mutation analysis, MAMA) in which chromosomes from affected patients are isolated in hybrid cells formed by fusing cells of the patient with a suitable rodent recipient. Since each allele can be examined independently, mutations are not obscured by the wild-type product from the normal allele, as is the case with standard analyses. With this new approach more than 95% of FAP patients were found to harbor constitutional mutations of the APC gene.

Management of Familial Adenomatous Polyposis

Management of FAP can be viewed as a multistep procedure which requires a close collaboration of several specialists (clinical geneticists, gastroenterologists and surgeons) within a multidisciplinary team. Several important decisions must be taken, including type and time of surgery, and whether or not to intervene with medical approaches. For these reasons, patients should be properly informed about the advantages and disadvantages of each procedure, and their full collaboration is a prerequisite for optimal treatment. Moreover, affected individuals should be aware that the disease concerns the family and not only themselves, with a consequent necessary extension of the traditional relationship between patient and physician.

The Role of Counseling in the Diagnosis and Surveillance of Adenomatosis Coli

In the process of counseling, the physician (the counselor) acquires all relevant information concerning the patient, the family and the disease, and subsequently suggests a given strategy, which may involve genetic testing, clinical investigations, changes of diet and lifestyle, medical and surgical interventions. The counselor should also communicate and interpret the results of DNA testing, with the possible implications for the management of the disease.

In patients with FAP, counseling begins with a detailed pedigree analysis from both sides of the proband's family. All cancer diagnoses should be confirmed by clinical charts, histological records or death certificates; in addition, current age and age at death should be ascertained for everyone in the family tree. In the presence of clinical features of polyposis and of an autosomal dominant type of inheritance (at least in segregating families, which represent 70% of all FAP), genetic testing is discussed with the patient, together with the need for endoscopy or other examinations. Moreover, individuals at risk in the pedigree should be identified and contacted. The decision to undergo genetic testing is strictly personal and is based on informed consent. The elements of informed consent include information on the gene being tested and the implications, limitations and impact of results for the proband and other family members at risk [147].

In collaborating families, screening and follow-up are currently based on the results of genetic testing. In the case of mutation-positive results, colonoscopy or flexible sigmoidoscopy are usually recommended starting at puberty, when polyps begin to develop in the colorectum of the majority of patients [148, 33]. Mutation carriers also require surveillance (by gastroduodenoscopy) for the possible development of polyps in the upper gastrointestinal tract [55, 61], though the age at which to begin with endoscopic surveillance has not been defined. When an APC gene constitutional mutation is identified in a family, direct gene testing of relatives who have not been assessed will distinguish those who carry the mutation and those who do not. In the case of new mutations (approximately 30% of FAP cases), parents and siblings are not at risk, while descendants of the proband carry a 50% risk – in accordance with autosomal dominant transmission – and should undergo genetic testing.

A negative test signifies that a given patient does not carry the specific APC mutation which has been detected in the family. In this instance, there is no increased risk of developing polyps and cancer compared with the general population, so that early endoscopic screening is not required. This situation is different from that of "no mutation detected", in which genetic tests failed to identify germline APC mutations in a patient with clinical features of FAP. When no mutation has been detected, APC gene testing loses any predictive value for asymptomatic relatives at risk of tumor development; in these families, therefore, first-degree relatives of affected individuals should continue close endoscopic surveillance between puberty and the fourth to fifth decade of life [149]. Caution should be used in interpreting APC gene analysis when a mutation has not been detected: in fact, there is evidence that the results can frequently be misinterpreted as negative. Giardello et al. [150] recently reported that misinterpretation of the test results was as high as 31.6% of the investigated cases and, consequently, that FAP patients who underwent genetic tests often received inadequate counseling. This occurred when an unaffected family member from a FAP family was tested for APC mutations without testing an affected individual. Many physicians did not realize that a test in which no mutation was detected could represent a false-negative result in a pedigree in which APC mutations had not been previously identified in affected members. These findings underline the concept that constitutional mutations of APC should first be searched for in affected patients, and that unaffected family members should be investigated only when the molecular alteration has been characterized.

Surgical Treatment of FAP

In most FAP patients the rectum and the sigmoid are usually involved by diffuse adenomatosis; it follows that sigmoidoscopy is sufficient for the initial diagnosis of FAP. Several polyps should be removed for morphologic examination in order to ascertain their adenomatous nature and the degree of differentiation. For subsequent surveillance and diagnostic evaluation, pancolonoscopy is the technique of choice for exploring the entire large bowel (and the terminal ileum) and taking multiple biopsies. Moreover, at the time of diagnosis the patient should also undergo upper endoscopy, for the possible development of gastric and duodenal lesions [25, 43].

Since surgery is the definitive treatment of FAP, after a proper diagnosis, the time and type of operation should be considered. For individuals with symptomatic disease – who are usually over the age of 25–30 years – surgery should be carried out as soon as possible. For adolescents and, in general, for asymptomatic subjects, the time of operation can be individualized, taking into account the endoscopic findings, the morphologic assessment, and the fact that it is probably better to proceed with the operation after complete physical, psychological and sexual maturation. However, as suggested by various authors [1, 25], the presence of large adenomas, rapidly growing polyps or severe dysplasia at repeated biopsies may indicate the need for an earlier intervention.

The main surgical procedures for treating patients with adenomatosis coli are colectomy with ileorectal anastomosis (IRA) and restorative proctocolectomy with ileal pouch and ileoanal anastomosis (IAA) [151]. In the past, permanent ileostomy was currently carried out, but at present this invalidating procedure is limited to the rare patients with infiltrating malignancy of the lower rectum. Over the past decades it has been discussed whether the optimal treatment for adenomatosis coli should be IRA or IAA, and this is not surprising, since both techniques present advantages and disadvantages. Temporal trends, however, favor a larger use of proctocolectomy with IAA versus the more traditional IRA [41,152].

Colectomy with IRA can be considered when (A) the number of rectal adenomas is limited, so that they can be removed without damaging anorectal function, (B) the rectum and the lower sigmoid do not show malignant lesions, (C) the patient is aware of the risk of cancer in the remaining rectum and, consequently, is prepared to undergo close endoscopic surveillance of the rectal stump, with removal and histological examination of all newly detected polyps. Given these conditions, most surgeons would consider colectomy with IRA as the preferred approach. The main advantages of this technique are that it is a one-step procedure, with few complications and good functional results in terms of stool frequency and incontinence [153]. The main problem with IRA is the risk of cancer in the rectal stump, which has varied from 3.6% to 32% in different investigations [154, 155], despite surveillance. Moreover, there is also a cumulative risk of 40%–70% after 20 years of secondary proctectomy owing to an increased, and untreatable, rectal polyposis [156, 157]. The Finnish experience [158] in this sense is rather suggestive: colectomy with IRA was the technique of choice up to the year 1992. With a longer follow-up of operated patients, however, rectal cancer was noted more frequently, and the rectal cancer excision rate increased. These findings prompted the authors to favor restorative proctocolectomy with IAA instead of colectomy and IRA.

Those authors preferring proctocolectomy with IAA claim that the risk of cancer is unacceptably high in patients operated on by colectomy and IRA [159]. Total proctocolectomy with mucosal proctectomy and IAA has the main advantages of removing all colorectal mucosa and preserving the natural route of defecation. However, the technique usually implies a 2-stage procedure, including a temporary ileostomy. Thus, the surgical procedure is more complex than IRA, postoperative complications are more frequent, and the accommodation period may require several months. In addition, this approach does not eliminate the need for endoscopic control of the ileal pouch, since multiple ileal adenomas and, more rarely, carcinomas of the pouch have been reported several years after restorative proctocolectomy [69, 70, 72].

In summary, the surgical approaches for FAP are still being debated; despite the risk of cancer development, many surgeons still prefer colectomy with IRA and close endoscopic surveillance. Many other surgeons recommend restorative proctocolectomy with IAA, especially for young patients whose rectum is carpeted with adenomas. In a recent study, Bulow and collaborators [157] defined a subset of FAP patients in whom IRA should be recommended as the optimal treatment; the subgroup included young individuals with few rectal adenomas and a family history of mild phenotype, and patients with attenuated polyposis, provided there is acceptance (and awareness) of life-long rectal surveillance. Finally, as already discussed, there is some evidence that the genotype of the patients might influence the choice of operation [127, 129]. However, there are still concerns towards this novel approach, especially considering the large phenotypic variation frequently observed among patients with identical germline mutations. Presumably, at present, molecular analysis is of limited value in predicting the course of the disease; it is likely that the issue will become clearer after the identification and characterization of possible APC modifier genes [160, 161], which should exert their effect by modulating the phenotypic expression of the disease.

Overall Prognosis and Follow-up

As expected, the presence of malignancy of the large bowel at diagnosis represents the most important determinant of prognosis. Various authors [25, 35] reported that the 10-year survival of FAP patients was only 40%–50% in the presence of cancer, but as good as 90% for call-up family members, whose disease was detected through screening. These findings underscore the clinical relevance of recognition and early endoscopic screening among family members at risk, a procedure that has been improved by the recent introduction and diffusion of genetic testing [148]. However, we should not forget that in single cases early diagnosis is virtually impossible, unless the subject presents with relevant symptoms before cancer occurrence, and single cases represent some 20%–30% of all FAP patients. It follows that almost inevitably the clinical diagnosis of FAP will continue to be delayed in a fraction of cases, and that cancer development cannot be prevented in all FAP patients. For patients successfully treated, the main causes of death remain periampullary carcinoma and desmoid tumors [81].

After the operation, patients with FAP should undergo regular surveillance virtually for the rest of their life. The main purpose of this close follow-up is the control of additional lesions in the remaining rectum (or in the ileal pouch, after restorative proctocolectomy), in the upper gastrointestinal tract and in the terminal ileum. Endoscopic examination of the rectal stump and terminal ileum should be carried out at 6-month intervals; newly developed polyps are removed and histological slides examined. In the presence of malignancy, a further operation may be required [25, 33]. The ileal pouch should theoretically eliminate the risk of cancer; however, recent studies documented a high prevalence of adenomas in the pouch 5–7 years after surgery [72], and the risk of cancer development – though much lower than in the rectal stump – cannot be ignored [162]. Considering the length of time taken by the adenoma-carcinoma sequence in the colon, annual controls are probably not necessary; however, surveillance at 3- to 4-year intervals should be recommended after IAA. If polyps are present, closer intervals could be required, with endoscopic removal of lesions larger than 5 mm [72, 163].

Medical Treatment

In past years, antioxidant vitamins (in particular, ascorbic acid) and wheat fiber have been used in clinical trials for inhibiting or preventing tumor occurrence in patients with FAP, but with rather discouraging results [164, 165]. In contrast, regression of rectal adenomas was reported with the administration of sulindac [27, 166], a non-selective inhibitor of prostaglandin synthesis commonly used as an anti-inflammatory drug. In a subsequent controlled crossover study, Labayle et al. [167] showed almost complete regression of rectal polyps in five patients with FAP and IRA treated for 4 months with sulindac at a daily dose of 300 mg. Other authors confirmed the efficacy of sulindac [168], though complete disappearance of polyps was not observed in any of the investigated patients. Moreover, the gastrointestinal toxicity associated with sulindac and other conventional anti-inflammatory compounds may limit their long-term use for tumor prevention. In a recent study [28], Steinbach et al. evaluated the effect of celecoxib (a selective cyclo-oxygenase-2 inhibitor, which should be devoid of adverse effects on the gastroenteric tract [169]) on colorectal polyps in FAP patients who had not had their colorectum removed. After 6 months of treatment (800 mg/day), the patients showed a 28.0% reduction in the mean number of colorectal polyps and a 30.7% reduction in the polyp burden (the sum of polyp diameter), as compared with a reduction of 4%–5% in the control group. Virtually no effect was observed with smaller doses of celecoxib. These preliminary investigations lend further support to the role of cyclooxygenase in colorectal tumor development and to the possibility of interfering with this process with selective inhibitors of the enzyme [170].

Although the results obtained with sulindac and celecoxib seem to suggest a possible medical approach to FAP, they should be interpreted with caution. Indeed, there are reports [171, 172] of cancer occurrence in the rectal stump of FAP patients treated with sulindac. These rare cases suggest that anti-inflammatory drugs may block the formation of polyps but may not interrupt the dysplasia-carcinoma sequence. Clearly, more studies are needed before introducing any routine medical therapy for FAP patients; in the meantime surgery remains the only available treatment.

Conclusions

There is no doubt that familial polyposis will continue to represent an excellent model for the study of colorectal tumorigenesis. The discovery of the underlying molecular lesions associated with FAP contributed significantly to understanding the basic mechanisms of sporadic colorectal malignancies; moreover, clinical studies in FAP patients confirmed the possible role of anti-inflammatory drugs in inhibiting colorectal tumor development. However, despite our increased knowledge of the disease and the remarkable improvements in prophylactic surgery, the life expectancy of FAP patients remains lower than that of the general population, owing to the occurrence of other malignancies (in the periampullary region and in the rectal stump), desmoid tumors and the long-term effects of colorectal surgery. Future research should further elucidate the genotype-phenotype correlations, the intimate mechanisms of the APC gene and protein in the development of adenomas and carcinoma, and the role of possible modifier genes.

References

1. Haggitt RC, Reid BJ. Hereditary gastrointestinal polyposis syndromes. Am J Surg Pathol 1986; 10(12):871-87.
2. Ponz de Leon M. Hereditary Gastrointestinal Polyposis Syndrome. In: "Familial and Hereditary Tumors". Springer-Verlag, Heidelberg, 1994; 238-64.
3. Alm T, Dencker H, Lunderquist A et al. Gardner's syndrome. Acta Chir Scand 1973; 139:660-5.
4. Ponz de Leon M, Benatti P, Percesepe A et al. Epidemiology of cancer of the large bowel – The 12-year experience of a specialized Registry in Northern Italy. Ital J Gastroenterol Hepatol 1999; 31:10-8.
5. Herrera L, Kakati S, Gibas L et al. Gardner syndrome in a man with an interstitial deletion of 5q. Am J Med Genet 1986; 25:473-6.
6. Bodmer WF, Bailey CJ, Bodmer J et al. Localization of the gene for FAP on chromosome 5. Nature 1987; 328:614-9.
7. Vogelstein B, Fearon ER, Hamilton SR et al. Genetic alterations during colorectal-tumor development. N Engl J Med 1988; 319-525:32.
8. Chung DC. The genetic basis of colorectal cancer: insights into critical pathways of tumorigenesis. Gastroenterology 2000; 119:854-65.
9. Nakamura Y. The role of the adenomatous polyposis coli (APC) gene in human cancers. Adv Cancer Res 1993; 621:65-87.
10. Radice P, Cama A, Mariani-Costantini R. Molecular genetics of polyposis and hereditary colorectal cancer. Forum Trends in Experimental and Clinical Medicine 1996; 6:275-91.
11. Lynch HT, Smyrk T, McGinn T et al. Attenuated familial adenomatous polyposis (AFAP). A phenotypically and genotypically distinctive variant of FAP. Cancer 1995; 76:2427-33.
12. Spirio L, Green J, Robertson J et al. The identical 5' splice-site acceptor mutation in five attenuated APC families from Newfoundland demonstrates a founder effect. Hum Genet 1999; 105:388-98.
13. Sklifasowski NW. Polyadenoma tractus intestinalis. Vrac 1881; 4:55-7.
14. Cripps WH. Two cases of disseminated polypus of the rectum. Trans Pathol Soc Lond 1882; 33:165-8.
15. Smith T. Three cases of multiple polyps of the large bowel occurring in one family. S Barth Hosp Rep 1887; 23:225-9.
16. Lockhart-Mummery P. Cancer and heredity. Lancet 1925; 1:427-9.
17. Cockayne EA. Heredity in relation to cancer. Cancer Rev 1927; 2:337-47.
18. Lockhart-Mummery JP. The causation and treatment of multiple adenomatosis of the colon. Ann Surg 1934; 99:178-84.
19. Gardner EJ. A genetic and clinical study of intestinal polyposis, a predisposing factor for carcinoma of the colon and rectum. Am J Hum Genet 1951; 3:167-76.
20. Gardner EJ, Plenk HP. Hereditary pattern for multiple osteomas in a family group. Am J Hum Genet 1952; 4:31-6.
21. Gardner EJ, Richards RC. Multiple cutaneous and subcutaneous lesions occurring simultaneously with hereditary polyposis and osteomatosis. Am J Hum Genet 1953; 5:139-47.
22. Parks AG, Nicholls RJ, Beliveau P et al. Proctocolectomy with ileal reservoir and anal anastomosis. Br J Surg 1980; 67:533-8.
23. Utsunomiya J, Iwama T, Imajo M et al. Total colectomy, mucosal proctectomy and ileal anastomosis. Dis Colon Rectum 1980; 23:459-66.
24. Alm T, Lieznerski G. The intestine polyposis. Clin Gastroenterol 1973; 2:577-602.
25. Bulow S. Familial adenomatous polyposis. Ann Med 1989; 21:299-307.
26. Naylor EW, Lebenthal E. Gardner's syndrome: recent developments in research and management. Dig Dis Sci 1980; 25:945-9.
27. Waddell WR, Longhry RW. Sulindac for polyposis of the colon. J Surg Oncol 1983; 24:83-7.

28. Steinbach G, Lynch PM, Phillips RKS et al. The effect of Celecoxib, a cyclooxygenase-2 inhibitor, in familial adenomatous polyposis. N Engl J Med 2000; 342:1946-52.
29. Kinzler KW, Nilbert MC, Su LK et al. Identification of FAP locus from chromosome 5q21. Science 1991; 253:661-5.
30. Groden J, Thliveris A, Samowitz W et al. Identification and characterization of the familial adenomatous polyposis gene. Cell 1991; 66:589-600.
31. Houlston R, Crabtree M, Phillips R et al. Explaining differences in the severity of familial adenomatous polyposis and the search for modifier genes. Gut 2001; 48:1-5.
32. Utsunomiya J, Iwama T. Adenomatosis coli in Japan. In: Winawer S, Schottenfeld D, Sherlock P (eds). "Colorectal cancer: prevention, epidemiology and screening". Raven, New York, 1980; 83-95.
33. Alm T. Hereditary adenomatosis of the colon and the rectum. In: Lynch HT, Lynch PM (eds). "Colon cancer genetics". Von Nostrand Reinhold, New York, 1985; 30-51.
34. Lipkin M, Winawer SJ, Sherlock P. Early identification of individuals at increased risk for cancer of the large intestine. Clin Bull 1981; 11:13-21.
35. Jarvinen HJ. Epidemiology of familial adenomatous polyposis in Finland: impact of family screening on the colorectal cancer rate and survival. Gut 1992; 33:357-60.
36. Bulow S, Holm NV, Hauge M. The incidence and prevalence of familial polyposis in Denmark. Scand J Soc Med 1986; 14:67-74.
37. Ponz de Leon M, Di Gregorio C, Roncucci L et al. Epidemiologia dei tumori del colon-retto. Incidenza, mortalità, familiarità e sopravvivenza nella ex USL di Modena, 1984-1995. Pagine 1-58. Università di Modena, 1998.
38. Mitry E, Benhamiche AM, Jouve JL et al. Colorectal adenocarcinoma in patients under 45 years of age: comparison with older patients in a well-defined French population. Dis Colon Rectum 2001; 44:380-7.
39. Naylor EW, Gardner EJ. Penetrance and expressivity of the gene responsible for the Gardner syndrome. Clin Genet 1977; 11:381-93.
40. Ponz de Leon M, Sassatelli R, Zanghieri G et al. Hereditary Adenomatosis of the colon and rectum. Clinical features of eight families from Northern Italy. Am J Gastroenterol 1989; 84:906-16.
41. De Pietri S. Sassatelli R, Roncucci L et al. Clinical and biological features of adenomatosis coli in Northern Italy. Scan J Gastroenterol 1995; 30:771-9.
42. Utsunomiya J, Murata M, Tanimura M et al. An analysis of the age distribution of colon cancer in adenomatosis coli. Cancer 1980; 45:198-205.
43. Bussey HJR, Morson BC. Familial polyposis coli. In: Lipkin M, Good RA (eds). "Gastrointestinal tract cancer". Plenum Medical, New York, 1978; 275-94.
44. Heiskanen I, Luostarinen T, Jarvinen HJ. Impact of screening examinations on survival in familial adenomatous polyposis. Scand J Gastroenterol 2000; 35:1284-7.
45. Bussey HJR. Familial polyposis coli. John Hopkins University Press, New York, 1975.
46. Lynch HT, Smyrk TC. Classification of familial adenomatous polyposis: a diagnostic nightmare. Am J Hum Genet 1998; 62:1288-9.
47. Muto T, Kamiya J, Sawada T et al. Mucin abnormality of colonic mucosa in patients with FAP. Dis Colon Rectum 1985; 28:147-8.
48. Deschner E, Lipkin M. Proliferative pattern in colonic mucosa in familial polyposis. Cancer 1975; 35:413-8.
49. Roncucci L, Stamp D, Medline A et al. Identification and quantification of aberrant crypt foci and microadenomas in the human colon. Hum Pathol 1991; 22:287-94.
50. Mark J, Mitelman F, Dencker H et al. The specificity of the chromosomal abnormalities in human colonic polyps; a cytogenetic study of multiple polyps in a case of Gardner's syndrome. Acta Pathol Microbiol Immunol Scand 1973; 81:85-90.
51. Mitelman F, Mark J, Nilsson PG et al. Chromosome banding pattern in human colonic polyps. Hereditas 1974; 78:63-8.
52. Parks TG. Extracolonic manifestations associated with familial adenomatous polyposis. Ann R Coll Surg Eng 1990; 72:181-4.

53. Spigelman AD, Williams GB, Talbot IC et al. Upper gastrointestinal cancer in patients with familial adenomatous polyposis. Lancet 1989; 2:783-5.
54. Jarvinen H, Nyberg M, Peltokallio P. Upper gastrointestinal tract polyps in familial adenomatosis coli. Gut 1983; 24:333-9.
55. Wallace MH, Phillips PKS. Upper gastrointestinal disease in patients with familial adenomatous polyposis. Br J Surg 1998; 85:742-50.
56. Ida M, Tsuneyoshi Y, Itoh H et al. Natural history of gastric adenomas in patients with familial adenomatosis coli/Gardner's syndrome. Cancer 1988; 61:605-11.
57. Iwama T, Mishima Y, Utsunomiya J. The impact of familial adenomatous polyposis on the tumorigenesis and mortality at the several organs. Its rational treatment. Ann Surg 1993; 217:101-8.
58. Zwick A, Munir M, Ryan CK et al. Gastric adenocarcinoma and dysplasia in fundic gland polyps of a patient with attenuated adenomatous polyposis coli. Gastroenterology 1997; 113:659-63.
59. Hofgärtner WT, Thorp M, Ramus MW et al. Gastric adenocarcinoma associated with fundic gland polyps in a patients with attenuated familial adenomatous polyposis. Am J Gastroenterol 1999; 94:2275-81.
60. Iida M, Ohsato K, Itoh H et al. Diagnostic value of intraoperative fibroscopy for small intestinal polyps in familial adenomatosis coli. Endoscopy 1989;12:161-5.
61. Watanabe H, Enjoji M, Yao T et al. Gastric lesions in familial adenomatosis coli. Hum Pathol 1978; 9:269-83.
62. Jagelman DG, DeCosse JJ, Bussey HJR et al. Upper gastrointestinal cancer in familial adenomatous polyposis. Lancet 1988; 1:1149-51.
63. Offerhaus G, Giardiello F, Krush A et al. The risk of upper gastrointestinal cancer in familial adenomatous polyposis. Gastroenterology 1992; 102:1980-2.
64. Sellner F. Investigations on the significance of the adenoma-carcinoma sequence in the small bowel. Cancer 1990; 66:702-15.
65. Van Stolk RU. Endoscopic surveillance for polyposis syndromes. Gastrointest Endosc Clin N Am 1992; 3:509-27.
66. Noda Y, Watanabe H, Iida M et al. Histologic follow-up of ampullary adenomas in patients with familial adenomatosis coli. Cancer 1992; 70:1847-56.
67. Burke CA, Beck GJ, Church JM et al. The natural history of untreated duodenal and ampullary adenomas in patients with familial adenomatous polyposis followed in an endoscopic surveillance program. Gastrointest Endosc 1999; 49:358-64.
68. Ross JE, Mara JE. Small bowel polyps and carcinoma in multiple intestinal polyposis. Arch Surg 1974; 108:736-8.
69. Myrhoj T, Bulow S, Mogensen AM. Multiple adenomas in terminal ileum 25 years after restorative proctocolectomy for FAP. Dis Colon Rectum 1989; 32:618-20.
70. Iida M, Itoh H, Matsui T. Ileal adenomas in postcolectomy patients with familial adenomatosis coli / Gardner's syndrome. Dis Colon Rectum 1989; 32:1034-8.
71. Wu JS, McGannon EA, Church JM. Incidence of neoplastic polyps in the ileal pouch of patients with familial adenomatous polyposis after restorative proctocolectomy. Dis Colon Rectum 1998; 41:552-7.
72. Thompson-Fawcett MW, Marcus VA, Redston M et al. Adenomatous polyps develop commonly in the ileal pouch of patients with familial adenomatous polyposis. Dis Colon Rectum 2001; 44:347-53.
73. Palkar VM, deSouza LJ, Jagannath P et al. Adenocarcinoma arising in "J" pouch after total proctocolectomy for familial polyposis coli. Indian J Cancer 1997; 34:16-9.
74. Bassuini MM, Billings PJ. Carcinoma in an ileoanal pouch after restorative proctocolectomy for familial adenomatous polyposis. Br J Surg 1996; 83:506.
75. Utsunomiya J, Nakamura T. The occult osteomatous changes in the mandible in patients with familial polyposis coli. Br J Cancer 1975; 62:45-51.
76. Offerhaus GJA, Levin LS, Giardiello FM et al. Occult radiopaque jaw lesions in FAP and hereditary nonpolyposis colorectal cancer. Gastroenterology 1987; 93:490-7.

77. Blair NP, Trempe CL. Hypertrophy of the retinal pigment epithelium associated with Gardner's syndrome. Am J Ophthalmol 1980; 90:661–7.
78. Traboulsi EI, Krush AJ, Gardner EJ et al. Prevalence and importance of pigmented ocular fundus lesions in Gardner's syndrome. N Engl J Med 1987; 316:661–8.
79. Heyen F, Jagelman DG, Romania A et al. Predictive value of CHRPE as a clinical marker for familial adenomatous polyposis. Dis Colon Rectum 1990; 33:1003–8.
80. Baba S, Tsuchiya M, Watanabe I et al. Importance of retinal pigmentation as a subclinical marker in familial adenomatous polyposis. Dis Colon Rectum 1990; 33:660–5.
81. Farmer KCR, Hawley PR, Phillips RKS. Desmoid disease. In: Phillips RKS, Spigelman AD, Thompson JPS, eds. "Familial adenomatous polyposis and other polyposis syndromes". London: Edward Arnold 1994; 128–42.
82. Naylor EW, Gardner EJ, Richards R. Desmoid tumors and mesenteric fibromatosis in Gardner syndrome. Arch Surg 1979; 114:1161–85.
83. Erbe RW. Current concepts in genetics: inherited gastrointestinal polyposis syndromes. N.Engl J Med 1976; 294:1101–4.
84. Rodriguez-Bigas MA, Mahoney MC, Karakousis CP et al. Desmoid tumors in patients with familial adenomatous polyposis. Cancer 1994; 74:1270–4.
85. Arvanitis ML, Jagelman DG, Fazio VW et al. Mortality in patients with familial adenomatous polyposis. Dis Colon Rectum 1990; 33:639–42.
86. Jones IT, Fazio VW, Weakley FL et al. Desmoid tumors in familial polyposis coli. Ann Surg 1986; 204:94–7.
87. Ponz de Leon M, Varesco L, Benatti P et al. Phenotype-genotype correlations in an extended family with FAP and an unusual APC mutation. Dis Colon Rectum (in press).
88. Grant D. Intestinal transplantation: 1997 report of the international registry. Transplantation 1999; 67:1061–4.
89. Chatzipetrou MA, Tzakis AG, Pinna AD et al. Intestinal transplantation for the treatment of desmoid tumors associated with familial adenomatous polyposis. Surgery 2001; 129:277–81.
90. Itoh H, Ikeda S, Oohata Y et al. Treatment of desmoid tumors in Gardner's syndrome. Dis Colon Rectum 1988; 31:459–61.
91. Seiter K, Kemeny N. Successful treatment of a desmoid tumor with doxorubicin. Cancer 1993; 71:2242–4.
92. Lewis JJ, Boland PJ, Leung DHY et al. The enigma of desmoid tumors. Ann Surg 1999; 229:866–73.
93. Thompson JS, Harned RK, Anderson JC et al. Papillary carcinoma of the thyroid and FAP. Dis Colon Rectum 1983; 26:583–5.
94. Plail RO, Bussey HJR, Glazer G et al. Adenomatous polyposis: an association with carcinoma of the thyroid. Br J Surg 1987; 74:377–380.
95. Civitelli S, Tanzini G, Cetta M et al. Papillary thyroid carcinoma in three siblings with familial adenomatous polyposis. Int J Colorect Dis 1996; 11:34–37.
96. Bulow S, Holm NV, Mellemgaard A. Papillary thyroid carcinoma in Danish patients with FAP. Int J Colorectal Dis 1988; 3:29–31.
97. Giardiello FM, Offerhaus GJA, Lee DH et al. Increased risk of thyroid and pancreatic carcinoma in familial adenomatous polyposis. Gut 1993; 34:1394–6.
98. Bell B, Mazzaferri E. Familial Adenomatous Polyposis (Gardner's Syndrome) and thyroid carcinoma. A case report and review of the literature. Dig Dis Sci 1993; 38:185–190.
99. Bulow C, Bulow S, Leeds Castle Polyposis Group. Is screening for thyroid carcinoma indicated in familial adenomatous polyposis? Int J Colorect Dis 1997; 12:240–2.
100. Bernstein IT, Bulow F, Mauritzen K. Hepatoblastoma in two cousins in a family with adenomatous polyps. Dis Colon Rectum 1992; 35:373–4.
101. Komorowski RA, Tresp MG, Wilson SD. Biliary neoplasia in Gardner's syndrome. Dis Colon Rectum 1986; 29:55–8.
102. Jarvinen H, Nyberg M, Peltokallio P. Biliary involvement in familial adenomatosis coli. Dis Colon Rectum 1983; 26:525–8.

103. Painter TA, Jagelman DG. Adrenal adenomas and adrenal carcinomas in association with hereditary adenomatosis of the colon and rectum. Cancer 1985; 55: 2001-4.
104. Johnson Smith TGP, Clark SK, Katz DE et al. Adrenal masses are associated with familial adenomatous polyposis. Dis Colon Rectum 2000; 43:1739-42.
105. Matsuo H, Kato T, Hirai T et al. A case of cancerous familial adenomatous polyposis in urinary bladder due to migration of colonic mucosa through rectovesical fistula. Am J Gastroenterol 2000; 95:1352-4.
106. Leppert M, Dobbs M, Scambler P et al. The gene for familial polyposis coli maps to the long arm of chromosome 5. Science 1987; 238:1411-3.
107. Joslyn G, Carlson M, Thliveris A et al. Identification and deletion mutations and three new genes at the familial polyposis locus. Cell 1991; 66:601-13.
108. Heppner Goss K, Groden J. Biology of the adenomatous polyposis coli tumor suppressor. J Clin Oncol 2000; 18:1967-79.
109. Varesco L, Gismondi V, Jamer R et al. Identification of APC gene mutations in Italian adenomatous polyposis coli patients by PCR-SSCP analysis. Am J Hum Genet 1993; 52:280-5.
110. Kinzler KW, Vogelstein B. Lessons from hereditary colorectal cancer. Cell 1996; 87: 159-70.
111. Rubinfeld B, Albert I, Porfiri E et al. Binding of GSK3β to the APC β-catenin complex and regulation of complex assembly. Science 1996; 272:1023-6.
112. He TC, Sparks AB, Rago C et al. Identification of c-MYC as a target of the APC pathway. Science 1998; 281:1509-12.
113. Testu O, McCormick F. Beta-catenin regulates expression of cyclin D1 in colon carcinoma cells. Nature 1999; 398:422-6.
114. Baeg GH, Matsumine A, Kuroda T et al. The tumor suppressor gene product APC blocks cell cycle progression from G0/G1 to S phase. EMBO J 1995; 14:5618-25.
115. Wong MH, Hermiston ML, Syder AJ et al. Forced expression of the tumor suppressor adenomatosis polyposis coli protein induces disordered cell migration in the intestinal epithelium. Proc Natl Acad Sci USA 1996; 93:9588-93.
116. Korinek V, Barker N, Moerer P et al. Depletion of epithelial stem-cell compartments in the small intestine of mice lacking Tcf-4. Nat Genet 1998; 19:379-83.
117. Morin PJ, Vogelstein B, Kinzler KW. Apoptosis and APC in colorectal tumorigenesis. Proc Natl Acad Sci USA 1996; 93:7950-4.
118. Smith KJ, Johnson KA, Bryan TM et al. The APC gene product in normal and tumor cells. Proc Natl Acad Sci USA 1993; 90:2846-50.
119. Heinimann K, Mullhapt B, Weber W et al. Phenotypic differences in familial adenomatous polyposis based on APC gene mutation status. Gut 1998; 43:675-9.
120. Rozen P, Samuel Z, Shomrat R et al. Notable intrafamilial phenotypic variability in a kindred with familial adenomatous polyposis and an APC mutation in exon 9. Gut 1999; 45:829-33.
121. Friedl W, Caspari R, Sengteller M et al. Can APC mutation analysis contribute to therapeutic decision in familial adenomatous polyposis? Experience from 680 FAP families. Gut 2001; 48:515-21.
122. Spirio L, Olschwang S, Groden J et al. Alleles of the APC gene: an atypical form of familial polyposis. Cell 1993; 75:951-7.
123. Marshall B, Isidro G, Carvalhas R et al. Three novel APC gene mutations in three Portuguese FAP kindreds. Hum Mutat 1996; 8:395-6.
124. Nasioulas S, Jones IT, St.John JB et al. Profuse familial adenomatous polyposis with an APC exon 3 mutation. Familial Cancer 2001; 1:3-7.
125. Presciuttini S, Gismondi V, Scarcello E et al. Different expressivity of two adjacent mutations of the APC gene. Tumori 1999; 85:28-31.
126. Caspari R, Friedl W, Mandl M et al. Familial adenomatous polyposis: mutation at codon 1309 and early onset of colon cancer. Lancet 1994; 343:629-32.

127. Vasen HFA, van der Luijt RB, Slors JFM et al. Molecular genetic tests as a guide to surgical management of familial adenomatous polyposis. Lancet 1996; 348:433-5.
128. Wu JS, Paul P, McGannon EA et al. APC genotype, polyp number, and surgical options in familial adenomatous polyposis. Ann Surg 1998; 227:57-62.
129. Bertario L, Russo A, Radice P et al. Genotype and phenotype factors as determinants for rectal stump cancer in patients with familial adenomatous polyposis. Ann Surg 2000; 231:538-43.
130. Giardiello FM, Petersen GM, Piantadosi S et al. APC gene mutations and extraintestinal phenotype of familial adenomatous polyposis. Gut 1997; 40:521-5.
131. Caspari R, Olschwang S, Friedl W et al. Familial adenomatous polyposis: desmoid tumors and lack of ophtalmic lesions (CHRPE) associated with APC mutations beyond codon 1,444. Hum Mol Genet 1995; 4:337-40.
132. Gebert JF, Dupon C, Kadmon M et al. Combined molecular and clinical approaches for the identification of families with familial adenomatous polyposis coli. Ann Surg 1999; 229:350-61.
133. Gismondi V, Bafico A, Biticchi R et al. 310 basepair APC deletion with duplication of breakpoint (4394ins15del310) in an italian polyposis patient. Hum Mut 1998; 1:S220-2.
134. Ponz de Leon M, Benatti P, Percesepe A et al. Clinical features and genotype-phenotype correlations in 41 italian families with adenomatosis coli. Ital J Gastroenterol Hepatol 1999; 31:850-60.
135. Eccles DM, van der Luijt R, Breukel C et al. Hereditary desmoid disease due to a frameshift mutation at codon 1924 of the APC gene. Am J Hum Genet 1996; 59:1193-1201.
136. Tops CMJ, Wijnen JT, Griffioen G et al. Presymptomatic diagnosis of FAP by bridging DNA markers. Lancet 1989; 2:1361-3.
137. Olschwang S, Weiffenbach B, Laurent-Puig P et al. Genetic characterization of the APC locus involved in FAP. Gastroenterology 1991; 101:154-60.
138. Spirio L, Nelson L, Ward K et al. A CA-repeat polymorphism close to the APC gene offers improved diagnostic testing for familial APC. Am J Hum Genet 1993; 52:286-96.
139. Burt RW, Groden J. The genetic and molecular diagnosis of FAP. Gastroenterology 1993; 104:1211-4.
140. Cottrell S, Bicknell D, Kaklamanis L et al. Molecular analysis of APC mutations in familial adenomatous polyposis and sporadic colon carcinomas. Lancet 1992; 340:626-30.
141. Olschwang S, Laurent-Puig P, Groden J et al. Germline mutations in the first 14 exons of the adenomatous polyposis coli (APC) gene. Am J Hum Genet 1993; 52:273-9.
142. Miyoshi Y, Ando H, Nagase H et al. Germ-line mutations of the APC gene in 53 familial adenomatous polyposis patients. Proc Natl Acad Sci USA 1992; 89:4452-6.
143. Friedl W, Mandl M, Sengteller M. Single-step screening method for the most common mutations in familial adenomatous polyposis. Hum Mol Genet 1993; 2:1481-2.
144. Van der Luijt R, Khan PM, Vasen H et al. Rapid detection of translation-terminating mutations at the adenomatous polyposis coli (APC) gene by direct protein truncation test. Genomics 1994; 20:1-4.
145. Varesco L, Groden J, Spirio LT et al. Rapid screening method to detect nonsense and frameshift mutations: identification of disease-causing APC alleles. Cancer Res 1993; 53:5581-4.
146. Laken SJ, Papadopoulos N, Petersen GM et al. Analysis of masked mutations in familial adenomatous polyposis. Proc Natl Acad Sci USA 1999; 96:2322-6.
147. Wong N, Lasko D, Rabelo R et al. Genetic counseling and interpretation of genetic tests in familial adenomatous polyposis and hereditary nonpolyposis colorectal cancer. Dis Colon Rectum 2001; 44:271-9.
148. Petersen GM. Genetic testing and counseling in familial adenomatous polyposis. Oncology 1996; 10:89-94.
149. Cromwell DM, Moore RD, Brensinger JD et al. Cost analysis of alternative approaches to colorectal screening in familial adenomatous polyposis. Gastroenterology 1998; 114:893-901.

150. Giardiello FM, Brensinger JD, Petersen GM et al. The use and interpretation of commercial APC gene testing for familial adenomatous polyposis. N Engl J Med 1997; 336:823-7.
151. Vasen HFA, Bulow S, the Leeds Castle Polyposis Group. Guidelines for the surveillance and management of familial adenomatous polyposis (FAP): a word wide survey among 41 registries. Colorectal Dis 1999; 1:214-21.
152. Nyam DCNK, Brillant PT, Dozois RR et al. Ileal pouch-anal canal anastomosis for familial adenomatous polyposis. Early and late results. Ann Surg 1997; 226:514-21.
153. Ambroze WJ Jr, Dozois RR, Pemberton JH et al. Familial adenomatous polyposis: results following ileal pouch-anal anastomosis and ileorectostomy. Dis Colon Rectum 1992; 35:12-5.
154. Slors JFM, den Hartog Jager FCA, Trum JW et al. Long-term follow-up after colectomy and ileorectal anastomosis in familial adenomatous polyposis coli. Hepato-Gastroenterol 1989; 36:109-12.
155. Iwama T, Mishima Y. Factors affecting the risk of rectal cancer following rectum-preserving surgery in patients with familial adenomatous polyposis. Dis Colon Rectum 1994; 37:1024-6.
156. DeCosse JJ, Bulow S, Neale K et al. Rectal cancer risk in patients treated for familial adenomatous polyposis. Br J Surg 1992; 79:1372-5.
157. Bulow C, Vasen H, Jarvinen H et al. Ileorectal anastomosis is appropriate for a subset of patients with familial adenomatous polyposis. Gastroenterology 2000; 119:1454-60.
158. Heiskanen I, Jarvinen HJ. Fate of the rectal stump after colectomy and ileorectal anastomosis for familial adenomatous polyposis. Int J Colorect Dis 1997; 12:9-13.
159. Bjork JA, Akerbrant HI, Iselius LE et al. Morbidity and mortality in patients with familial adenomatous polyposis after colectomy and ileorectal anastomosis. Dis Colon Rectum 2000; 43:1719-25.
160. Moser AR, Luongo C, Gould KA et al. APC^{Min}: a mouse model for intestinal and mammary tumorigenesis. Eur J Cancer 1995; 31 A:1061-4.
161. Smits R, van der Houven van Oordt W, Luz A et al. APC1638 N: a mouse model for familial adenomatous polyposis-associated desmoid tumors and cutaneous cysts. Gastroenterology 1998; 114:275-83.
162. Von Herbay A, Stem J, Herfarth C et al. Pouch-anal cancer after restorative proctocolectomy for familial adenomatous polyposis. Am J Surg Pathol 1996; 20:995-9.
163. Bertoni G, Sassatelli R, Nigrisoli E et al. First observation of microadenomas in the ileal mucosa of patients with familial adenomatous polyposis. Gastroenterology 1995; 109: 374-80.
164. Bussey HJR, DeCosse JJ, Deschner EE et al. A randomized trial of ascorbic acid in polyposis coli. Cancer 1982; 50:1434-9.
165. DeCosse JJ, Miller HH, Lesser ML. Effect of wheat fiber and vitamins C and E on rectal polyps in patients with FAP. JNCI 1989; 81:1290-7.
166. Waddell WR, Ganser GF, Cerise EJ et al. Sulindac for polyposis of the colon. Am J Surg 1989; 157:175-9.
167. Labayle D, Fischer D, Vielh P et al. Sulindac causes regression of rectal polyps in FAP. Gastroenterology 1991; 101:635-9.
168. Giardiello FM, Hamilton SR, Krush AJ et al. Treatment of colonic and rectal adenomas with sulindac in FAP. N Engl J Med 1993; 328:1313-6.
169. Emery P. Cyclooxygenase-2: a major therapeutic advance? Am J Med 2001; 110: 42S-5S.
170. Taketo MM. Cyclooxygenase-2 inhibitor in tumorigenesis. J Natl Cancer Inst 1998; 90:1609-20.
171. Niv Y, Fraser GM. Adenocarcinoma in the rectal segment in familial polyposis coli is not prevented by sulindac therapy. Gastroenterology 1994; 107:854-7.
172. Lynch HT, Thorson AG, Smyrk T. Rectal cancer after prolonged sulindac chemoprevention. Cancer 1995; 75:936-8.

12 Other Polyposis of the Large Bowel

Introduction

Besides classical adenomatosis coli, many other polyposis syndromes of the large bowel have been described and characterized. Common features of the syndromes include the development of polyps in the intestine, an autosomal dominant type of genetic transmission, and the presence of various extraintestinal manifestations, which characterize each specific phenotype.

Just as the study of inborn errors of metabolism improved our understanding of many normal metabolic pathways, it is certain that the polyposis syndromes together with familial adenomatous polyposis (FAP) contain clues concerning the pathogenesis of colorectal cancer. Thus, to biologists and geneticists, study of the polyposis syndromes, despite their rare occurrence, is yielding greater knowledge of carcinogenesis, although there is also some evidence implicating a role of environmental factors in the causative chain leading to the various phenotypes.

Recently, the molecular defects responsible for the development of some of these polyposis syndromes have been partially characterized [1]. Several genes have been identified, and various metabolic pathways leading to cancer were defined. These new findings contributed to reinforce the concept that the polyposis syndromes represent a superb model for the study of colorectal tumorigenesis; moreover, the available evidence suggests that there are several molecular pathways that can explain the passage from a highly replicative colorectal mucosa to polyps of various dimensions and eventually to infiltrating carcinoma [2]. This may imply the existence of colorectal carcinomas with a different biological nature and, presumably, a different clinical behavior.

Table 12.1 summarizes the main polyposis syndromes, their clinical spectrum of neoplastic and non-neoplastic lesions, and the associated molecular defects identified so far.

Peutz-Jeghers Syndrome

As reported by McGarrity et al. [3], "The initial observation of Peutz-Jeghers syndrome was reported by J. R. T. Conner to the Aesculapio Society of London in 1895 [4]. He presented two sisters, age 12 years, with unique ink-black pigmentations of the lips and mouth. He noted that the patients were of dark complexion and anemic. The Conner twins were brought to the attention of the eminent

Table 12.1. Main clinical and biologic features of polyposis syndromes (*FAP* familial adenomatous polyposis, *GI* gastrointestinal)

Disease	Genetic transmission	Main clinical features	Responsible genes	Ref.
FAP	Autosomal dominant	Diffuse adenomatous polyposis, desmoids, gastric and duodenal polyps	APC (5q21)	[1, 2]
Peutz-Jeghers syndrome	Autosomal dominant	Melanin spots in skin and mucosae; hamartomatous polyps in the GI tract; risk of gastrointestinal and extra-intestinal malignancies.	STK11 (19p13)	[13 to 34]
Juvenile polyposis	Sporadic, autosomal dominant	Hamartomatous polyps in the colorectum, stomach and small bowel; risk of colorectal cancer	PTEN, SMAd4 (18q21)	[35 to 58]
Cowden's disease	Autosomal dominant	Facial lesions; skin and mucous lesions; hamartomatous polyps of the GI tract; risk of breast cancer	PTEN (10q22–23)	[59 to 77]
Turcot's syndrome	Autosomal dominant, recessive (?)	Adenomas of the large bowel; brain tumors (medulloblastoma, glioma, glioblastoma, astrocytoma)	APC, MLH1, MSH2, PMS2	[78 to 91]
Muir-Torre syndrome	Autosomal dominant	Sebaceous adenomas and carcinoma of the face, scalp and trunk; colorectal, endometrial and other visceral cancers	MLH1, MSH2	[92 to 108]
Cronkhite-Canada syndrome	Sporadic	Hamartomatous polyps of the GI tract; alopecia, skin pigmentation, nail, dystrophy protein-losing enteropathy	–	[109 to 116]
Bannayan-Riley-Ruvalcaba syndrome	Sporadic, autosomal dominant	Hamartomatous polyps of the large bowel, mental retardation, microcephaly, visceral lipomas, pigmented macula of the penis	PTEN 10q22–23	[117 to 121]

Peutz-Jeghers Syndrome 255

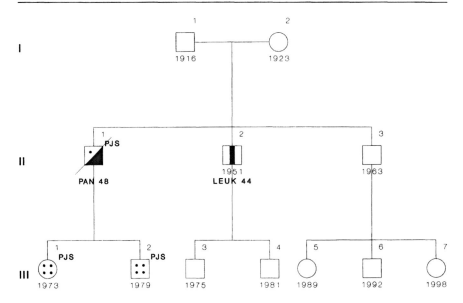

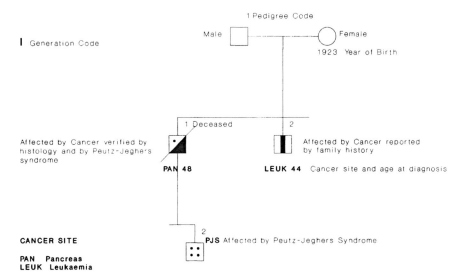

Fig. 12.1. Pedigree of a family with Peutz-Jeghers syndrome. Two siblings developed classical features of the disease from infancy, and one of them (III-1) was operated on several times for bowel intussusception. The father (II-1) died at age 48 years of pancreatic cancer, which is included in the tumor spectrum of the syndrome

physician Sig. Jonathan Hutchinson who commissioned an illustration [5]". After more than 20 years, the Dutch physician Peutz described the association of gastrointestinal polyps with melanin spot of the mouth and lips in 3 young siblings [6]. The father, who had no symptoms, was found to have some pigmented spots in the buccal mucosa. On the basis of these observations, Peutz suggested the existence of an autosomal dominant syndrome characterized by gastrointestinal polyposis and mucocutaneous pigmentations. Since Jeghers described 10 additional cases in 1942 [7], the disease is now known as Peutz-Jeghers syndrome. A representative pedigree of a family with PJS is shown in Fig. 12.1.

Clinical Manifestations and Morphology

PJS is characterized by the presence of hamartomatous polyps of the gastrointestinal tract, melanin spot of the lips and buccal mucosa, and an autosomal dominant mode of genetic transmission [8,9]. The morphological appearance of polyps is rather peculiar. Hamartomas (from the ancient Greek for "errors") show a complex branching pattern of smooth muscle supporting normal lamina propria and glands; thus, these lesions are composed of normal elements indigenous to the site in which they appear, although their general architecture is markedly abnormal [3, 10]. The recognition of epithelium misplacement, the presence of various normal-appearing cells, lack of nuclear atypia and of lymphatic invasion are all findings supporting the hamartomatous (and intrinsically benign) nature of PJS polyposis [11]. Hamartomatous polyps are found more frequently in the small bowel but are also present in the stomach, colon and, more rarely, other mucosal surfaces, such as the upper respiratory and urinary tracts [12]. The polyps can grow to very large size (several centimeters) and, combined with their pedunculated nature, are a frequent cause of recurrent intussusception, one of the main clinical symptoms of PJS patients, which can lead to bleeding and abdominal pain.

The pigmented lesions of PJS are characterized by increased melanocytes at the epidermal-dermal junction, with an excess of melanin in the basal cells [13]. No malignant changes have been associated with these pigmented macules. The spots are typically "peri-orificial", since they cluster primarily around the mouth, eyes, nostrils, and sometimes also in the perianal area [14]. They may develop at birth or in infancy, and have been described in all races and skin types [3]. Melanin spots can fade or even disappear with age, though they tend to persist in the buccal mucosa, and this is an important element for establishing the diagnosis in individuals with suspected PJS [13].

Although hamartomatous polyps are commonly not considered precancerous lesions, various studies in the last two decades documented an increased occurrence of gastrointestinal malignancies in patients with PJS [15, 16]. In contrast, other authors minimized the risk of gastrointestinal cancer and cautioned surgeons to maintain a conservative approach in dealing with PJS patients [17, 18]. In the Johns Hopkins experience [15], cancer occurred in 15 of 31 patients with PJS after an average follow-up of 25 years; however, only four of these tumors were localized in the gastrointestinal tract, whereas most neoplasms occurred in other organs, such as pancreas, breast, lung and ovary. More recent observations stressed the increased risk of cancer in patients with PJS. Boardman et al. [19] reported 10 cases of gastrointestinal cancer and 16 of extraintestinal cancer among 34 patients with PJS over a period of 40 years, for a relative risk of 18.3 in women and 6.2 in men. Similarly, Giardiello et al. [20], in a meta-analysis of 210 patients with PJS described in 6 publications, found a relative risk (RR) for all cancers of 15.2, and RR as high as 57 for esophageal cancer, 213 for gastric cancer, 520 for neoplasms of the small bowel and 84 for colorectal carcinoma. Interestingly, RR for tumors of several other organs were also significantly elevated: 132 for pancreatic cancer, 17 for lung tumors, 15.2 for breast cancer and 27.0 for ovarian malignancies. The authors concluded that patients with PJS are at very high relative and absolute risk for developing gastrointestinal and non-gastrointestinal cancer.

The causes of this increased risk of cancer remain unclear; however, large hamartomas may contain foci of adenomatous changes, and there is evidence favoring the existence of a hamartoma-adenoma-carcinoma sequence in the stomach [21], small bowel [22] and colorectum [23]. Moreover, there is also evidence that patients with PJS are prone to develop adenomatous as well as hamartomatous polyps, especially in the large bowel [24]. As far as the risk of other malignancies is concerned, the excess of extraintestinal tumors in PJS families clearly suggests that the gene responsible for the disease (STK11, see below) might be of importance in the tumorigenesis of other organs. From the clinical point of view, these studies raise concerns about the most appropriate surveillance program in PJS patients; indeed, the results place the risk of breast, gynecological, colorectal, stomach and pancreatic cancer in the range of risk in which screening and follow-up programs have been advocated for other conditions [20].

Molecular Biology of PJS

Genetic linkage analysis in families with PJS demonstrated the presence of a highly penetrant gene located at chromosome 19p13.3 [25, 26]. More recently, the responsible gene – called STK11 – was identified by positional cloning, and truncating germline mutations of STK11 have been reported in PJS patients [27, 28]. The STK11 gene is identical to the previously cloned LKB1 gene, which encodes a serine/threonine kinase with high homology to the *Xenopus* kinase XEEK1 [29]. STK11 extends over 23 kb, is composed of nine exons and is ubiquitously expressed in various human tissues. Somatic mutations in the STK11 gene were detected in several sporadic tumors, including colorectal and gastric carcinomas and malignant melanoma [30, 31]. These findings suggest that STK11 is probably a tumor suppressor gene, and that alterations to it play an important role in tumor development and in the pathogenesis of PJS. Moreover, the identification of constitutional mutations in the STK11 gene in an index patient offers the possibility of a predictive diagnosis and the initiation of specific screening and surveillance programs in genetically affected families.

In a recent investigation, Gruber et al. [30] tried to characterize the various genetic alterations implicated in the development of hamartomas and carcinomas in PJS. Inactivating mutations of the STK11 gene were found in hamartomatous lesions of all investigated families and appeared necessary and sufficient to initiate the phenotypic expression of the disease. This is a further confirmation that STK11 acts as a tumor suppressor gene involved in the very early phases of the development of hamartomas and, subsequently, carcinomas. Since no alterations in the APC gene were detected, STK11 presumably plays a "gate-keeper" role similar to that of APC in FAP, regulating the formation of hamartomatous lesions. Moreover, none of the tumor samples showed mutations of the *k-ras* gene, thus suggesting that alterations of this commonly mutated (in tumors) oncogene do not play a determinant role in PJS. In contrast, loss of heterozygosity was detected in carcinomas (but not in hamartomas) especially at 17p and 18q. These findings – together with positive immunostaining for p53 – suggest that p53 and, presumably, other tumor suppressor genes – such as DCC – might be involved at a later stage of tumorigenesis in PJS.

Management

PJS may run for several years without presenting relevant difficulties for the patients. Most of them, however, develop abdominal symptoms, such as pain, diarrhea and bleeding, usually due to intussusception and obstruction. Moreover, by the age of 40 years, the risk of cancer becomes relevant. The two main objectives in managing these patients are, therefore, the treatment of hamartomas (especially those of the small bowel) and the prevention of carcinomas in various target organs.

Since the main problem is small-bowel polyposis, the clinician may take advantage of new techniques – such as small-bowel enteroscopy and polypectomy – which allow for greater surveillance and removal of these lesions. To survey the distal small bowel, barium studies every 2 years have been suggested: individuals with polyps larger that 1.5 cm should undergo laparotomy with intraoperative endoscopy, since the risk of serious complications is relevant [32]. While small polyps can be treated by electrocautery snare, large lesions may require enterotomy; the enteroscope can be advanced through the enterotomy site to allow examination of the entire small bowel. In many patients the formation of new polyps tends to diminish with age, so the intervals between radiographic examinations may increase [33]. The management of the risk of gastrointestinal malignancies ties in closely with the management of polyps in general.

As far as the risk of tumors of other organs is concerned, the optimal strategy has not yet been defined. Some authors agree on routine breast and pelvic examination and palpation of the testes [34]. Other authors advocated mammography by the age of 25 years, and abdominal ultrasound (especially to survey ovary, uterus and pancreas) by the age of 20–30 years, at 1- to 3-year intervals [3].

These recommendations, however, should be revised periodically, as new and more detailed information from studies on cancer risk and genetics in PJS becomes available.

Juvenile Polyposis

Juvenile polyposis (JP) is a distinct form of intestinal polyposis characterized by the presence of multiple polyps (from a few to hundreds) occurring primarily in the colorectum but occasionally in the small bowel and stomach. The disease may arise sporadically, but 30%–50% of these patients show a strong family history for the same type of polyposis and features of autosomal dominant transmission (familial juvenile polyposis). Patients with JP are at increased risk of cancer, especially of the colorectum [35].

Phenotypic Characteristics, Genetics and Cancer Risk

In JP, polyps are considered a subgroup of hamartomas; their number varies between 10 and 200, and can be found in the large bowel (where they are more common and numerous), stomach and small bowel. Histological examination shows dilated and elongated glands with slightly irregular contours set in an abundant stromal tissue; the glands are lined by normal colonic epithelial cells, and the stroma is frequently inflamed and edematous and contains dilated mucus-filled cysts [36]. Mixed polyps are not rare in JP; in this type of polyp, adenomatous areas can be recognized in the context of a hamartomatous lesion. Since adenomas are prone to malignant transformation, their occurrence may explain the frequency of carcinomas reported in JP [36].

The first description of familial JP is a further contribution of the St. Mark's team to our understanding of polyposis syndromes [37, 38]. In this case, the disease is transmitted from one generation to the next with high penetrance and in accordance with an autosomal dominant mode of inheritance. Non-familial cases might simply be phenocopies or can be due to new mutations of the responsible genes (see below). Rather interestingly, birth defects – such as craniomegaly, intellectual handicap, cryptorchidism, malrotation of the bowel and cardiac lesions – are relatively frequent in apparently sporadic JP, but rare in familial JP [39, 40].

While juvenile polyps do not confer an increased risk of cancer [41], patients with JP (both sporadic and familial) have an increased incidence of colorectal neoplasia, and carcinoma may develop in up to 20% of them at a relatively young age [42, 43]. Thus, Jarvinen et al. [44] reported 9 cases of colorectal cancer among 102 patients with JP, and a positive family history for this tumor (usually occurring at an early age of onset) in the majority of the investigated kindreds. Similarly, Jass et al. [36] could demonstrate that 18 of 87 JP patients observed at St. Mark's developed cancer of the large bowel during the follow-up. The excess risk for cancer seems to be limited to the colorectum, though gastric, duodenal and pancreatic carcinoma have been reported in JP families [41]. It is likely that some hamartomatous lesions evolve into adenomas of various degrees of dysplasia and subsequently undergo malignant changes. Because of this risk, prophylactic subtotal colectomy has been advocated, especially for familial JP cases with numerous polyps [44]; as an alternative, life-long endoscopic surveillance is recommended [45, 46].

Individuals with JP may remain asymptomatic for many years; when the disease becomes manifest, patients usually present with rectal bleeding and iron-deficiency anemia. Less frequently, diarrhea, abdominal pain and evidence of protein-losing enteropathy can be noted [47].

Molecular Biology and Genetic Heterogeneity of JP

The molecular basis of JP is rather complex, and the available evidence suggests the existence of genetic heterogeneity. Among the reasons for this complexity, there is the fact that hamartomatous juvenile polyps may occur as a manifestation of Cowden disease and of Bannayan-Ruvalcaba-Riley syndrome (see below), two inherited conditions associated with constitutional mutations of specific genes. Thus, germline mutations in PTEN, the gene responsible for Cowden disease, have been described in patients with JP [48]. PTEN is a protein tyrosine phosphatase gene which has been located at 10q22-23 and is somatically inactivated in a large spectrum of human tumors, acting as a tumor suppressor gene [49, 50]. It is possible that JP families with constitutional mutations of PTEN represent a phenotypic variant of Cowden disease. However, the recent description of a JP family with a constitutional deletion of five bases in exons 4, and without clinical features of Cowden disease, clearly suggests that there is phenotypic heterogeneity in JP, Cowden disease or Bannayan-Ruvalcaba-Riley syndrome [51].

During the same period, another gene was found to be mutated in many families with JP; SMAD4 (DPC4) – located at chromosome 18q21 – was identified by studying homozygous deletions in pancreatic and colorectal carcinomas [52]. The gene encodes for a protein involved in transforming growth factor β signal transduction, which mediates growth inhibitory signals from the cell surface to the nucleus [53]. Six other members of the SMAD family have been characterized in humans; each of them is a homologue of the others and plays a different role in signal transduction. Howe et al. [54, 55] reported constitutional mutations of SMAD 4 in families with JP. Subsequent studies confirmed these observations and detected truncating or missense mutations in up to 21% of patients and families with JP [56, 57]; in contrast, no germline alterations of SMAD1, SMAD2, SMAD3 and SMAD5 genes could be detected in JP [58].

The available evidence, therefore, indicates that different molecular mechanisms (many of which remain to be elucidated) are associated with hamartomatous juvenile polyps of identical appearance.

Management of JP

After the identification of a patient with JP, a detailed pedigree should be traced, with particular attention paid to neoplastic and colorectal diseases. Then the entire gastrointestinal tract of the index case should be examined for polyps, while colonoscopy is probably sufficient to confirm or exclude the diagnosis among siblings. Since the evolution of hamartomas and transformation into adenomatous polyps and carcinomas is a slow process, the patient's care may initially be conservative and is based on periodic endoscopic examinations and biopsies. Treatment strategies for JP patients need to be individualized according to the number, size and location of polyps, as well as the patient's clinical status. While surgery is the obvious treatment for malignancy, some authors advocate prophylactic colectomy with ileorectal anastomosis for patients at high risk (dysplastic adenomatous polyps) of an evolving carcinoma sequence [35].

Cowden's Disease

Cowden's disease (CD) is a genodermatosis characterized by multiple hamartomas, neoplasms of ectodermal, mesodermal and endodermal origin, and an autosomal dominant type of transmission. CD was first reported by Lloyd and Dennis in 1963, who named the syndrome after their patient Rachel Cowden [59]. In a successive report [60], Weary et al. proposed the name of "multiple hamartoma syndrome".

Clinical Manifestations and Morphology

CD is a rare disease comprising a mixture of lesions affecting the skin, mucous membranes, breast and thyroid gland. Several genetic studies confirmed the autosomal dominant pattern of inheritance with a high penetrance in both sexes and moderate interfamilial and intrafamilial differences in the expressivity of several symptoms [59, 61]. Facial lesions are the most typical and distinctive features of CD and occur in the majority of these patients; these consist of multiple, small and keratotic papules concentrated around the orifices and associated with hair follicles. Hyperkeratotic and verrucous lesions are usually found on the dorsal surface of the hands and feet, together with palmoplantar keratosis. Moreover, oral mucosal lesions are present in up to 80% of these individuals and consist of small verrucous papulae on the gums and lips [47, 60, 62]. Additional extraintestinal manifestations include a broad range of lesions, such as lipomas, haemangiomas, ganglioneuromas, cysts of the breast and ovary, colloid goiter, adenomas of the thyroid gland, craniomegaly, arched palate, adenoid facies and female genital tract neoplasms [47, 59, 63].

The primary gastrointestinal involvement in CD is represented by isolated or clustered polyps of various histological types. These can be seen from the esophagus to the rectum, and their frequency is of the order of 60%–80% of all cases

[47]. Gastrointestinal lesions in CD are characterized by fibrosis of the lamina propria, cystic dilation of glands, extension of the muscularis mucosae into the lamina propria, accumulation of adipose tissue and lymphoid follicles [59, 64]. These hamartomatous polyps seem to possess little potential for malignant degeneration [65]; however, adenomatous and carcinomatous changes have also been reported [62, 66] in association with hamartomas, though the precise risk of colon cancer in these subjects is still unclear. Patients with CD are at high risk for other neoplasms, in particular breast and thyroid carcinomas; the risk of breast cancer is so high that some authors [65] recommended prophylactic mastectomy by the age of 30 years. Polyp-like lesions have also been found, by ultrasound, in the gallbladder of CD patients; their hamartomatous origin has been suspected [67].

Molecular Basis of CD

The gene responsible for Cowden's disease has recently been localized to chromosome 10q22-23 and subsequently identified as PTEN (or MMAC1), encoding a dual-specificity phosphatase which functions as a tumor suppressor [68-70]. Constitutional alterations of PTEN – including missense, nonsense and single splice site mutations – have been detected in several CD families [71]; moreover, loss of heterozygosity and deletions of PTEN were found in fibroadenomas of the breast, thyroid adenomas and various hamartomatous tissues [72]. It is likely, therefore, that tumorigenesis in CD follows the two-hit model suggested by Knudson [73] and well documented in several familial cancer syndromes, such as retinoblastoma, Wilms' tumor and adenomatosis coli [74]. According to this model, the first mutation in a tumor suppressor gene occurs in the germline cells; subsequently, a second somatic mutation arises in the other allele of the same gene and causes its complete loss of function. Inactivation of a tumor suppressor gene leads to uncontrolled cell replication, clonal expansion and eventually cancer. The development of carcinoma in CD presumably requires additional genetic and epigenetic events, which remain to be elucidated [65]. Finally, recent studies support the hypothesis that abnormal DNA methylation may play a role in the transcriptional suppression of PTEN [75, 76].

Management of CD

Owing to the infrequent development of malignancy of the gastrointestinal tract in CD, close endoscopic surveillance is usually not recommended, and clinical investigations are mainly based on the occurrence of symptoms, such as bleeding, abdominal pain or discomfort [65]. The excess risk of breast cancer requires mammography by the age of 30 years every 1-2 years, with biopsy of suspected lesions. As an option, prophylactic mastectomy can be proposed to patients unwilling to undergo regular surveillance [77]. The frequency of thyroid alterations suggests screening by thyroid function tests, thyroid scanning and fine needle aspiration biopsy of any suspected anatomic abnormality.

Turcot Syndrome

Turcot syndrome (TS) was described by Turcot and colleagues in 1959, when they reported two siblings with numerous polyps in the large bowel, one of whom developed a medulloblastoma of the spinal cord and the other a glioblastoma of the frontal lobe [78]. No other member of this family showed intestinal or brain tumors. After other reports of similar cases or families, the eponym "Turcot syndrome" was used to denote the association of colorectal polyposis with tumors of the central nervous system. To date, more than 120 cases of TS have been reported, in which tumors such as glioma, medulloblastoma and astrocytoma have been associated with a broad spectrum of colorectal lesions, from adenoma to diffuse polyposis [79]. Many clinical and biological aspects of TS remain undefined, and the available evidence suggests the presence of genetic heterogeneity, with different molecular mechanisms associated with a similar phenotypic expression of the disease.

Clinical and Morphologic Aspects of TS

The number of colorectal lesions in TS is variable; however, in a few cases polyps have been found to be as numerous as in FAP, while in most families colorectal adenomas tend to be larger than in FAP, but they often number less than 100 [80]. At histological examination, tubular or villous adenomas are found, with varying degrees of dysplasia and with a strong propensity for malignant transformation. This, however, does not occur in most of the patients, since they frequently die of brain tumors before the age of 30 years. Indeed, affected individuals may not live long enough to have children and, thus, to reveal the genetic nature of the disease [81]. Several types of brain tumors have been reported in TS, including glioma, medulloblastoma, astrocytoma, neuroblastoma and glioblastoma; they become manifest with typical neurological symptoms and signs, usually by the second or third decade of life. Once these tumors develop, the clinical course is usually rapid, and the prognosis extremely severe; however, unusually long survival has been reported in a few patients whose tumors showed microsatellite instability (see below) [82].

Complex Genetic and Molecular Basis of TS

The type of genetic transmission of TS remains controversial; this should not be surprising since the early occurrence of highly malignant brain tumors prevents the study of large families in many cases, and the transmission of a given phenotype through several generations. Moreover, controversies also reign with regard to whether TS has to be considered a genetic disorder distinct from familial polyposis, or whether it represents a random association between FAP and gliomas. The situation became even more complex after evidence was found of an involvement of DNA mismatch repair genes in the pathogenesis of a subset of TS [82].

Lewis and co-workers [83] suggested that TS patients could be classified into three groups. Type I families transmit the disease according to an autosomal recessive transmission; the parents of affected individuals do not show colonic lesions or brain tumors. Type II families appear to have an autosomal dominant polyposis syndrome in which one or more members also have tumors of the central nervous system; the parents of these patients have colonic polyposis. Type III are cases of TS with no familial history of polyposis or brain tumors, and should be considered sporadic. Itoh et al. [84] analyzed 72 families with features of TS and concluded that the syndrome followed an autosomal recessive inheritance. Other authors [85, 86] were led to different conclusions and suggested that TS and FAP may have a common autosomal dominant type of transmission, with a pleiotropic effect and variable expressivity. More recent family studies supported the autosomal dominant basis of TS [87].

Hamilton and colleagues [82] tried to elucidate the molecular basis of TS by evaluating 14 families identified in two cancer registries together with the kindred originally described by Turcot. Genetic alterations were detected in 13 of the 14 registry families. Constitutional mutations of the APC gene could be found in 10 of these families, in whom the most frequent brain tumor was medulloblastoma. In three of the other families and in the original family described by Turcot, microsatellite instability could be detected, and constitutional mutations in the DNA mismatch repair gene MLH1 and PMS2 were found in two families. The authors concluded that TS may result from two distinct germline abnormalities: mutation of the APC gene, as is usually found in FAP, and mutation of a DNA mismatch repair gene, that is usually found in hereditary non-polyposis colorectal cancer (Lynch syndrome) [88]. Since both FAP and HNPCC are characterized by autosomal dominant transmission, these results favor the dominant hypothesis for TS. In addition, tumor development in FAP and HNPCC has been related to the two-hit inactivation of a tumor suppressor gene; it is therefore likely that the Knudson hypothesis may also explain tumor occurrence in TS [73].

In a recent investigation, De Rosa et al. [89] reported a TS family in which two sisters – with no history of tumor occurrence in their parents and other family members – were affected by primary brain tumor (an oligodendroglioma and a neuroblastoma). In one of the two patients, carcinoma of the splenic flexure developed at age 18 years, together with multiple polyps. Two constitutional mutations within the PMS2 gene were detected: a G deletion in exon 11 and a four base-pair deletion in exon 14, which were both inherited from the patient's unaffected parents and induced a generalized microsatellite instability. Both mutations gave rise to stop codons and truncated proteins. Since carriers of one mutation were healthy (the father, the mother and the two younger brothers of the affected sisters), and the disease became manifest only when both mutations were inherited, the transmission of TS in this family seems to be autosomal recessive.

Management of TS

The rarity of TS and its variable phenotypic expression do not allow firm recommendations for management and surveillance. Given the clinical suspicion of TS, constitutional mutations of APC and of the main DNA mismatch repair genes (MLH1, MSH2 and PMS2) should be searched for. In the presence of APC mutations or with clinical features of adenomatosis coli, sigmoidoscopic surveillance is required, with biopsy of the largest lesions and prophylactic colectomy to prevent cancer occurrence, as for classical FAP [90]. Patients with features of HNPCC or germline mutations of DNA mismatch repair genes and microsatellite instability should undergo complete colonoscopy, owing to the risk of proximal colonic neoplasms; in addition, surveillance of some extracolonic sites (i.e. endometrium and stomach) may be advisable [91].

The early diagnosis and prevention of brain tumors remain elusive. However, symptoms and signs of central nervous system impairment should not be ignored and require careful clinical investigation in all families with clinical characteristics of FAP or HNPCC. The value of periodic neurological evaluation of high-risk asymptomatic individuals (or gene carriers) has still to be demonstrated.

Muir-Torre Syndrome and Other Rare Polyposis

The Muir-Torre syndrome (MTS) is a rare autosomal dominant disease characterized by the association of multiple keratoacanthomas and sebaceous tumors of the skin with visceral malignancies. Because of the preponderance of early onset colorectal cancer in these families, the disease is now considered a different phenotypic variant (or a subtype) of the more common HNPCC.

Clinical and Morphologic Features of MTS

In 1967, Torre [92] reported the clinical case of a 57-year-old individual in whom, over a period of several years, more than 100 cutaneous papular lesions had appeared on the scalp, face and trunk. These lesions were classified as sebaceous adenomas and carcinomas, or as sebaceous basal cell epitheliomas. The patient had previously been operated on for carcinoma of the Vater ampulla (age 50) and for a primary colorectal cancer (age 35). Also in 1967, Muir et al. [93] reported the case of a patient with numerous cutaneous lesions on the face in association with multiple primary carcinomas of the colorectum, duodenum and larynx. Since then, this new clinical entity has been denominated Muir-Torre syndrome.

Since the original descriptions, more than 150 patients with MTS have been reported in the world literature [94, 95]. The age at diagnosis ranges from 30 to 90 years, with a median of about 50, and a male:female ratio of 2:1. Among visceral malignancies, primary colorectal carcinoma represented 55% of the total, and cancer of the urogenital system (endometrium, ovary, bladder, kidney and ureter) approximately 25%. It should be noted that cancer sites and proportions correspond closely to those reported for HNPCC [96]. Nearly half of the MTS patients thus far reported had two or more visceral malignancies, and 10% had more than four.

The location of colorectal cancer in patients with MTS tends to differ from that seen in the general population. In fact, the majority of these tumors are located in the proximal colon (from the caecum to the splenic flexure), as opposed to the prevalent distal location (70% or more) of common sporadic neoplasms [94, 97]. Moreover, the average age of onset of colorectal tumors in MTS patients (50 years) anticipates by 15-20 years the median age of occurrence in the general population. Again, the location of tumors and early age of onset in MTS correspond closely to those reported in HNPCC [96]. Finally, adenomatous polyps were found in approximately one-third of MTS patients.

Skin lesions in MTS tend to appear before or concurrently with visceral malignancies in about 30% of the patients [98], while in 50% sebaceous tumors develop after an internal neoplasm. The defining skin lesions of MTS are sebaceous adenomas, carcinomas or epitheliomas; in addition, sebaceous hyperplasia, keratoacanthoma, basal cell carcinoma and squamous cell cancer may frequently occur in MTS. Since sebaceous lesions are relatively rare in the general population, any patient found to have one of these skin lesions should be evaluated for internal malignancies associated with MTS [98]. It has been suggested [99] that tumors of sebaceous glands in MTS represent the cutaneous expression of an individual and familial predisposition to develop carcinomas of the gastrointestinal tract and of other visceral organs.

Sporadic cases of MTS may occur, and it is likely that they represent first mutations in a given kindred [100]; the disease, however, usually shows an autosomal dominant type of transmission, with variable penetrance [101]. Lynch et al. described several patients with features of MTS among their families with HNPCC [102]. On a clinical basis – and some 10 years before the discovery of the human DNA mismatch repair genes – they interpreted MTS as an extended manifestation of the gene responsible for HNPCC, resulting in a more complete phenotypic expression.

Molecular Biology of MTS

Initial molecular studies in patients with MTS revealed microsatellite instability in both sebaceous gland tumors and colorectal carcinomas [103]. Subsequent investigations led to the detection of constitutional mutations in the main DNA mismatch repair genes – MLH1 and MSH2 – in MTS patients, thus lending further support to the view that the disease might be a clinical variant of HNPCC [104, 105]. However, as opposed to the common forms of HNPCC, for which no clinical clear-cut features exist, rendering the diagnosis of individual cases rather difficult, MTS presents characteristic clinical traits. In fact, the association of specific skin lesions with colorectal and other internal neoplasms may allow the physician to reach a correct diagnosis even in the absence of a clear family history. This has important implications for the offspring of the affected individual and for other relatives at risk.

In a recent study, Entius et al. [106] evaluated microsatellite instability and the expression of MLH1 and MSH2 genes in 13 patients with MTS and in individuals with sporadic sebaceous gland carcinoma. Microsatellite instability could be detected in 69% of MTS-related neoplasms, but in none of the sporadic cases. Eight of the 9 patients with instability showed loss of expression of either MLH1 or MSH2 gene. The authors concluded that loss of immunohistochemical expression of mismatch repair genes and microsatellite instability can be used as markers of an underlying MTS in individuals with sebaceous gland tumors. Moreover, the observed findings suggest the existence of at least two variants of MTS; the majority of cases seem to be related to DNA mismatch repair, whereas in approximately 30% other molecular mechanisms could be involved.

Management of MTS

The treatment and surveillance of MTS patients closely correspond to those of individuals with the more common HNPCC [107]. At least 50% of patients ultimately diagnosed with MTS present with an internal malignancy (especially colorectal cancer) before the appearance of skin lesions. This observation strongly suggests initiating screening of subjects at risk of MTS at an early age, usually around 25–30 years.

The initial approach includes a detailed clinical history of the proband and the definition of an extended pedigree. Analysis of microsatellite instability in skin or visceral tumors followed by a search for mutations in the DNA mismatch repair genes may allow the identification of gene carriers, whose risk of developing cancer is of the order of 80%–100% [107]. In gene carriers and in high-risk individuals in affected branches of the family, the entire large bowel should be examined by lower endoscopy, starting at age 25–30 years and repeating the test every 2–3 years [94, 100]. Considering that visceral malignancies other than colorectal cancer represent nearly 35% of those found, computed tomography scanning of the abdomen and pelvis has been recommended [108]. The test should parallel colonoscopic surveillance every 2–3 years. Skin lesions are relatively easy to detect; after biopsy and diagnosis of sebaceous gland tumors, these should be removed by an expert dermatologist. Thus, the diagnosis and management of MTS requires a multidisciplinary approach, including primary care physician, geneticist, biologist, dermatologist, gastroenterologist and surgeon.

Cronkhite-Canada Syndrome

Cronkhite-Canada Syndrome (CCS) was described in 1955 by L.W. Cronkhite and W.J. Canada [109]. The disease is characterized by gastrointestinal polyposis associated with alopecia, skin hyperpigmentation, nail dystrophy and protein-losing enteropathy. The disease has a poor prognosis owing to malnutrition resulting from altered absorption in the gastrointestinal tract [110]. A few patients, however, may respond to enteral nutrition and corticosteroids [111, 112]. Polyps of the gastrointestinal tract tend to appear in adults; histologically, these lesions reveal hyperplastic and hamartomatous changes and are similar to those observed in JP [113, 114]. No genetic basis has been documented for CCS, whose pathogenesis is unknown. Adenomatous and carcinomatous degeneration of colorectal polyps can occur [115, 116], and this suggests initiating endoscopic surveillance of affected individuals. Surgical treatment of CCS is reserved for patients with colorectal malignancies; it is not an effective treatment of protein-losing enteropathy [110].

Bannayan-Riley-Ruvalcaba Syndrome

Bannayan-Riley-Ruvalcaba syndrome (BRRS) (also called Ruvalcaba-Myhre-Smith syndrome, Riley-Smith syndrome and Bannayan-Zonana syndrome) is a rare congenital disorder characterized by hamartomatous polyps of the large bowel associated with mental retardation, macrocephaly, subcutaneous and visceral lipomas, haemangiomas, lipid storage myopathy and pigmented macules of the penis [117, 118]. Cases of BRRS reported in the literature number about 50 [119, 120] and include sporadic cases as well as families in which the disease seems to be transmitted through an autosomal dominant type of inheritance.

The close histological similarity of polyps in BRRS and JP and the frequency of congenital abnormalities in patients with JP suggest that the disease could be a variant of JP. In accordance with this view, linkage studies localized the gene responsible for BRRS to chromosome 10q22–23 [121], where the PTEN gene was mapped and characterized in families with JP and Cowden disease [48, 51]. Thus, it is likely that the three hamartomatous polyposis syndromes – JP, CS and BRRS – may share the same genetic defect (i.e. constitutional mutations of the PTEN gene).

Conclusions

The polyposis syndromes of the large bowel form an interesting group of diseases whose main features include the occurrence of polyps usually not limited to the large bowel and the presence of a variety of clinical signs and symptoms in other organs and systems. Despite their rarity, the molecular basis of many of these syndrome has been partially clarified with the identification of the responsible genes. These new findings contributed – in most cases – to supporting the importance of the Knudson's two-hit hypothesis in the pathogenesis of inherited tumors and shed further light on the intimate mechanisms implicated in colorectal tumorigenesis.

References

1. Ponz de Leon M, Percesepe A. Pathogenesis of colorectal cancer. Digest Liver Dis 2000; 32:807-21.
2. Chung DC. The genetic basis of colorectal cancer: insights into critical pathways of tumorigenesis. Gastroenterology 2000; 119:854-65.
3. McGarrity TJ, Kulin HE, Zaino RJ. Peutz-Jeghers syndrome. Am J Gastroenterol 2000; 95:596-604.
4. Connor JT. Aesculapian Society of London. Lancet 1895; 2:1169.
5. Hutchinson J. Pigmentation of lips and mouth. Vol. VII, Archives of Surgery. London: West, Newman, 1896.
6. Peutz JLA. Over een merkwaardige, gecombineerde familiaire polyposis van de slijmliezen van den tractus intestinalis met die van di neuskeelholte en gepaard met eigenaardige pigmentaties van huid-en slijmvliezen. Ned Maandschr v Gen 1921; 10:134-46.
7. Jeghers H, McKusick VA, Katz KH. Generalized intestinal polyposis and melanin spots of the oral mucosa, lips and digits; a syndrome of diagnostic significance. N Engl J Med 1949; 241:1031-6.
8. Linder NM, Greene MH. The concise handbook of family cancer syndrome. J Natl Cancer Inst 1998; 90:1039-71.
9. Dormandy TL. Gastrointestinal polyposis with mucocutaneous pigmentation (Peutz-Jeghers syndrome). N Engl J Med 1957; 256:1186-90.
10. Spigelman AD, Arese P, Phillips RKS. Polyposis: the Peutz-Jeghers syndrome. Br J Surg 1995; 82:1311-4.
11. Estrada R, Spjut HJ. Hamartomatous polyps in Peutz-Jeghers syndrome. Am J Surg Pathol 1983; 7:747-54.
12. Sommerhaug RG, Mason T. Peutz-Jeghers syndrome and ureteral polyposis. Jama 1970; 211:120-122.
13. Farmer RG, Hawk WA, Turnbull RB. The spectrum in the Peutz-Jeghers syndrome. Report of three cases. Am J Dig Dis 1963; 8:953-61.
14. Touraine A, Couder F. Lentiginose peri-orificielle et polypose viscerale. Presse Med 1946; 54:405.
15. Giardiello F, Welsh SB, Hamilton SR et al. Increased risk of cancer in the Peutz-Jeghers syndrome. N Engl J Med 1987; 316:1511-4.
16. Sligelman AD, Murday V, Phillips RKS. Cancer and the Peutz-Jeghers syndrome. Gut 1989; 30:1588-90.
17. Burdick D, JT, Scanlon GT. Peutz-Jeghers syndrome. A clinical-pathological study of a large family with a 10-year follow-up. Cancer 1963; 16:854-67.
18. Morson B. Precancerous lesions of upper gastrointestinal tract. Precancerous lesions of the colon and rectum. JAMA 1962; 179:311-5, 316-21.
19. Boardman LA, Thibodeau SN, Schaid DJ et al. Increased risk for cancer in patients with Peutz-Jeghers syndrome. Ann Intern Med 1998; 128:896-899.
20. Giardiello FM, Brensinger JD, Tersmette AC et al. Very high risk of cancer in familial Peutz-Jeghers syndrome. Gastroenterology 2000; 119:1447-53.
21. Foley TR, McGarrity TJ, Abt A. Peutz-Jeghers syndrome: a 38 year follow up of the "Harrisburg Family". Gastroenterology 1988; 95:1535-40.
22. Perzin KH, Bridge MF. Adenomatous and carcinomatous changes in hamartomatous polyps of the small intestine (Peutz-Jeghers syndrome). Report of a case and review of the literature. Cancer 1982; 49:971-83.
23. Narita T, Eto T, Ito T. Peutz-Jeghers syndrome with adenomas and adenocarcinomas in colonic polyps. Am J Surg Pathol 1987; 11:76-81.
24. Bartholomew LG, Dahlin DC, Waugh JM. Intestinal polyposis associated with mucocutaneous melanin pigmentation (Peutz-Jeghers syndrome). Review of the literature and report of six cases with special reference to pathologic findings. Gastroenterology 1957; 32:434-51.

25. Hemminki A, Tomlinson I, Markie D et al. Localization of a susceptibility locus for Peutz-Jeghers syndrome to 19p using comparative genomic hybridization and targeted linkage analysis. Nature Genet 1997; 15:87-90.
26. Amos CI, Bali D, Thiel TJ et al. Fine mapping of a genetic locus for Peutz-Jeghers syndrome on chromosome 19p. Cancer Res 1997; 57:3653-6.
27. Hemminki A, Markie D, Tomlinson I et al. A serine/threonine kinase gene defective in Peutz-Jeghers syndrome. Nature 1998; 391:184-7.
28. Jenne DE, Reimann H, Nezu J et al. Peutz-Jeghers syndrome is caused by mutation in a novel serine threonine kinase. Nature Genet 1998; 18:38-43.
29. Su JY, Erikson E, Maller JL. Cloning and characterization of a novel serine/threonine protein kinase expressed in early Xenopus embryos. J Biol Chem 1996; 271: 14430-7.
30. Gruber SB, Entius MM, Petersen GM et al. Pathogenesis of adenocarcinoma in Peutz-Jeghers syndrome. Cancer Res 1998; 58:5267-70.
31. Guldberg P, thor Straten P, Ahrenkiel V et al. Somatic mutation of the Peutz-Jeghers syndrome gene, LKB1/STK11, in malignant melanoma. Oncogene 1999; 18: 1777-80.
32. Panos RG, Opelka FG, Nogueras JJ. Peutz-Jeghers syndrome. A call for intraoperative endoscopy. Am Surg 1990; 56:331-3.
33. Paterlini A, Huscher C, Saline A. Jejunal endoscopic polypectomy in Peutz-Jeghers syndrome. Endoscopy 1983; 15:82-4.
34. Rebsdorf Pedefrsen I, Hartvigsen A, Fischer Hansen B et al. Management of Peutz-Jeghers syndrome. Experience with patients from the Danish Polyposis Register. Int J Colorect Dis 1994; 9:177-9.
35. Longo WE, Touloukian RJ, West AB et al. Malignant potential of juvenile polyposis coli. Report of a case and review of the literature. Dis Colon Rectum 1990; 33:980-4.
36. Jass JR, Williams CB, Bussey HJR. Juvenile polyposis – a precancerous condition. Histopathol 1988; 13:619-30.
37. McColl I, Bussey HJR, Veale AMO et al. Juvenile polyposis coli. Proc R Soc Med 1964; 57:896-7.
38. Bussey HJR, Veale AMO, Morson BC. Genetics of gastrointestinal polyposis. Gastroenterology 1978; 74:1325-30.
39. Walpole IR, Cullity G. Juvenile polyposis: a case with early presentation and death attributable to adenocarcinoma of the pancreas. Am J Med Genet 1989; 32:1-8.
40. Cox KL, Frates RC, Wong A et al. Hereditary generalized juvenile polyposis associated with pulmonary arteriovenous malformation. Gastroenterology 1980; 70: 1566-70.
41. Giardiello FM, Offerhaus JGA. Phenotype and cancer risk of various polyposis syndromes. Eur J Cancer 1995; 31:1085-7.
42. Giardiello FM, Hamilton SR, Kern SE et al. Colorectal neoplasia in patients with juvenile polyposis or juvenile polyps. Arch Childhood Dis 1991; 66:971-5.
43. Grotsky HW, Rickert RR, Smith WD et al. Familial juvenile polyposis coli: a clinical and pathological study of a large kindred. Gastroenterology 1982; 82:494-501.
44. Jarvinen H, Franssila KO. Familial juvenile polyposis coli: increased risk of colorectal cancer. Gut 1984; 25:792-800.
45. Saul SH, Raffensperger E. Juvenile polyposis: intramucosal signet-cell adenocarcinoma arising in a polyp at a gastrojejunostomy site. Surg Pathol 1988; 1:159-64.
46. Subramony C, Scott-Conner CEH, Skelton D et al. Familial juvenile polyposis. Study of a kindred: evolution of polyps and relationship to gastrointestinal carcinoma. Am J Clin Pathol 1994; 102:91-7.
47. Haggitt RC, Reed BJ. Hereditary gastrointestinal polyposis syndromes. Am J Surg Pathol 1986; 12:871-87.
48. Olschwang S, Serova-Sinilnikova OM, Lenoir GM et al. PTEN germ-line mutations in juvenile polyposis coli. Nature Genet 1998; 18:12-4.

49. Tashiro H, Blazes MS, Wu r et al. Mutations in PTEN are frequent in endometrial carcinoma but rare in other common gynecological malignancies. Cancer Res 1997; 57: 3935–40.
50. Rasheed BK, Stenzel TT, McLendon RE et al. PTEN gene mutations are seen in high-grade but not in low-grade gliomas. Cancer Res 1997; 57:4187–90.
51. Huang SC, Chen CR, Lavine JE et al. Genetic heterogeneity in familial juvenile polyposis. Cancer Res 2000; 60:6882–5.
52. Thiagalingam S, Lengauer C, Leach F et al. Evaluation of candidate tumor suppressor genes on chromosome 18 in colorectal cancers. Nature Genet 1996; 13:343–6.
53. Eppert K, Scherer SW, Ozcelik H et al. Madr2 maps to 18q21 end encodes a TGF-beta-regulated Mad-related protein that is functionally mutated in colorectal carcinoma. Cell 1996; 86:543–52.
54. Howe JR, Roth S, Ringold JC et al. Mutations in the SMAD4/DPC4 gene in juvenile polyposis. Science 1998; 280:1086–8.
55. Howe JR, Ringold JC, Hughes JH et al. Direct genetic testing for Smad4 mutations in patients at risk for juvenile polyposis. Surgery 1999; 126:162–70.
56. Roth S, Sistonen P, Salovaara R et al. SMAD genes in juvenile polyposis. Genes Chrom Cancer 1999; 26:54–61.
57. Woodford-Richens K, Bevan S, Churchman M et al. Analysis of genetic and phenotypic heterogeneity in juvenile polyposis. Gut 2000; 46:656–60.
58. Bevan S, Woodford-Richens K, Rozen P et al. Screening SMAD1, SMAD2, SMAD3, and SMAD5 for germline mutations in juvenile polyposis syndrome. Gut 1999; 45: 406–8.
59. Starink TM, van der Veen JPW, Arwert F et al. The Cowden syndrome: a clinical and genetic study in 21 patients. Clinical Genet 1986; 29:222–33.
60. Weary PE, Gorlin RJ, Gentry WC et al. Multiple hamartoma syndrome (Cowden's disease). Arch Dermatol 1972; 106:682–90.
61. Salem OS, Steck WD. Codwen's disease (multiple hamartoma and neoplasia syndrome). J Am Acad Dermatol 1983; 8:686–96.
62. Marra G, Armelao F, Vecchio FM et al. Cowden's disease with extensive gastrointestinal polyposis. J Clin Gastroenterol 1993; 16:1–6.
63. Brownstein MH, Mehregan AM, Bikowski JB et al. The dermatopatnology of Cowden's syndrome. Br J Dermatol 1979; 100:667–73.
64. Gorenšek M, Matko I, Škralovnik A et al. Disseminated hereditary gastrointestinal polyposis with orocutanenous hamartomatosis (Cowden's disease). Endoscopy 1984; 16:59–63.
65. Williard W, Borgen P, Bol R et al. Cowden's disease. A case report with analyses at the molecular level. Cancer 1992; 69:2969–74.
66. Hover AR, Cawthern T, McDanial W. Cowden's disease: a hereditary polyposis syndrome diagnosable by mucocutaneous inspection. J Clin Gastroenterol 1986; 8: 576–9.
67. Christensen AH, Ishak KG. Benign tumors and pseudotumors of the gallbladder. Report of 180 cases. Arch Patol 1970; 90:423–32.
68. Frayling IM, Bodmer WF, Tomlinson IPM. Allele loss in colorectal cancer at the Cowden Disease/Juvenile polyposis locus on 10q. Cancer Genet Cytogenet 1997; 97:64–9.
69. Li J, Yen C, Liaw D et al. PTEN, a putative protein tyrosine phosphatase gene mutated in human brain, breast, and prostate cancer. Science 1997; 275:1943–7.
70. Steck PA, Pershouse MA, Jasser SA et al. Identification of a candidate tumour suppressor gene. MMAC1, at chromosome 10q23.2 that is mutated in multiple advanced cancers. Nature Genet 1997; 15:356–62.
71. Eng C, Peacocke M. PTEN and inherited hamartoma-cancer syndromes. Nature Genet 1998; 19:223.
72. Marsh DJ, Dahia PLM, Coulon V et al. Allelic imbalance, including deletion of PTEN/MMACI, at the Cowden Disease locus on 10q22–23, in hamartomas from

patients with Cowden Syndrome and germline PTEN mutation. Genes Chrom Cancer 1998; 21:61–9.
73. Knudson AG. Mutation and cancer: statistical study of retinoblastoma. Proc Natl Acad Sci USA 1971; 68:820–3.
74. Knudson AG. Hereditary cancer, oncogenes and antioncogenes. Cancer Res 1985; 45: 1437–43.
75. Whang YE, Wu X, Suzuki H et al. Inactivation of the tumor suppressor PTEN/MMAC1 in advanced human prostate cancer through loss of expression. Proc Natl Acad Sci USA 1998; 95:5246–50.
76. Chi SG, Kim HJ, Park BJ et al. Mutational abrogation of the PTEN/MMAC1 gene in gastrointestinal polyps in patients with Cowden disease. Gastroenterology 1998; 115: 1084–9.
77. Walton BJ, Morain WB, Baughman RD et al. A further indication for prophylactic mastectomy. Surgery 1986; 99:82–6.
78. Turcot J, Depres JP, St Pierre F. Malignant tumors of the central nervous system associated with familial polyposis of the colon: report of two cases. Dis Colon Rectum 1959; 2:465–8.
79. Jarvis L, Bathurst N, Mohan D et al. Turcot's syndrome: a review. Dis Colon Rectum 1988; 31:907–14.
80. Newton HB, Rosenblum MK, Malkin MG. Turcot's syndrome. Flow cytometric analysis. Cancer 1991; 68:1633–9.
81. Kropilak M, Jagelman MD, Fazio VW et al. Brain tumors in familial adenomatous polyposis. Dis Colon Rectum 1989; 32:778–82.
82. Hamilton SR, Liu B, Parsons RE et al. The molecular basis of Turcot's syndrome. N Engl J Med 1995; 332:839–47.
83. Lewis JH, Ginsberg AL, Toomey KE. Turcot's syndrome: evidence for autosomal dominant inheritance. Cancer 1983; 51:524–8.
84. Itoh H, Ohsato M, Yao T et al. Turcot's syndrome and its mode of inheritance. Gut 1979; 20:414–9.
85. Smith WG, Kern BB. The nature of the mutation in familial multiple polyposis: papillary carcinoma of the thyroid, brain tumors, and familial multiple polyposis. Dis Colon Rectum 1973; 16:264–71.
86. Costa OL, Silva DM, Colnago FA et al. Turcot syndrome: autosomal dominant or recessive transmission? Dis Colon Rectum 1987; 30:391–4.
87. Matsui T, Hayashi N, Yao K et al. A father and son with Turcot's syndrome: evidence for autosomal dominant inheritance. Report of two cases. Dis Colon Rectum 1998; 41: 797–801.
88. Chung DC, Rustgi AK. DNA mismatch repair and cancer. Gastroenterology 1995; 109: 1685–99.
89. De Rosa M, Fasano C, Panariello L et al. Evidence for a regressive inheritance of Turcot's syndrome caused by compound heterozygous mutations within the PMS2 gene. Oncogene 2000; 19:1719–23.
90. Rustgi AK Hereditary gastrointestinal polyposis and nonpolyposis syndromes. N Engl J Med 1994; 331:1694–702.
91. Lynch HT, Smyrk TC, Watson P et al. Genetics, natural history, tumor spectrum, and pathology of hereditary nonpolyposis colorectal cancer: an updated view. Gastroenterology 1993; 104:1535–49.
92. Torre D. Multiple sebaceous tumors. Arch Dermatol 1968; 98:549–51.
93. Muir EG, Belly AJY, Barlow KA. Multiple primary carcinomata of the colon, duodenum and larynx associated with kerato-acanthomata of the face. Br J Surg 1967; 54: 191–5.
94. Cohen PR, Kohn SR, Davis DA et al. Muir-Torre syndrome. Dermatol Clin 1995; 13: 79–89.
95. El Nakadi B, Nouwynck C, Salhadin A. Combined therapeutic approach for extraorbital sebaceous carcinoma in a Torre's syndrome. Eur J Surg Oncol 1995; 321:321–2.

96. Lynch HT, Watson P, Kriegler M et al. Differential diagnosis of hereditary nonpolyposis colorectal cancer (Lynch syndrome I and Lynch syndrome II). Dis Colon Rectum 1988; 31:372-7.
97. Ponz de Leon M, Sassatelli R, Scalmati A et al. Descriptive epidemiology of colorectal cancer in Italy: the 6-year experience of a specialised registry. Eur J Cancer 1993; 29: 367-71.
98. Wyman A, Brown JN, Zeiderman MR et al. Multiple sebaceous neoplasms and visceral carcinoma: Torre's syndrome. Eur J Surg Oncol 1990; 16:74-6.
99. Alessi E, Brambilla L, Luporini G et al. Multiple sebaceous tumors and carcinomas of the colon. Torre syndrome. Cancer 1985; 55:2566-74.
100. Cohen PR, Kohn SR, Kurzrock R. Association of sebaceous gland tumors and internal malignancy: the Muir-Torre syndrome. Am J Med 1991; 90:606-13.
101. Fathizahed A, Medenica MM, Soltani K et al. Aggressive keratoacanthoma and internal malignant neoplasm. Arch Dermatol 1982; 118:112-4.
102. Lynch HT, Fusaro RM, Roberts C et al. Muir-Torre syndrome in several members of a family with a variant of the cancer family syndrome. Br J Dermatol 1985; 113:295-301.
103. Honchel R, Halling KC, Schaid DJ e3 t al. Microsatellite instability in Muir-Torre syndrome. Cancer Res 1994; 54:1159-63.
104. Kruse R, Rutten A, Lamberti C et al. Muir-Torre phenotype has a frequency of DNA mismatch-repair-gene mutations similar to that in hereditary nonpolyposis colorectal cancer families defined by the Amsterdam criteria. Am J Hum Genet 1998; 63: 63-70.
105. Bapat B, Xia L, Madlensky L et al. The genetic basis of Muir-Torre syndrome includes the hMLH1 locus. Am J Hum Genet 1996; 59:736-9.
106. Entius MM, Keller JJ, Drillenburg P et al. Microsatellite instability and expression of hMLH1 and hMSH2 in sebaceous gland carcinomas as markers for Muir-Torre syndrome. Clinical Cancer Res 2000; 6:1784-9.
107. Lynch HT, Smyrk T, Watson P et al. Hereditary colorectal cancer. Semin Oncol 1991; 18:337-66.
108. Serleth HJ, Kisken WA. A Muir-Torre syndrome family. Am Surg 1998; 64:365-9.
109. Cronkhite LW Jr, Canada WJ. Generalized gastrointestinal polyposis: an unusual syndrome of polyposis, pigmentation, alopecia and onychatrophia. N Engl J Med 1955; 252:1011-5.
110. Hanzawa M, Yoshikawa N, Tezuka T et al. Surgical treatment of Cronkhite-Canada syndrome associated with protein-losing enteropathy. Report of a case. Dis Colon Rectum 1998; 41:932-4.
111. Russell DM, Bhathal PS, St John DJ. Complete remission in Cronkhite-Canada syndrome. Gastroenterology 1983; 85:180-5.
112. Yamashita T, Miyazawa M, Suzuki T et al. A case of Cronkhite-Canada syndrome improved markedly with antiplasmin agent and steroid. Gastroenterol Endosc 1996; 38:45-50.
113. Daniel ES, Ludwig SL, Lewin KS et al. The Cronkhite-Canada syndrome: an analysis of clinical and pathologic features and therapy in 55 patients. Medicine 1974; 61:293-308.
114. Burke AP, Sobin LH. The pathology of Cronkhite-Canada polyps: a comparison to juvenile polyposis. Surg Pathol 1989; 13:940-6.
115. Katayama Y, Kimura M, Konn M. Cronkhite-Canada syndrome associated with a rectal cancer and adenomatous changes in colonic polyps. Am J Surg Pathol 1985; 9: 65-61.
116. Marhotra R, Sheffield A. Cronkhite-Canada syndrome with colon carcinoma and adenomatous changes in C-C polyps. Am J Gastroenterol 1988; 83:772-6.
117. Ruvalcaba RHA, Myhre S, Smith DW. Sotos syndrome with intestinal polyposis and pigmentary changes of the genitalia. Clin Genet 1980; 18:413-6.

118. Gorlin RJ, Cohen MM Jr, Condon LM et al. Bannayan-Riley-Ruvalcaba syndrome. Am J Med Genet 1992; 44:307-14.
119. Fargnoli MC, Orlow SJ, Semel-Conception J et al. Clinico-pathologic findings in the Bannayan-Riley-Ruvalcaba syndrome. Arch Dermatol 1996; 132:1214-8.
120. Hayashi Y, Ohi R, Tomita Y et al. Bannayan-Zonana syndrome associated with lipomas, hemangiomas, and lymphangiomas. J Pediatr Surg 1992; 6:722-3.
121. Zigman AF, Lavine JE, Jones MC et al. Localization of the Bannayan-Riley-Ruvalcaba syndrome gene to chromosome 10q23. Gastroenterology 1997; 113:1433-7.

13 Carcinoid Tumors of the Large Bowel

Introduction

Carcinoid tumors (CT) are neuroendocrine neoplasms derived from enterochromaffin cells [1]. The main histological characteristic of CT is the positive reaction to silver stain and to other markers of neuroendocrine tissue, such as neuron-specific enolase and chromogranin; consequently, it has been suggested to replace the term "carcinoid" with "neuroendocrine" tumors [2]. Despite the soundness of this proposal, the term carcinoid has persisted even in the most recent articles and reviews [3] and will be used in the present chapter.

CT may arise in many organs and tissues. In 1963, William and Sandler [1] classified CT according to their presumed embryological origin: thus, foregut carcinoids originate in the lung, bronchus and stomach; midgut carcinoids in the small intestine, appendix and proximal colon (from caecum to the splenic flexure); and hindgut carcinoids in the distal colon and rectum. The incidence of CT is difficult to evaluate owing to the frequent lack of relevant symptoms. Large clinical investigations estimated an incidence rate of the order of 1–2 cases/100,000/year [4, 5], while autopsy studies [6] revealed a frequency as high as 8–9 cases/100,000.

Various studies indicate that the appendix is the most frequent site of CT, followed by the rectum, ileum, bronchi and stomach [4, 5, 7]. Carcinoid tumors of the colon seem to be rare neoplasms, diagnosed in the late phases of the disease, and often with a poor prognosis [8]. Finally, data from a specialized cancer registry show that CT represent approximately 1% of all registered neoplasms of the large bowel [9].

Brief History

The term "carcinoid" was introduced by Oberndorfer [10] in 1907 to define a distinct class of intestinal tumors with a clinical behavior less aggressive than the more common colorectal adenocarcinoma. The microscopic examination of these tumors showed the absence of glandular structures, thus suggesting that the lesions developed from epithelial cells within the crypts of Lieberkuhn. A few years before, the first carcinoid syndrome was described in a patient with ileal carcinoma and multiple liver metastases who experienced diarrhea and dyspnea after eating [11]. The first carcinoid of the colon was described by Saltycow [8] in 1912, while Gosset and Masson [12], using silver impregnation techniques, showed that carcinoids might arise from "enterochromaffin cells", so called because they stained with potassium chromate. Since these cells take up and reduce silver, they are also known as "argentaffin", and their possible endocrine origin was proposed [12, 13]. In 1953, Lemback [14] demonstrated the presence of serotonin in CT, and in 1954 the new entity "carcinoid syndrome" was established. This is an argentaffin gastrointestinal tumor causing diarrhea, flushing, asthma, cyanosis and right-sided valvular heart disease [15]. In the following years the development of new immunohistochemical techniques led to the identification of several other hormonal substances contained in CT, such as histamine, dopamine, neurotensin, prostaglandins and kallikrein [3, 16]. As already mentioned, some authors proposed using the general terms of "neuroendocrine tumors" for these neoplasms [2].

Biology and Pathology of CT

At the present time, the term carcinoid is used to describe tumors – both intestinal and extra-intestinal – with characteristic functional, morphological and staining patterns. Macroscopically, these lesions are solid and yellowish, owing to the high lipid content. Upon microscopic observation, CT are trabecular, glandular, or form rosettes in their pattern of growth. The tumor cells are rather similar, with faint pink granular cytoplasm and round nuclei with a few mitoses [17]. These cells – called argentaffin or enterochromaffin – possess the ability to take up and decarboxylate amine precursors and thus are also known as APUD cells (for Amine Precursor Uptake and Degradation). Cytoplasmic granules contain hormones which can be identified and measured by immunohistochemistry, thus confirming the diagnosis of CT. In particular, the ability of these cells to synthesize 5-hydroxytryptamine (serotonin) from the tryptophan contained in food is pathognomonic for the diagnosis of CT [18]. Serotonin is synthesized by the enzyme aromatic acid decarboxylase and is subsequently metabolized by monoamine oxidase to 5-hydroxy-indolacetic acid, which is excreted in the urine. In addition to serotonin, CT have been found to secrete histamine, corticotropin [19], dopamine [20], substance P [21], neurotensin [16], prostaglandins [22] and kallikrein [23]. The release of serotonin and of other vasoactive compounds into the circulation is associated with the clinical features of carcinoid syndrome [15].

Carcinoid tumors – especially of the stomach and bronchi, but rarely of the large bowel – are part of the spectrum of multiple endocrine neoplasia type 1 (MEN-1) in approximately 10% of cases [24]. MEN-1 is an autosomal dominant genetic disorder associated with loss of Men-1, a putative tumor suppressor gene located on chromosome 11q13 [25]. The disease is characterized by tumors of the pituitary gland, pancreatic islet cells and parathyroid gland [26].

In normal individuals, the large majority of tryptophan is used to synthesize nicotinic acid, and 1% or less is converted into serotonin. In contrast, in patients with CT, the production of serotonin (and of its metabolite 5-hydroxy-indoacetic acid) predominate, and the metabolite appears in the urine of most patients. Serotonin and other secretory products of CT are usually secreted into the portal system and reach the liver, where they are degraded and inactivated. In this case, CT do not cause any signs or symptoms. However, when liver metastases are present, serotonin and other vasoactive substances may reach the systemic circulation, and features of carcinoid syndrome become evident [27].

The classical carcinoid syndrome can be associated with tumors of the stomach and of the upper intestinal tract but is extremely rarely associated with CT of the large bowel [3]. The syndrome is characterized by cutaneous flushing, diarrhea, wheezing and heart-valve dysfunction. The symptoms result from synergistic interactions between serotonin metabolites, various kinins and prostaglandins released by the tumors into the systemic circulation [23, 27] and appear in the presence of massive metastatic liver involvement from CT. Carcinoid heart disease is usually a late manifestation of the disease and is the consequence of continuously high concentrations of circulating amines [28].

Clinical Features of Colorectal CT

The appendix is the main site of CT occurrence in the large bowel (Fig. 13.1). Carcinoids are the most common neoplasms of the appendix, are more often diagnosed in the fourth or fifth decade of life, and seem to be more frequent in women than in men (Table 13.1) [5]. The large majority of CT of the appendix

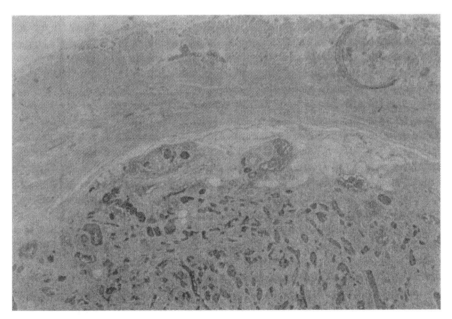

Fig. 13.1. Carcinoid tumor of the appendix. Malignant cells are identified by immunohistochemistry for chromogranin. Around the tumor is the muscular wall of the appendix

Table 13.1. Main clinical features of carcinoid tumors of the large bowel

Tumor site	Appearance (age in years)	Symptoms	Dimensions (average)	Prognosis
Appendix	30–50	Acute appendicitis	<2 cm	Usually good
Colon	60–70	Liver metastasis	~5 cm	30%–40% overall survival at 5 years
Rectum	60–70	Rectal bleeding, abdominal pain	>2 cm	40%–50% overall survival at 5 years

do not cause symptoms and are detected as an unexpected finding during surgery for acute appendicitis [29]. When symptoms occur, they can mimic appendicitis. The size of the tumor is the best predictor of the clinical outcome in patients with appendiceal CT. Over 95% of these lesions are less than 2 cm in diameter and are associated with a favorable prognosis [30]. In the small fraction of cases with lesions of 2 cm or more, nodal or distant metastases can be found in approximately one-third [31]. In a recent study, Sandor et al. [7] analyzed, retrospectively, 1,570 appendiceal carcinoids. They found that these tumors represent about 19% of all CT and show a marked female predominance. The overall 5-year survival for localized lesions was 94%, in case of local invasion 84.6%, and for distant metastasis 33.7%. Rather unexpectedly, in about 15% of all cases, tumors (non-carcinoid) at other sites could be detected.

CT represent less than 1% of all colonic tumors [5, 9]. In most cases, the disease manifests in the sixth or seventh decade of life, with symptoms such as anorexia, abdominal pain and weight loss [3, 32], while the carcinoid syndrome is present in less than 5% of these patients. The lesions are more frequent in the proximal portions of the large bowel, in particular the caecum [33, 34]. Symptoms usually develop in the late phases of the disease, and the average tumor diameter at presentation is 5 cm, with approximately two-thirds of patients demonstrating nodal or distant metastases [32]. The 5-year survival is approximately 70% for patients with localized disease, but as low as 20% if distant metastasis is present [3, 5]. In a population-based study of 36 patients with CT of the colon, Spread et al. [8] reported that the average age at diagnosis was 68.4 years. Symptoms occurred late in the course of the disease; 64% of the lesions were in Dukes' D stage and 22% in Dukes' C at diagnosis. Only one patient presented with a malignant carcinoid syndrome. The average tumor size was 5–8 cm, and most lesions had invaded the pericolic fat. Overall survival at 5 years was only 26%, which was significantly lower than that with rectal or appendiceal carcinoid tumors and common colonic adenocarcinomas. Survival was closely related to the stage at diagnosis, degree of differentiation, histological pattern and mitotic rate. The authors concluded that CT of the colon are rare neoplasms which are diagnosed late in the course of the disease and frequently carry a bad prognosis.

Rectal CT account for 1%-2% of all rectal neoplasms and are most frequent in the sixth decade of life (Table 13.1) [5]. At variance with other gastrointestinal CT, rectal carcinoids usually contain glucagon- and glicentin-related peptides rather than serotonin [35]. About one-half of rectal CT do not produce symptoms and are detected on routine endoscopy carried out for various reasons; in patients with symptoms, the disease usually manifests with rectal bleeding, abdominal pain or constipation [36, 37]. The carcinoid syndrome is rare. As for most colorectal tumors, regional lymph nodes and the liver are the main sites of metastatic involvement. Metastases are rare in patients with CT of less than 1 cm in diameter, but occur in the majority of cases in which lesions are more than 2 cm in diameter [3, 38]. The 5-year survival is about 80% for patients with localized disease, 50% for patients with nodal involvement and 18% for subjects with liver metastasis [5, 39].

If metastatic CT are suspected, liver ultrasound and computed tomography should be carried out to confirm or exclude liver involvement. Liver function tests, including alkaline phosphatase, are of little help. Since liver metastases from CT are often hypervascular and may appear isodense relative to the liver after intravenous contrast material, computed tomography should be done both before and after the administration of contrast agents [40]. Measurement of the serotonin metabolite 5-hydroxy-indolacetic acid in a 24-h or 48-h urine collection is of help in confirming the diagnosis of metastatic CT and in the subsequent monitoring of these patients. Feldman et al. [16] showed that an elevated urinary excretion of 5-hydroxy-indolacetic acid predicted the presence of CT with a sensitivity of 73% and a specificity of 100%. Moreover, Eriksson et al. [41], using a polyclonal antiserum against chromogranin A and B, suggested that serum chromogranin levels might represent a sensitive marker for detecting neuroendocrine tumors. The clinical course of patients with metastatic CT is extremely variable, and it is not infrequent to observe patients with a severe liver involvement who remain free of symptoms for years [4, 5]. Various authors have attempted to identify possible indicators of the clinical outcome – such as plasma chromogranin A levels, 5-hydroxy-indolacetic acid urinary excretion, carcinoembryonic antigen and some histological parameters – but the results have been unsatisfactory so far [42, 43].

Diagnosis and Treatment of CT of the Large Bowel

Patients with advanced CT are relatively uncommon, and optimum management should therefore be done in centers of expertise. The increasing number of investigative procedures and therapeutic options available to diagnose and treat complex CT has suggested the institution of specialized and multidisciplinary teams and clinics [27].

Diagnosis of CT

Appendiceal carcinoids tend to present with the clinical signs and symptoms of acute appendicitis; they are therefore diagnosed at surgery or during histological examination of a removed appendix. CT of the colon and rectum are best seen at endoscopy, though endoscopic ultrasound might be even more sensitive [44]. Barium enema and computed tomography can be useful for the detection of polypoid lesions of the large bowel but are less sensitive than colonoscopy. Angiography can be used to show a tumor blush, but this is an invasive examination and should be considered in the clinical context of its effect on management [45]. Since CT may express several neuroendocrine peptide receptors, this can be used for scintigraphic imaging with labeled somatostatin or octreotide [46]. More sophisticated techniques – such as single-photon-emission computed tomography – have also been proposed for the diagnosis of CT [47].

Treatment of the Primary Tumor

For appendiceal CT of less than 2 cm in diameter, simple appendicectomy is the treatment of choice, provided there is no macroscopic evidence of local spread [31]. Patients with tumors larger than 2 cm are usually treated with right hemicolectomy, since local recurrence after simple appendicectomy has been reported [3]. This type of operation is also suggested for lesions located at the base of the appendix [27]. CT of the colon are treated with standard right or left hemicolectomy; in the rare case of patients with early stage disease, local excision can also be effective [48]. For lesions of the rectum, local excision can be proposed when the tumors are less than 1 cm in diameter; for larger lesions, the two main options are low anterior resection or abdominoperineal resection [49, 50].

Treatment of Metastatic CT

In dealing with CT with liver metastases and carcinoid syndrome, one of the main aims is the control of symptoms (especially flushing, diarrhea and dyspnea). Changes of lifestyle can be important, and patients should be aware of precipitating factors such as alcohol, spicy foods and vigorous exercise. At present, treatment with inhibitors of serotonin release is the best strategy. Somatostatin and its analogues octreotide and lanreotide are highly effective in controlling flushing and diarrhea in approximately 70% of the treated patients [51]. In addition, there is evidence that these compounds can exert an inhibitory effect on tumor growth [52]. Octreotide should be started at small doses (50 µg subcutaneously, three times per day) and then progressively increased up to 200 µg three times daily. In a recent study, Rubin et al. [53] evaluated the effect of a microencapsulated long-acting formulation of octreotide acetate which was given subcutaneously every 4 weeks. In a large series of investigated patients, the new formulation was as effective as daily octreotide in controlling symptoms of carcinoid syndrome.

As with any other similar condition, the treatment of liver metastasis is difficult and rarely successful. Surgical resection can be attempted in patients with limited hepatic involvement, which has resulted in the long-term relief of symptoms and prolonged survival in highly selected individuals [54, 55]. Alternative treatments include hepatic-artery occlusion, embolization or chemoembolization [56, 57], but unfortunately the duration of the clinical response after these approaches is usually short, ranging between 7 and 20 months [3]. Liver transplantation has also been proposed for metastatic CT, but despite some encouraging results [58], the number of treated patients is too small to assess the real value of this novel approach.

The combination of interferon-alpha and somatostatin analogues has shown some efficacy not only for controlling symptoms of carcinoid syndrome but also as a possible medical therapy for metastatic CT [59]. However, the low rate of tumor regression and the high incidence of side-effects (fever, fatigue, anorexia, weight loss, hair loss, insomnia) has limited the use of interferon for metastatic CT. Moreover, chemotherapy with classic cytostatic chemical compounds (such as 5-fluorouracil, streptozocin, doxorubicin, cisplatin and cyclophosphamide) has been used in the treatment of metastatic CT, but with limited success [60-62]. Finally, the use of radiolabelled somatostatin analogues [63] revealed some efficacy in inducing tumor shrinkage and clinical improvement in a small number of patients with metastatic CT. Clearly, more studies are needed to establish the role of various medical treatments for advanced CT.

Conclusions

CT have long been a source of clinical interest. Although the large bowel is one of the main sites of CT occurrence, these lesions can be detected in several other digestive organs, even outside the gastrointestinal tract. The term "carcinoid" was initially used to define a tumor that, although resembling an adenocarcinoma, behaved in a more benign fashion. Since then, it has become clear that this more benign phenotype was not always clinically evident. Thus, the biology and the behavior of these poorly understood lesions remained a source of considerable debate [3, 5]. The term carcinoid may now be regarded as obsolete, since it fails to represent the spectrum of tumors that originate from different neuroendocrine cells and produce a variety of biologically active agents. It is likely that in the future the more appropriate term "neuroendocrine" will be used instead of "carcinoid" for designating these tumors [64].

References

1. Williams ED, Sandler M. The classification of carcinoid tumors. Lancet 1963; i:238-9.
2. Capella C, Heitz PU, Hofler H et al. Revised classification of neuroendocrine tumors of the lung, pancreas and gut. Digestion 1994; 50 S 2:11.
3. Kulke MH, Mayer RJ. Carcinoid tumors. N Engl J Med 1999; 340:858-68.
4. Godwin J. Carcinoid tumors: an analysis of 2837 cases. Cancer 1975; 36:560-9.
5. Modlin IM, Sandor A. An analysis of 8305 cases of carcinoid tumors. Cancer 1997; 79:813-29.
6. Berge T, Linell F. Carcinoid tumours: frequency in a defined population during a 12-year period. Acta Pathol Microbiol Scand 1976; 84:322-30.
7. Sandor A, Modlin IM. A retrospective analysis of 1570 appendiceal carcinoids. Am J Gastroenterol 1998; 93:422-8.
8. Spread C, Berkel H, Jewell L et al. Colon carcinoid tumors. A population-based study. Dis Colon Rectum 1994; 37:482-91.
9. Ponz de Leon M, Di Gregorio C, Roncucci L et al. Epidemiology of tumours of the colon and rectum: incidence, mortality, familiality and survival in the Health Care District of Modena. University of Modena, 1988; pages 1-58.
10. Oberndorfer S. Karzinoide tumoren des Dunndarms. Frankfort Z Pathol 1907; 1:426.
11. Ranson WB. A case of primary carcinoma of the ileum. Lancet 1890; 2:1020.
12. Gosset A, Masson P. Tumeurs endocrine de l'appendice. Presse Med 1914; 22:237.
13. Ciaccio C. Sur une nouvelle espece cellulaire dans les glandes de Lieberkuhn. C R Soc Biol 1906; 1:76.
14. Lembeck F. 5-hydroxytryptamine in a carcinoid tumor. Nature 1953; 172:910.
15. Thorson A, Bjork G, Bjorkman G et al. Malignant carcinoid of the small intestine with metastases to the liver, valvular disease of the right heart (pulmonary stenosis and tricuspid regurgitation without septal defect) peripheral vasomotor symptoms, bronchoconstriction and an unusual type of cianosis. Am Heart J 1954; 47:795.
16. Feldman JM, O'Dorisio TM. Role of neuropeptides and serotonin in the diagnosis of carcinoid tumors. Am J Med 1986; 81 S:41-8.
17. Soga J, Tazawa K. Pathologic analysis of carcinoids. Cancer 1971; 28:990-8.
18. Norheim I, Norheim-Theodorsson E, Brodin E et al. Tachykinins in carcinoid tumours: their use as a tumour marker and possible role in the carcinoid flush. J Clin Endocrinol Metab 1986; 64:605-12.
19. Limper AH, Carpenter PC, Scheithauer B et al. The Cushing syndrome induced by bronchial carcinoid tumors. Ann Intern Med 1992; 117:209-14.
20. Feldman J. Increased dopamine production in patients with carcinoid tumors. Metabolism 1985; 34:255-60.
21. Skrabanek P, Cannon D, Kirrane J et al. Substance P secretion by carcinoid tumors. Ir J Med Sci 1978; 147:47-9.
22. Sandler M, Karin SM, Williams ED. Prostaglandins in amine-peptide-secreting tumours. Lancet 1968; 2:1053-4.
23. Lucas KJ, Feldman JM. Flushing in the carcinoid syndrome and plasma kallikrein. Cancer 1986; 58:2290-3.
24. Lehy T, Mignon M, Cadiot G et al. Gastric endocrine cell behaviour in Zollinger-Ellison patients on long term potent antisecretory treatment. Gastroenterology 1989; 96:1029-40.
25. Chandrasekharappa SC, Guru SC, Manickam P et al. Positional cloning of the gene for multiple endocrine neoplasia-type 1. Science 1997; 276:404-7.
26. Lehy T, Cadiot G, Mignon M et al. Influence of multiple endocrine neoplasia type I on gastric endocrine cells in patients with Zollinger-Ellison syndrome. Gut 1992; 33:1275-9.
27. Caplin ME, Buscombe JR, Hilson AJ et al. Carcinoid tumours. Lancet 1998; 352:799-805.

28. Creutzfeldt W. Carcinoid tumours: development of our knowledge. World J Surg 1996; 20:126-31.
29. Roggo A, Wood WC, Ottinger LW. Carcinoid tumors of the appendix. Ann Surg 1993; 217:385-90.
30. Anderson JR, Wilson BG. Carcinoid tumours of the appendix. Br J Surg 1985; 72: 545-6.
31. Moertel CG, Weiland LH, Nagorney Dm et al. Carcinoid tumor of the appendix: treatment and prognosis. N Engl J Med 1987; 317:1699-701.
32. Rosenberg JM, Welch JP. Carcinoid tumors of the colon: a study of 72 patients. Am J Surg 1985; 149:775-9.
33. Berardi RS. Carcinoid tumors of the colon (exclusive of the rectum): review of the literature. Dis Colon Rectum 1972; 15:383-91.
34. Ballantyne GH, Savoca PE, Flannery JT et al. Incidence and mortality of carcinoids of the colon. Data from the Connecticut Tumor Registry. Cancer 1992; 69:2400-5.
35. Capella C, Heitz PU, Hofler H et al. Revised classification of neuroendocrine tumors of the lung, pancreas and gut. Virchows Arch 1995; 425:547-60.
36. Jetmore AB, Ray JE, Gathright JB Jr et al. Rectal carcinoids: the most frequent carcinoid tumor. Dis Colon Rectum 1992; 35:717-25.
37. Soga J. Carcinoids of the rectum: tumors of the carcinoid family – hindgut endocrinomas. Acta Med Biol 1982; 29:157-201.
38. Naunheim KS, Zeitels J, Kaplan EL et al. Rectal carcinoid tumors – treatment and prognosis. Surgery 1983; 94:670-6.
39. Crocetti E. Gastrointestinal carcinoid tumours. A population-based study. Ital J Gastroenterol Hepatol 1997; 29:135-7.
40. Woodard PK, Feldman JM, Paine SS et al. Midgut carcinoid tumors: CT findings and biochemical profiles. J Comput Assist Tomogr 1995; 19:400-5.
41. Eriksson B, Arnberg H, Oberg K et al. A polyclonal antiserum against chromogranin A and B – a new sensitive marker for neuroendocrine tumors. Acta Endocrinol 1990; 122:145-55.
42. Engstrom PF, Lavin PT, Moertel CG et al. Streptozocin plus fluorouracil versus doxorubicin therapy for metastatic carcinoid tumor. J Clin Oncol 1984; 2:1255-9.
43. Federspiel BH, Burke AP. Shekitka KM et al. Carcinoembryonic antigen and carcinoids of the gastrointestinal tract. Mod Pathol 1990; 3:586-90.
44. Giovanni M, Seitz JF, Thomas P et al. Electronic sectorial ultrasound endoscopy in benign and malignant tumoral pathology of the stomach: results in 30 patients. Gastroenterol Clin Biol 1993; 17:26-32.
45. Aspestrand F, Kolmannskog F, Jacobsen M. CT, MR imaging and angiography in pancreatic apudomas. Acta Radiol 1993; 34:468-73.
46. Kwekkeboom DJ, Krenning EP. Somatostatic receptor scintigraphy in patients with carcinoid tumours. World J Surg 1996; 20:157-61.
47. Perault C, Schvartz C, Wampach H et al. Thoracic and abdominal SPECT-CT image fusion without external markers in endocrine carcinomas. J Nucl Med 1997; 38: 1234-42.
48. Koura AN, Giacco GG, Curley SA et al. Carcinoid tumors of the rectum: effect of size, histopathology, and surgical treatment on metastasis free survival. Cancer 1997; 79:1294-8.
49. Sauven P, Ridge JA, Quan SH et al. Anorectal carcinoid tumors: is aggressive surgery warranted? Ann Surg 1990; 211:67-71.
50. Burke M, Sheperd N, Mann CV. Carcinoid tumours of the rectum and anus. Br J Surg 1987; 74:358-61.
51. Arnold R, Frank M, Kajdan U. Management of gastroenteropancreatic endocrine tumours: the place of somatostatin analogues. Digestion 1995; 55:107-13.
52. Arnold R, Trartmann ME, Creutzfeldt W et al. Somatostatin analogue octreotide and inhibition of tumours growth in metastatic endocrine gastroenteropancreatic tumours. Gut 1996; 38:430-8.

53. Rubin J, Ajani J, Schirmer W et al. Octreotide acetate long-acting formulation versus open-label subcutaneous octreotide acetate in malignant carcinoid syndrome. J Clin Oncol 1999; 17:600-6.
54. Que FG, Nagorney DM, Batts KP et al. Hepatic resection for metastatic neuroendocrine carcinomas. Am J Surg 1995; 169:36-43.
55. Dousset B, Saint-Marc O, Pitre J et al. Metastatic neuroendocrine tumors: medical treatment, surgical resection, or liver transplantation. World J Surg 1996; 20:908-15.
56. Ruszniewski P, Rougier P, Roche A et al. Hepatic arterial chemoembolization in patients with liver metastases of endocrine tumors: a prospective phase II study in 24 patients. Cancer 1993; 71:2624-30.
57. Carrasco CH, Charnsangavej C, Ajani J et al. The carcinoid syndrome: palliation by hepatic artery embolization. Am J Roentgenol 1986; 147:149-54.
58. Lang H, Oldhafer KJ, Weimann A et al. Liver transplantation for metastatic neuroendocrine tumors. Ann Surg 1997; 225:347-54.
59. Janson ET, Oberg K. Long-term management of the carcinoid syndrome: treatment with ocreotide alone and in combination with alpha-interferon. Acta Oncol 1993; 32:225-9.
60. Bukowski RM, Johnson KG, Peterson RF et al. A phase II trial of combination chemotherapy in patients with metastatic tumors: a Southwest Oncology Group study. Cancer 1987; 60:2891-5.
61. Moertel CG, Hanley JA. Combination chemotherapy trials in metastatic carcinoid tumor and the malignant carcinoid syndrome. Cancer Clin Trials 1979; 2:327-34.
62. Moertel CG, Kvols LK, O'Connell MJ et al. Treatment of neuroendocrine carcinomas with combined etoposide and cisplatin: evidence of major therapeutic activity in the anaplastic variants of these neoplasms. Cancer 19921; 68:227-32.
63. Otte A, Mueller-Brand J, Dellas S et al. Yttrium-90-labelled somatostatin-analogue for cancer treatment. Lancet 1998; 351:417-8.
64. Corleto VD, Angeletti S, Panzuto F et al. Digestive neuroendocrine tumours: diagnosis and treatment in Italy. A survey by the Oncology Study Section of the Italian Society of Gastroenterology (SIGE). Digest Liver Dis 2001; 33:217-21.

14 Colorectal Cancer at the Beginning of the New Millennium

Research in colorectal cancer has evolved remarkably during the past century and, in particular, in the last 20-30 years. The intimate mechanisms of the disease have been partially clarified by the tremendous advances in molecular biology. Similarly, the genetic nature of a fraction of colorectal malignancies has been documented, and the responsible genes identified and characterized. In parallel, endoscopy became an established procedure for removing precancerous lesions of the large bowel, and careful clinical investigations revealed that adjuvant chemotherapy can be of benefit for many patients. Moreover, mass screening procedures have been proposed and validated, and sophisticated new surgical approaches have been developed.

However, these and many other advances should be considered with caution and with a constructive but critical attitude. In fact, the available evidence indicates that colorectal tumors are not "under control" (as in the case, for instance, of neoplasms of the cervix), and this despite the enormous amount of new knowledge accumulated in the last 2-3 decades. Indeed, the prevention and early detection of colorectal carcinoma remain difficult, and mass screening can hardly be implemented in the general population. Even more relevant, surgery was basically the only hope for cure at the end of 19th century, and surgery is still at present the only option for the large majority of colorectal cancer patients.

In these concluding remarks, I would like to focus on three main aspects of colorectal cancer research: trends of incidence, gene-environment interaction, and the problems of dealing with patients in the new "Molecular Era".

The Colorectal Cancer Epidemic

In Western society, colorectal cancer is the third leading cause of cancer-related deaths [1]. Crude incidence rates are of the order of 50-80 new cases/100,000/year, and this corresponds to approximately 160,000 diagnoses of colorectal cancer every year in the USA, and some 30,000 in countries such as Britain or Italy [2, 3]. Nearly 40% of affected patients are going to die of this disease. Incidence rates are increasing in most European countries and in Japan [4, 5], whereas they tend to maintain stable in the USA [6, 7]. Thus, in the immediate future we should expect stable or slightly rising rates, at least in well developed countries. But what about colorectal cancer in emerging countries?

From the few available data, colorectal cancer shows very low incidence rates in most of the Third World, about 2-10 new cases/100,000/year [8-10]. More than 50% of these patients die of the disease, because of late diagnosis and limited clinical resources. However, many things are changing in emerging countries. Gradually, Western technology (computer, television, and many other modern devices) is changing the aspect of populations used to living from agriculture and sheep farming for centuries. With the technology, Western lifestyle and dietary habits will be adopted by a progressively larger number of people, who will become more sedentary (spending more time watching a monitor), less used to physical activity, and will eat more meat and animal fat. These changes will probably lead to a reduction of the impact of old enemies of underdeveloped countries – such as malaria, trachoma, tuberculosis, leprosy and yellow fever – but undoubtedly will expose the populations to an increased risk of colorectal malignancies, either because the Western diet and lifestyle are closely associated with colorectal cancer, or because life expectancy will rise, and aging is another strong risk factor for these tumors.

Thus, as a "side effect" of this recent tendency called "globalization", we should expect a progressive spreading of the colorectal cancer epidemic to most of the emerging countries. The same reasoning can be applied to other malignancies – such as breast, lung and prostate carcinomas – strongly related to the Western diet and habits [11-13].

Gene-Environment Interaction

The environment has been considered for many years as the main cause of human neoplasms [14]. However, the role of exogenous factors cannot explain many common observations. For example, why will only 1 of 5 or 6 heavy smokers develop lung cancer, and only a fraction of persons chronically infected with hepatitis B or C virus develop liver cancer? A superficial observer might simplify the issue by saying that this is due to chance, but an alternative and more likely explanation is that the genetic susceptibility to cancer (as well as for many other conditions) is different from person to person.

Genetic background and environmental agents appear now as the two fundamental "actors" in the process of tumorigenesis [15, 16]. Until 2-3 decades ago, much more attention was usually given to exogenous factors (such as cigarette smoking, diet or alcohol abuse), the effects of which seemed sufficient to explain tumor development in most cases. The trend seems to have reversed in the last decade, and rather paradoxically, at present the risk is that of interpreting tumor occurrence only as a sequence of genetic events, thus underevaluating the role of the environment [17].

What is becoming more and more apparent is that tumor development is closely dependent on the interaction between environmental agents and genetic factors. In other words, the genetic background determines, in a given population, those individuals who are particularly prone to cancer; subsequently – and usually over the course of many years – exogenous factors interact with genes, causing the appearance of the neoplastic phenotype in individuals not only exposed but also genetically predisposed [15, 16].

Considering colorectal malignancies, a close gene-environment interaction can be suspected in many areas of investigation. Thus, for instance, though individuals living in Western countries share the most common environmental risk factors, only a fraction of them (4%-6%) develop colorectal carcinoma, presumably those who are somehow predisposed. But the relevance of this interaction becomes even clearer if one considers families with hereditary nonpolyposis colorectal cancer [18]; in this case, constitutional mutations of the responsible genes have been identified, so that individuals at high risk can be recognized and kept under surveillance. In these families, cancer is never present at birth but develops in some subjects after the age of 20-30 years, in others in their 50s or 60s, and does not appear at all in others. Since all high-risk individuals in a given family are carriers of the same mutation, the interval of time before cancer occurrence should depend on the impact of exogenous factors, though the role of modifier genes cannot be excluded "a priori". This concept is of great practical importance, since environmental factors could – at least in theory – be controlled through a more appropriate diet, a healthier lifestyle, or chemoprevention.

Thus, studies on the gene-environment interaction will become one of the major objectives of cancer research in the new millennium. Though these investigations are still in their infancy, the study of enzymes involved in carcinogen metabolism (*N*-acetyltransferase, cytochrome P450, glutathione transferase and others) represents an excellent model and a suitable tool for this purpose [19].

Dealing with Colorectal Cancer Patients in the "Molecular Era"

During the past 2-3 decades, molecular biology has led to the discovery of genes that are responsible – when mutated – for a number of hereditary cancers. The identification of these "cancer genes" stressed the relevance of primary genetic factors in a variety of cancer syndromes and largely contributed to an increasing interest in the genetic etiology of cancer by basic investigators and clinicians.

We feel we are in a transitional phase between traditional medicine – based on the clinical diagnosis, with the aid of laboratory tests and imaging techniques – and a new "Era" that can be defined as "Molecular Medicine", in which the traditional approach will be partially replaced by the new diagnostic tools offered by molecular biology [20, 21].

These new techniques can determine – without uncertainties – the presence or absence of genetic alterations in an affected patient or in an individual at risk. Moreover, a correct molecular diagnosis can be reached many years before the appearance of symptoms and may help the clinician to distinguish between different disorders with identical phenotypes. To identify a specific mutation in a deleterious gene may also be of prognostic relevance or may suggest a more appropriate treatment [22]. Finally, genetic tests are usually carried out on constitutional DNA, which can be easily obtained from peripheral blood cells or urinary sediment, thus avoiding the need for biopsy or other invasive techniques.

These concepts are exemplified in Lynch syndrome (HNPCC), one of the most common hereditary cancer syndromes [23, 24]. When a germline mutation is detected in an affected individual in a HNPCC family, all unaffected family members at risk can be tested for the presence of that specific heterozygote mutation, so that we can discover how many of them carry the mutated allele and – consequently – are at an extremely high risk of developing cancer at a very early age. Asymptomatic carriers will be informed about this risk and invited to undergo a close surveillance or, as an option, prophylactic surgery. Moreover, in the same subjects it would be prudent to reduce the impact of exogenous factors – such as an inappropriate diet and physical inactivity – which are thought to increase the risk of colorectal malignancy [25]. When – despite surveillance – a colorectal tumor develops in a gene carrier, treatment should be designed not only to remove the neoplasm, but also to prevent further metachronous lesions, which are particularly frequent in HNPCC; thus, the possibility of subtotal colectomy with ileorectal anastomosis versus traditional hemicolectomy should be discussed with the patient. In any case, the remaining tract of the large bowel should be examined with frequent endoscopic controls. In other words, the molecular diagnosis of HNPCC has a profound effect on the diagnosis, treatment, prognosis and surveillance of both affected patients and gene carriers.

Besides the undoubted scientific interest in these new concepts, patients and physicians are becoming aware of the many ethical, social, economic and psychological problems that could result from the knowledge of a cancer risk confirmed by molecular genetic testing. How should we define (and consider) an apparently normal individual who is a carrier of a genetic alteration associated with tumor development? Can we use the term "patient" even when the disease has not yet manifested, but the risk approaches 100% (as in the case of familial adenomatous polyposis)? How can we help these patients to deal with psychological problems deriving from the awareness of being highly susceptible to tumor development? How should we manage the information (about their status) of healthy carriers of a potentially lethal mutation? These and many other problems will represent formidable challenges for oncologists in the new millennium.

References

1. Wingo P, Tong T, Bolden S. Cancer statistics 1995. CA Cancer J Clin 1995; 45:8–30.
2. Levi F, Te VC, Randimbison L et al. Trends in cancer incidence and mortality in Vaud, Switzerland, 1974–1993. Ann Oncol 1996; 7:497–504.
3. Inciardi JF, Lee JG, Stijnen T. Incidence trends for colorectal cancer in California: implications for current screening practices. Am J Med 2000; 109:277–81.
4. Capocaccia R, De Angelis R, Frova L et al. Estimation and projections of colorectal cancer trends in Italy. Int J Epidemiol 1997; 26:1–9.
5. Black RJ, Bray F, Ferlay J et al. Cancer incidence and mortality in the European Union: Cancer Registry data and estimates of national incidence for 1990. Eur J Cancer 1997; 33:1075–1107.

6. Cooper GS, Yuan Z, Landefeld S et al. A national population-based study of incidence of colorectal cancer and age. Cancer 1995; 75:775-81.
7. Troisi RJ, FreedmanAN, Devesa SS. Incidence of colorectal carcinoma in the U.S. An update of trends by gender, race, age, subsite, and stage, 1975-1994. Cancer 1999; 85:1670-6.
8. Al-Jaberi TM, Ammari F, Gharieybeh K et al. Colorectal adenocarcinoma in a defined Jordanian population from 1990 to 1995. Dis Colon Rectum 1997; 40:1089-94.
9. Tovar-Guzman V, Flores-Aldana M, Salmeron-Castro J et al. Epidemiologic panorama of colorectal cancer in Mexico, 1980-1993. Dis Colon Rectum 1998; 41:225-31.
10. Segal I, Edwards CA, Walker ARP. Continuing low colon cancer incidence in African populations. Am J Gastroenterol 2000; 95:859-60.
11. Chlebowski RT. Reducing the risk of breast cancer. N Engl J Med 2000; 343:191-8.
12. Smart CR. Prostate cancer facts and fiction. J Surg Oncol 1997; 66:223-9.
13. Travis WD, Travis LB, Devesa SS. Lung cancer. Cancer 1995; 75:191-202.
14. Peto J. Cancer epidemiology in the last century and the next decade. Nature 2001; 411:390-5.
15. Balkwill F, Mantovani A. Inflammation and cancer: back to Virchow? Lancet 2001;3 57:539-45.
16. Ponz de Leon M. Genetic basis of tumour development. Ital J Gastroenterol 1996; 28:232-45.
17. Lairmore TC, Norton JA. Advances in molecular genetics. Am J Surg 1997; 173:37-41.
18. Lynch HT, Smyrk T, Lynch J. An update of HNPCC (Lynch syndrome). Cancer Genet Cytogenet 1997; 93:84-99.
19. Mucci LA, Wedren S, Tamimi RM et al. The role of gene-environment interaction in the aetiology of human cancer: examples from cancers of the large bowel, lung and breast. J Intern Med 2001; 249:477-93.
20. Collins FS. Shattuck lecture - Medical and societal consequences of the human genome project. N Engl J Med 1999; 341:28-37.
21. Lynch HT, Fusaro RM, Lemon SJ et al. Survey of cancer genetics. Genetic testing implications. Cancer 1997; 80:523-32.
22. Meijers-Heijboer H, van Geel B, van Putten WLJ et al. Breast cancer after prophylactic bilateral mastectomy in women with a BRCA1 or BRCA2 mutation. N Engl J Med 2001; 345:159-64.
23. Lynch HT, Watson P, Shaw TG et al. Clinical impact of molecular genetic diagnosis, genetic counseling, and management of hereditary cancer. Part II: Hereditary Nonpolyposis Colorectal Carcinoma as a model. Cancer 1999; 86:1637-43.
24. Emery J, Lucassen A, Murphy M. Common hereditary cancers and implications for primary care. Lancet 2001; 358:56-63.
25. Shike M. Diet and lifestyle in the prevention of colorectal cancer: an overview. Am J Med 1999; 106:11S-5S.

Subject Index

A
abdomen/abdominal
- abscess 88
- cancer of the stomach 200
- discomfort 81
- distension 80
- pain 80-81, 256, 260, 279
- ultrasound 104

abdominoperineal resection 139, 185-186, 280
aberrant crypt foci (AFC) 24, 26, 52-54, 67, 231
abscess, abdominal 88
acetylcysteine 123
adenoma/adenomatous/adenomatosis 23-25, 55-60, 102, 118-119, 126, 127, 207, 231, 241-242, 253
- aggressive 200
- coli (see FAP)
- de novo carcinogenesis vs. adenoma-carcinoma sequence 66-67
- degeneration 268
- depressed 63, 67
- duodenal adenoma 106, 231
- dysplastic 103
- flat (see there) 63, 67
- large 23, 26
- lesion 121
- metachronous 173
- microadenoma 54, 67
- microadenomatosis 31
- polyp/polyposis (see there) 1, 4, 6, 24, 28, 31, 52, 54, 60-63, 81, 82, 95, 101, 118, 120, 125, 195, 200, 226, 229, 238, 253, 261, 266
- recurrent 118
- removal 120-121
- sebaceous 266
- serrated 61-62
- small 23, 26
- syndrome 225
- tubular or tubulovillous 229, 263

adenoma-carcinoma sequence 8-10, 55, 59-60, 63, 117, 120, 232, 243
adhesion 28
adjuvant
- chemotherapy 145, 148, 154, 171
- irradiation (see there) 145, 185-186
- radiotherapy 145
AFAP (attenuated familial adenomatous polyposis) 226
AFC (aberrant crypt foci) 24, 26, 52-54, 67, 231
AgNOR (agyrophilic nucleolar organizer region) 167, 201
AIDS 181, 183
- epidemic 181
alcoholic beverage 6-7
alopecia, mild 142
α-fetoprotein 81
amine
- heterocyclic 14
- precursor uptake and degeneration (APUD) 276
Amsterdam criteria of HNPCC 192, 207-208, 212
anal canal, cancer of 181-186
- clinical features and pathology 184
- epidemiology 181-182
- receptive anal intercourse 182
- risc factors 182-183
- treatment 185-186
anastomosis/anastomotic
- anal 226
- anastomotic dehiscence 166
- ileorectal/ileoanal anastomosis (IRA/IAA) 8, 13, 105, 122, 126, 138, 214, 233, 237, 241-244
- subtotal colectomy with ileorectal anastomosis 138, 261
anemia, iron-deficiency 80, 260
aneuploidy 7, 38, 167
angiogenesis 125
angioma 66

Subject Index

anorexia 80
antibodies
- monoclonal (*see there*) 153
- radiolabelled 153
antiinflammatory
- compound 7
- drug 7, 234
antioxidant vitamin 14, 24, 60, 118, 123, 126, 243
APC gene 7, 9, 14, 25–32, 40–41, 100, 101, 106, 121, 125, 225–227, 230, 231, 235–241, 253, 258, 264–265
- 311.8-KDa protein 236
- attenuated 237
- and its function 235–236
- I1307 K 10, 40–41, 101
- modifier genes 243
- mutation 53, 238
apoptosis 125, 168, 236
appendectomy 280
appendicitis 278
argentaffin 276
ascorbic acid 126, 234, 243
aspirin 25, 123, 126
asthma 276
astrocytoma 263
Auerbach plexus 51
autoradiography 40
autosomal
- co-dominant transmission 195
- dominant
- - condition 59
- - disease 107, 240
- - fashion 106
- - gene 195
- - model 1, 23
- - polyposis syndrome 256, 264
- - type of genetic transmission 33, 122, 195, 227, 240, 253, 259, 261
- monogenic model 11
- recessive inheritance 264
azoxymethane 52

B

Bannayan-Ruvalcaba-Riley syndrome (BRRS) 260, 268
Bannayan-Zonana syndrome 268
barium enema 81–82, 84, 99, 102, 173
basal cell carcinoma 266
BAX 37, 38, 206
β-catenin 28, 236
β-carotene 123
Bethesda criteria of HNPCC 207
big killers 172

biliary tract, carcinoma of 235
bleeding, rectal 81, 164, 234, 256, 260, 279
bowel disease
- carcinoid tumors of large bowel 275–281
- hyperplastic 8
- inflammatory (*see there*) 7, 8, 38–40, 52, 65–66, 125, 128, 182
- other polyposis of large bowel 253–268
- irritable bowel syndrome 88
brain tumor 201
BRCA1 and BRCA2 41, 101
breast cancer 41, 70, 98, 200, 262
- hereditary 41
bromodeoxyuridine 40, 52, 167
bryostatin 1 151

C

calcium 25, 60, 118, 123, 126–127
- folinate 150
capecitabine 150, 151
carboplatin 150
carcinoembryonic antigen (*see* CEA) 81, 84, 85, 146, 170, 173–174, 279
carcinoid
- appendiceal 278
- syndrome 277–278
- tumor 66, 70
- - of large bowel 275–281
- - - biology and pathology 276–277
- - - brief history 275–276
- - - carcinoid syndrome 276, 280
- - - clinical features of colorectal carcinoid tumors 277–279
- - - definiton "carcinoid" 281
- - - diagnosis 279–280
- - - rectal 279
- - - treatment 279–281
carcinoma in situ 57
carcinomatous degeneration 268
β-carotene 118, 123, 126
CAT scanning 85, 86, 88
catenin
- β-catenin 28, 236
- γ-catenin 236
CDX-2 206
CEA (carcinoembryonic antigen) 81, 84, 146, 170, 173–174, 279
- serum level 85
celecoxib 226, 244
cell
- differentiation 127
- proliferation 52
- replication 167

Subject Index 293

c-erb β_2 168
cervical carcinoma 181
chemoembolization 281
- drugs 152
chemoprevention 49, 122, 123-128
- of CC 117-128
- colorectal tumor, main compounds 125-128
- general concepts 123-125
chemotherapy 141, 143-145, 148-153, 164-165, 185-186, 234
- adjuvant 145, 148, 154, 171
- for advanced CC 148-151
- doxorubicin-based 234
- 5-fluorouracil-based 141-143, 145, 148-151, 214
- toxicity and costs 151
chromogranin 70, 275, 279
chromosome/chromosomal
- aberrations 231
- chromosome 5 235
- 1 deletion 28
- 5q 26, 27, 28
- 17p 26, 27, 28
- 18q 26, 27, 28
- instability 40
CHRPE (congenital hypertrophy of the retinal pigment epithelium) 13-14, 233-234, 237-238
cisplatin 150, 152, 281
c-jun 236
clinical finding: symptom and sign 80-89
c-myc 168, 236
codon 1307 41
colectomy 8, 105
- hemicolectomy, right or left 138, 214, 280
- subtotal 126, 214
- - prophylactic 214
- - with ileorectal anastomosis 138, 261
colitis ulcerative/*Crohn's* colitis 7, 25, 38, 40, 100, 104, 122, 182
colonoscopy 81-84, 96-99, 102-104, 108-109, 117, 121, 173-174, 240, 280
- surveillance 108
- virtual (computed tomography) 83
colorectal cancer (*see* CC)
- familial CC 10-11
colostomy 185, 186
combination therapy 141-143, 149-150, 185
computed tomography (CT) 83, 146, 173-174
- liver 174

constipation 80, 88, 279
constitutional mutation 202
corticosteroid 7
costs of chemotherapy in advanced CC 151
counseling 106, 212
- FAP 240-241
- HNPCC 212
Cowden disease 25, 31, 33, 105, 261-262
- clincial manifestations and morphology 261-262
- management 26
- molecular basis 262
CRAC1 208-209
Crohn's disease/ulcerative colitis 7, 25, 38, 40, 100, 104, 105, 122, 182
- lymphoid response, *Crohn's*-like 201
- - peritumoral 215
Cronkhite-Canada syndrome (CCS) 25, 267-268
cyanosis 276
cyclin D1 236
cyclooxygenase 1 and 2 inhibitor 7, 125, 226, 244
cyclophosphamide 281
cyst, epidermoid 13, 106
cytokeratin 170
- immunohistochemical staining 137
cytostatic coumpounds 141
cytotoxic coumpounds 141
- arterial infusion of cytotoxic drugs 152

D
DALM (dysplasia associated lesion or mass) 65, 105
DCC gene 9, 28, 31, 33, 60, 137, 168, 253
de novo carcinogenesis vs. adenoma-carcinoma sequence 66-67
degree of tumor differentiation 146, 166
denaturing gradient gel electrophoresis 239
dental
- abnormalities 236
- line 184
dentigerous cyst 233
deoxycholic acid 127
depressed adenoma 63, 67
dermatitis 142
desmoid
- epidermoid 13
- tumor 14, 25, 106, 226, 231, 234, 238, 243, 244
diabetes mellitus 15

diagnosis and clinical future 79–89
- imaging studies in diagnosis of recurrent or metastatic disease 85–88
diarrhea 80, 142, 260, 275–277, 280
diet 3–5, 118–119
- and micronutrient 3–5, 15, 118, 127
differentiated lesions/carcinoma 69, 201, 236
- moderately differentiated 69
- poorly differentiated carcinoma 198
- well differentiated 69, 137
difluoromethylornithine 123
digital rectal examination 173
diminutive 102
- polyps 102
diploid tumor 201
disease (*see* syndrome)
distribution 55
diverticula 97
DNA
- hypermethylation 28
- hypomethylation 5, 9
- methylation 5, 26, 28, 127
- - abnormal 262
- repair/repair system 14, 30, 38, 193
- - mismatch repair gene 25, 107, 125, 169, 191–193, 198, 200, 204, 206, 212–213, 263–264, 267
dopamine 276
doxorubicin-based chemotherapy 234, 281
DPC4 (SMAD4) gene 28, 33, 65, 260
drug(s) 7–8
- anti-inflammatory 7, 15, 234, 244
- non-steroidal anti-inflammatory (NSAID) 15, 123, 125
Dukes' staging 70, 81, 136, 163
duodenal adenoma/lesions 231–232
- periampullary 106, 232
- polyp 232
dysplasia/dysplastic 53, 56–58, 105, 122, 200, 232, 260
- alteration 14
- DALM (dysplasia associated lesion or mass) 65, 105
- in inflammatory bowel disease 65–66
- high-grade 28
- severe 39, 57, 241
dyspnea 275, 280

E
E2F-4 206
E-cadherin 28
electromagnetic energy 85

embolization 152, 281
- chemoembolization 281
- hepatic artery 152
endoluminal ultrasound 84, 86
endometrial cancer/carcinoma 108, 200, 207
endorectal sonography/ultrasound 84, 146
endoscopy/endoscopic
- lower 85
- polypectomy 137–138
- screening 108
- surveillance after endoscopic polypectomy 102–103
end-points 124
- intermediate 124
- surrogate 124
energy imbalance 5–6
eniluracil 151
enterochromaffin cells 275, 276
environmental factor 3–4
eosinophil 51
- cell infiltration 166
epidemiology 2–3
- descriptive 54
epidermoid
- cyst 13, 106, 225, 226
- desmoid 13
ethnic differences in CC survival 171–172
EX01 208–209
expression/expressivity of oncogene 124, 227
- clinical 210
extracolonic manifestations 198, 231–235
extraintestinal manifestations 253

F
familial/familiality 100
- CC 10
- factor 10–14
- familial adenomatous polyposis (*see* FAP)
family G 192
FAP (familial adenomatous polyposis) 1, 10–14, 25, 30–32, 40–41, 52, 63, 105–107, 117, 121–126, 138, 191, 225–244, 253, 258–259, 263–265
- adenoma 59
- APC gene and its functions 235–236
- attenuated type 31, 229–230
- colorectal lesions 229–231
- counseling in diagnosis and surveillance 240–241
- definition and historical overview 226–227

- diagnosis, clinical features
  and morphology 229
- epidemiology and formal genetics
  227–229
- extracolonic manifestations 231–235
- genotype-phenotype correlations
  236–238
- management 239–240
- medical treatment 243–244
- molecular biology 235
- overall prognosis and follow-up 243
- single cases 229
- surgical treatment 241–243
- tumorigenesis 31
fatique 80, 142
FDG (fluorodeoxyglucose) 88
fecal occult blood test 96–99, 109, 173
FHIT gene inactivation 28
fibroblast 51
fibroma 66
fibrosis, extent of 69
fissure 184
fistulae 182, 184, 234
flat adenoma 63, 67
- hereditary flat adenoma syndrome 63
flavonoids 5, 14, 123
floxuridine 152
fluorescence of in situ hybridization 38
fluorodeoxyglucose (FDG) 88
fluoropyrimidine-based regimen 149, 150
5-fluorouracil 152, 281
- chemotherapy, 5-fluorouracil-based
  141–143, 145, 148–151, 185–186, 215
- - infusional 5-fluorouracil regimen 149
- - irinotecan and 5-fluorouracil
    combination 149, 150
- - leucovorin and 5-fluorouracil
    combination 149, 150
- - levamisole and 5-fluorouracil
    combination 141–143, 214
- - methotrexat and 5-fluorouracil
    combination 149
- - mitomycin C and 5-fluorouracil
    combination 185–185
flushing 276–277, 280
focal carcinoma 57
folate 5, 14, 25, 60, 118, 123, 127
folinic acid 127, 143, 215
follow-up of CC patients 172
- controlled studies evaluating the
  effectiveness of follow-up 174
fra-1 236
fundic gland hyperplasia 231

G
GADD45 30
γ-catenin 236
γ-emitting radionuclide 84
ganglioneuroma 33, 261
Gardner syndrome 225–226, 233, 238
gastric
- cancer 200
- erosion 126
- polyp 106, 231
gastrin 6
gastroduodenoscopy 240
gate-keeper gene 28, 32, 258
genetic
- counseling 106
- - FAP 240–241
- - HNPCC 212
- heterogeneity 260
genital warts 184
genodermatosis 261
genomic instability 184, 200
genotype-phenotype correlations, FAP
  236–238
germline mutations 213, 237
gland, fundig gland hypoplasia 231
glicentin-related peptides 279
glioblastoma 263
glucagon-related peptides 279
glucose 6, 119
goblet cell 50–51
grading of CC 69
growth factor 6
- insulin-like 128
GTBP 204
- hMSH6/GTBP 35
guaiac impregnated slide 97

H
H^3-thymidine 52
haemangioma 261
haematogenous metastasis 69
haematologic malignancy 201
haemoccult test/screening study 81, 96–99
haemorrhoidal
- plexus 50
- superior 69
hamartoma/hamartomatous lesion 31, 33, 64–65, 256–261
- carcinoma 64
- changes 268
- hamartoma-adenoma-carcinoma
  sequence 64
- multiple hamartoma syndrome 261
- polyp 8, 31, 64–65, 256–257, 262, 268

Subject Index

Hartmann procedure 140
hBUB1 38
heart disease
- heart-valve dysfunction 277
- ischaemic 15
hemicolectomy, right or left 138, 214, 280
hemorrhoid 80, 88, 97, 182, 184
hepatic artery ligation or embolization 152
hepatitis B and C virus 123
hepatobiliary tract tumor 200
hepatoblastoma 13, 25, 235
hepatocellular carcinoma 123
hereditary
- breast cancer 41, 70, 98
- cancer syndrome, surveillance in 105-106
- factor 10-14
- - hereditary non-polyposis CC/*Lynch* syndrome (*see* HNPCC)
heteroduplex analysis 239
heterozygote 195
- loss of heterozygosity 9, 28, 62
histamine 276
- histamine H_2 antagonist 128
histocytoma 200
histology/histological
- feature and grading 67-69
- venous or perineural invasion 146
histopathology 56-58
HIV infection 181, 183
hMLH1 35, 107, 204, 207
hMSH2 35, 107, 206, 207
hMSH6 206, 207
- hMSH6/GTBP 35
HNPCC (hereditary non-polyposis CC)/*Lynch* syndrome 1, 5, 10-15, 25, 35-38, 40-41, 59, 82, 101, 105-108, 117, 121-122, 125, 138, 169, 191-216, 264-267
- age at diagnosis and referential location in the right colon 198
- Amsterdam criteria 192, 207-208, 212
- Bethesda criteria 207
- brief history 191-192
- clinical features 197-198
- colorectal tumorigenesis 35-38
- diagnosis 209
- DNA mismatch repair in bacteria 203
- epidemiology and frequency 192-194

- extracolonic tumor spectrum 198
- formal genetics and the role of family history 195-197
- frequency of mutations in HNPCC families 207-208
- genetic counseling 212-213
- human mismatch repair genes 203-205
- identification 209-210
- management and survival 213
- microsatellite instability
- - and cancer development 206
- - the MSI + phenotype 205
- molecular biology 202-203
- multiple tumors 199-200
- new genes predisposing to 208-209
- pathology 201-202
- phenotype 201
- screening 215
- survival 215-216
- suspected 207, 210-212
- treatment and follow-up 214-215
- tumor spectrum 200-201
homosexuality 181-182
hormonal factor 6
hPMS1 and hPMS2 gene 204, 207
HPV (human papillomavirus) infection 181-184, 186
- HPV-16 183
h-ras oncogene 168
Huntington chorea 212
hydrocarbon, polycyclic 14
hydrocolonic sonography 83-84
5-hydroxy-indolacetic acid 276, 279
5-hydroxytryptamine (serotonin) 70, 276-279
hypermethylation
- of DNA 28
- of MLH1 promoter region 37, 205
hyperplastic
- changes 268
- polyp 61, 98
hypertension 15
hypogastric
- nerves 141
- plexus, inferior 141
hypomethylation of DNA 5, 9
hysterectomy, prophylactic 214

I

IGF2R 206
ileal/ileorectal/ileoanal
- anastomosis (IRA/IAA) 8, 13, 105, 122, 126, 138, 214, 233, 237, 241-244

Subject Index   297

– – colectomy with IRA   242
– pouch   241, 243
– reservoir   226
ileus, postoperative   166
iliac lymph nodes, superficial   69
imaging study
– in diagnosis of recurrent or metastatic disease   85–88
– in primary cancer   82–85
immunohistochemical staining for cytokeratin   137
in situ hybridization, fluorescence   38
^{111}indium   84
inflammation   97
inflammatory bowel disease   7, 8, 52, 65–66, 125, 128, 182
– CC development   38–40
– polyp and dysplasia in   65–66
– surveillance   104–105
informed consent   106
initiation   23
insulin   6, 119
insulin-like growth factor   128
interferon-α 281
intermediate end-points   124
interstitial irradiation   185
intestinal
– obstruction   234
– transplantation   234
– vasoactive intestinal peptide   70
intraepithelial neoplasia   183
intramucosal carcinoma   57
invasion
– lymphatic   137–138
– vascular   137
^{123}iodine   84
irinotecan   149
– and 5-fluorouracil combination   149–150
– and oxaliplatin combination   150
iron-deficiency anemia   80, 260
irradiation, adjuvant   145, 185–186
– external beam irradiation   185
– interstitial   185
– postoperative   145
– preoperative   145
– sandwich   145
irritable bowel syndrome   88
ischaemic heart disease   15

J
JP (juvenile polyposis)   25, 31, 33, 65, 259–261, 268
– management   261
– molecular biology and genetic heterogeneity of JP   260–261
– surveillance   260

K
kallikrein   276
Kaposi sarcoma   183
keratinizing squamous cell carcinoma   181, 184
keratoacanthoma   265, 266
Ki67   40, 167
kinin   277
Knudson hypothesis / two-hit hypothesis   31, 106, 205, 262, 264, 268
k-ras oncogene   28, 31, 32, 40, 60, 62, 100, 137, 168–169

L
laboratory investigation   81
laparoscopy/laparoscopic surgery   135, 138–139
laryngeal carcinoma   200
leucovorin and 5-fluorouracil combination   149, 150
levamisole and 5-fluorouracil combination   141–143, 215
lifestyle   119–120
Li-Fraumeni syndrome   169, 212
ligation, hepatic artery   152
lipoma   33, 66, 261
liver
– computer tomography   174
– transplantation   151, 152, 281
– ultrasound   173
LKB1/STK11   64, 257–258
lobectomy, radical   148
lung cancer   123
lymph nodes, superficial iliac   69
lymphadenectomy   139
lymphatic
– follicle   51, 66
– invasion   69, 137–138
– microinvasion   166
– tissue   71
lymphocyte/lymphocytic   51
– *Crohn's*-like lymphoid response (*see there*)   201, 215
– infiltration   69
lymphoid
– hyperplasia   33
– polyp   66
lymphoma, non-*Hodgkin*   71
Lynch syndrome/hereditary non-polyposis CC (*see* HNPCC)

M

macrophage 51
malignant/malignancy
- polyp 55
- prevention 4
MAMA (monoallelic mutation analysis) 239
mandible osteoma 225
mast cell 51
- cell infiltation 166
mastectomy, prophylactic 262
MCC gene 9, 28
Mdm-2 30
MED1 208-209
medicalization 54, 163, 172
- of Western society 54
medullary or undifferentiated lesion 201
medulloblastoma 263
Meissner plexus 51
melanin spot 256
MEN-1 (multiple endocrine neoplasia type 1) 276
mesalazine 7
mesorectal excision 140, 145-146, 154, 166
- total 145
metachronous
- adenoma 173
- colorectal
- - lesion 59, 104, 107, 125, 199
- - tumor 173
metastasis and staging, pattern of 69-70, 137
- metastatic burden 148
- micrometastasis (*see there*) 137, 170-171
- surgical treatment of metastatic CC 147-148
methotrexate and 5-fluorouracil combination 149
methylation of DNA 5, 26, 28
microadenoma/microadenomatosis 31, 54, 67
microinvasation, lymphatic 166
micrometastasis 137
- and prognosis 170-171
micronutrient and diet 3-5, 15, 118, 125
microsatellite 41, 101, 107, 124, 169
- instability (MSI) 9, 13, 14, 35, 37, 38, 40-41, 53, 59, 62, 107, 168-170, 191-194, 198, 201, 205-215, 267
- loci 35
microscopic appearance 67
Miles operation 140, 147
MIN gene 14
- MOM1 (for modifier of MIN) 14

miscellaneous 123
mismatch repair gene 25, 107, 125, 169, 191-193, 198, 200, 204, 206, 212-213, 263-264, 267
mitomycin C 186
- and 5-fluorouracil combination 185-186
mitotic checkpoint 38
MLH1 gene 37, 60, 101, 122, 193-194, 198-201, 205, 208-213, 264-267
- hypermethylation 37
MLH3 gene 204
MMAC1/PTEN 33, 260, 262, 268
molecular
- markers of prognosis 168-170
- staging 137
MOM1 (for modifier of MIN) 14
monoallelic mutation analysis (MAMA) 239
monoclonal antibody 153-154
- recombinant monoclonal antibody (C30.6) 153
MRI (magnetic resonance imaging) 85, 86, 88, 173
MSH2 gene 37, 38, 60, 101, 122, 193-194, 198-201, 208-212, 265-267
MSH3 gene 37
MSH6 gene 37, 38, 101, 204, 208
MSI (microsatellite instability) 9, 13, 14, 35, 37, 38, 40-41, 53, 59, 62, 107, 168-170, 191-194, 198, 201, 205-215, 267
- phenotype 205-206
mucin/mucinous lesion/carcinoma 53, 67, 169, 198, 201
- histological type 37, 146, 215
mucocutaneous
- papillomatous papule 33
- pigmentations 256
mucosa/mucosal
- colorectal 50-52
- intramucosal carcinoma 57
- proctectomy 242
Muir-Torre syndrome (MTS) 25, 200, 265-267
- clinical and morphologic features 265-266
- management 267
- molecular biology 266-267
- surveillance 267
multiple endocrine neoplasia type 1 (MEN-1) 276
multiplicity 55
muscularis mucosae 50-51, 57, 137
mut H 203

mut L   203, 204
mut S   203, 204
mutator
– gene   1, 23, 35, 203–205
– phenotype   37
myoma   66

N
N-acetylcysteine   127
nervi erigentes   141
neuroblastoma   263–264
neuroendocrine
– carcinoma   70
– neoplasm   275
– peptide receptor   280
– tumor   276, 279, 281
neurofibroma/neurofibromatosis   66, 200
neurotensin   276
nitrosamine   14
NMR (nuclear magnetic imaging)   146
non-*Hodgkin* lymphoma   71
non-keratinizing squamous cell carcinoma   181, 184
non-malignant precursor lesion   98
non-polyposis CC, hereditary/*Lynch* syndrome (*see* HNPCC)
non-steroidal anti-inflammatory drugs (NSAID)   15, 123, 125
n-ras oncogene   168
NSAID (non-steroidal anti-inflammatory drugs)   15, 123, 125
nuclear
– ploidy   167
– polarity   69

O
obesity   5–6
obligate carrier   195
obstruction   164
– intestinal   234
occult blood test   96–99, 109, 173
octreotide   280
odontoma   106
oestrogen   128
oligodendroglioma   264
oncogene   1, 9, 23, 26, 40, 153
– *c-erb* β_2 168
– *c-myc*   168, 236
– *c-jun*   236
– *fra-1*   236
– *h-ras*   168
– *k-ras*   28, 31, 32, 40, 60, 62, 100, 137, 168–169
– *n-ras* oncogene   168

– expression   124
osteoma   13, 25, 106, 233
– mandibular   225–226
– skull   225
oxaliplatin   150
– irinotecan and oxaliplatin combination   150

P
p53 gene   7, 9, 28–31, 33, 40, 60, 62, 100, 137, 153, 168–170, 258
pain, abdominal   80–81, 256, 260, 279
pancolonoscopy   214
pancreas, carcinoma of   235
Paneth cells   51
papillomatous papule, mucocutaneous   33
papillomavirus infection (*see* HPV)   181–183
parasympathetic nerve   50
pathogenesis   23–42
pathology   49–72
PCNA   40, 167
PCR (poymerase chain reaction)   100
pedigree analysis   209
penetrance   210
peptic ulcer   126
perforation of tumor   146
periampullary carcinoma   106, 232
– carcinoma of the periampullary region   13, 243
perineural or venous invasion at histology   146
peroxidase-like activity   97
PET (positron-emission tomography)   88, 173
– PET scanning   104
Peutz-Jeghers syndrome   25, 31, 64, 105, 253–261
– clinical manifestations and morphology   256–257
– juvenile polyposis (JP)   259–261, 268
– management   258–259
– molecular biology   257–258
– phenotypic characteristics, genetics and cancer risk   259–260
– surveillance   258
phenocopies, HNPCC   194, 198, 210
phenotype/phenotypic
– expression   243
– genotype-phenotype correlations, FAP   236–238
– mild   242
– MSI + phenotype   205–206
– mutator phenotype   37

physical activity   5–6
plasma cell   51
platinum drugs   150
plexus
- *Auerbach*   51
- *Meissner*   51
PMS1 and PMS2 gene   101, 264–265
polymorphism analysis   239
polyp/polyposis, colorectal   8–10, 54, 60–66, 101–103, 268
- adenomatous   1, 4, 6, 24, 28, 31, 52, 60, 82, 95, 101, 118, 120, 125, 195, 200, 206, 238, 261, 266, 268
- - attenuated adenomatous polyposis 229–230
- - etiology   60
- - familial adenomatous polyposis (see FAP)
- - premalignant lesion (adenomatous polyp)   81, 95
- - upper gastrointestinal polyp   238
- diminutive   102
- dysplastic   64
- gastric   106, 231
- hamartomatous polyp   8, 31, 64–65, 256–262, 268
- hyperplastic   61, 98
- in inflammatory bowel disease 65–66
- juvenile polyposis (see JP)   25, 31, 33, 65, 259–261
- lymphoid   66
- malignant   55–58
- - endoscopic treatment   137–138
- mixed   61–64, 259
- other type   82
- - other polyposis of large bowel 253–268
- syndrome   225, 253
polypectomy   99
- endoscopic   137
- - surveillance after   102–103
pouch, ileal   241, 243
poymerase chain reaction (PCR)   100
PPP2R1B gene   28
precancerous lesion   2
precursor lesion, non-malignant   98
premalignant lesion (adenomatous polyps) 81, 95
prevention and chemoprevention of CC 117–128, 213
- under special conditions   121
prevention of colorectal malignancy   4
proctitis   88

proctocolectomy
- restorative   8, 13, 226, 233, 237, 241–243
- - with ileorectal anastomosis   138
- total   242
prognosis
- micrometastasis   170–171
- molecular markers   168–170
progression   23, 123
promotion   23, 123
prophylactic surgery   214, 244
prostaglandin   276–277
prostate specific antigen   81
protein
- kinase C   127
- truncation tests   239
provitamin   126
PTEN/MMAC1   33, 260, 262, 268
pyridoxine   151

R
radiofrequency   85
radioimmunodetection   84–86
radioimmunoscintigraph   86
radiolabelled antibodies   153
radionuclide, γ-emitting   84
radiotherapy   141, 144–146, 152, 164, 171, 185–186
- adjuvant   145
ras oncogene family   7, 9, 27, 168–170
- *h-ras*   168
- *k-ras*   28, 31, 32, 40, 60, 62, 100, 137, 168–169
- *n-ras*   168
receptive anal intercourse   182
recombinant monoclonal antibody (C30.6) 153
rectosigmoid cancer, recurrence   86
rectosigmoidoscopy   82
rectum/rectal
- bleeding   81, 164, 234, 256, 260, 279
- surgical treatment of resectable tumor 139–141
recurrence
- local/locoregional   85, 103–104, 125, 135, 137, 140, 141, 145–147, 154, 172, 186
- - management   146–147
- rate   174
- of rectosigmoid cancer   86
- reliable predictor of   170
removal of adenoma   120–121
renal pelvis, transitional cell carcinoma 200

Subject Index

resection
- abdominoperineal 139, 185–186
- anterior 140
- colorectal tumor treatment, resectable 137–141
- – segmental resection 138
- proposed surveillance programs after CC resection 173

retina/retinal
- CHRPE (congenital hypertrophy of the retinal pigment epithelium) 13–14, 233–234, 237–238
- spots 25, 106, 226

retinoic acid 126
retinoid 123
retinol 126
ring cell carcinoma, signet 201
RNAse protection assay 239
Ruvalcaba-Mirhe-Smith syndrome 25, 268

S

scopolamine 83
screening (*see also* surveillance) 95–109, 163, 172, 174
- endoscopic 108
- HNPCC 215
- in individuals with familial CC 100
- media, society and CC screening 108–109
- new screening procedure based on molecular analysis 100
- prophylactic 229
- recommendations for individuals with familial risk 102

sebaceous
- adenoma 266
- carcinoma 266
- epithelioma 266
- hyperplasia 266
- tumor 265–267
- – gland tumor 267

segregation
- analysis 195
- family 240

selenium 118, 123
semustine-based chemotherapy 143
- vincristine and semustine combination 143

serotonin (5-hydroxytryptamine) 70, 276–279
serrated adenoma 61–62
sexual promiscuity 182
sexually transmitted disease 182

sigmoidoscopy 82, 96, 98–99, 102, 103, 109, 121, 173–174
- flexible 98, 240
signet ring cell carcinoma 201
single strand conformation polymorphism 239
size 55
skull osteoma 225
SMAD4 (DPC4) gene 28, 33, 65, 260
small bowel tumors 200
smoking beverage 6–7
soft-tissue tumor 13, 200, 225
somatostatin 280
sonography (*see also* ultrasound) 83–88
- endorectal 146
- endosonography 84
- hydrocolonic 83–84
squamous cell carcinoma 67, 266
- keratinizing 181, 184
- non-keratinizing 181, 184
SRC gene 28
staging
- colorectal neoplasm 136–137
- *Dukes'* staging 70, 81, 136, 163
- metastasis and staging, pattern of 69–70, 137
- molecular 136
stapling device 146
STK11/LKB1 31–32, 64, 257–258
stomach, cancer of 200
stomatitis 142
streptozocin 281
substance P 276
sulfasalazine 7
sulindac 8, 25, 121–123, 125, 126, 226, 244
superficial iliac lymph nodes 69
surgical treatment of metastatic CC 147–148
surrogate end-points 124
surveillance (*see also* screening) 95–109, 121, 173–175, 213, 232, 242, 258
- after endoscopic polypectomy 102–103
- after surgery for CC 103–104
- colonoscopy 108, 121
- in hereditary cancer syndrome 105–106
- HNPCC, surveillance program 207
- *Muir-Torre* syndrome 267
- in patients with inflammatory bowel disease 104–105
- *Peutz-Jeghers* syndrome 258
- proposed surveillance programs after CC resection 173–174
- *Turcot* syndrome 265

survival and follow-up of CC   163–175
- ethnic differences in CC survival
  171–172
- factors influencing   164
- HNPCC   215–216
- temporal trends in CC survival
  171–172
suspected HNPCC   207, 210–212
synchronous colorectal lesion   59, 107, 199
syndrome/disease (named only)
- *Bannayan-Ruvalcaba-Riley*   260, 268
- *Bannayan-Zonana*   268
- *Cowden*   25, 31, 33, 105, 261–262
- *Crohn*   7, 25, 38, 40, 100, 104, 105, 122, 182
- *Cronkhite*-Canada   25, 267–268
- *Gardner*   225–226, 233, 238
- *Knudson*   31, 106, 205, 262, 268
- *Li-Fraumeni*   169, 212
- *Lynch* (see HNPCC)
- *Muir-Torre*   25, 200, 265–267
- non-*Hodgkin*   71
- *Peutz-Jeghers*   25, 31, 64, 105, 253–261
- *Ruvalcaba-Mirhe-Smith*   25, 268
- *Turcot*   13, 105, 263–265
- *Zollinger-Ellison*   6

T
TAG-72   84
tamoxifen   234
^{99}technetium   84
teeth, supernumerary   25, 233
tegafur and uracil combination   150
TGF (tumor necrosis factor)
- TGFα 65, 168
- TGFβ 33, 168, 206
- TGFβII receptor gene   37, 38
therapy (see treatment)
thymidine   142
- tritiated   167
thymidylate synthase   142–143
thyroid cancer/carcinoma   25, 226, 234, 262
TNM system   70, 136
tocophenol   126
toxicity and costs of chemotherapy in advanced CC   151
transitional cell carcinoma   200
- renal pelvis   200
- ureter   200
transplantation, intestinal   151–152, 234
- liver   151, 152, 281
treatment of CC   135–154
- advanced colorectal tumor   147

- anal cancer   185–186
- chemotherapy (see there)   141, 143–145, 148–153, 164–165, 171, 185–186, 234
- combination therapy   141–143, 149–150, 185
- FAP, surgical treatment   241–243
- HNPCC   214–215
- innovative treatments   152–153
- irradiation (see there)   145, 185–186
- medical treatment   141–144
- metastatic CC, surgical treatment   147–148
- radiotherapy (see there)   141, 144–146, 151, 164, 171, 185–186
- resectable colorectal tumor   137–141
- - endoscopic   137
trends in CC survival   171–172
triacylglycerol level   6, 119
trichilemmoma   33
tryptophan   276
tubular or tubulovillous adenoma   229, 263
tubulin   236
tumor
- carcinoid   66
- degree of tumor differentiation   146, 166
- desmoid   14, 25, 106, 226, 231, 234, 238, 243, 244
- growth, pattern of   69
- metachronous   173
- multiple   199–200
- necrosis factor β (see TGFβ)   33
- neuroendocrine   276, 279, 281
- perforation   146
- sebaceous   265–267
- soft tissue   13–14
- suppressor gene   1, 9, 23, 26, 40, 153, 257, 264
- - DDC   9
Turcot syndrome   13, 105, 263–265
- clinical and morphologic aspects   263
- complex genetic and molecular basis of   263–264
- management   265
- surveillance   265

U
ulcerative or *Crohn's* colitis   7, 25, 38, 40, 100, 104, 105, 122, 182
ultrasound   83–88
- abdominal   104
- CAT scanning   85, 88
- endoluminal   84, 86

- endorectal 84
- intraoperative 85
- liver 173
- PET scanning 104
- rectal 173
- standard 85

undifferentiated or medullary lesion 201
upper gastrointestinal polyp 238
uracil and tegafur combination 150
ureter, transitional cell carcinoma 200
urinary tract infection 166
ursodeoxycholic acid 123, 127

V

vascular or lymphatic invasion 137
vasoactive
- intestinal peptide 70
- substances 277

venous invasion at histology 146, 166
vincristine and semustine combination 143

virtual (computed) colonoscopy 83
vitamins 5, 14, 24–25, 118, 123
- antioxidant 14, 24, 60, 118, 123, 126, 243
- carotene 118, 123, 126
- provitamin 126
- vitamin A 5, 14, 25, 118
- vitamin C 5, 14, 25, 118
- vitamin D 123, 127
- vitamin E 5, 14, 25, 118, 123

W

weight loss 80
well-differentiated carcinoma 69, 137
wheezing 277
Wilm's tumor 262

X

X-linked modifier gene 227

Z

Zollinger-Ellison syndrome 6